Basic Medical Language

SIXTH EDITION

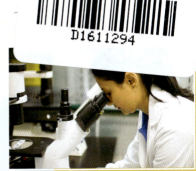

DANIELLE LAFLEUR BROOKS, MED, MA

Faculty, Medical Assisting and Allied Health and Science
Community College of Vermont
Montpelier, Vermont

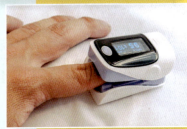

MYRNA LAFLEUR BROOKS, RN, BED

Founding President
National Association of Health Unit Coordinators
Faculty Emeritus
Maricopa Community College District
Phoenix, Arizona

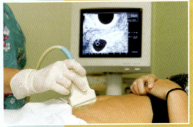

DALE LEVINSKY, MD

Clinical Associate Professor
Department of Family and Community Medicine
University of Arizona College of Medicine
Tucson, Arizona

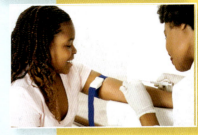

ELSEVIER

ELSEVIER

3251 Riverport Lane
St. Louis, Missouri 63043

ISBN: 978-0-323-59600-8
Set ISBN: 978-0-323-53319-5

Library of Congress Control Number: 2018955334

Publishing Director: Kristin Wilhelm
Senior Content Strategist: Linda Woodard
Content Development Manager: Luke Held
Publishing Services Manager: Julie Eddy
Project Manager: Abigail Bradberry
Design Direction: Renee Duenow

Printed in China

Last digit is the print number: 9 8 7 6 5 4 3 2

Working together to grow libraries in developing countries

www.elsevier.com • www.bookaid.org

For our students, who continue to inspire us with their dedication to learning while balancing life's other demands. Every page is for you.

Contents

Preface, vi   *Features, vii*

How Will I Learn?, xiv

Dear Instructor, xv

Online Teaching Resources, xv

LESSON 1   Introduction to Medical Language, Body Structure, and Oncology, 1

LESSON 2   Directional Terms, Positions, and Imaging, 29

LESSON 3   Integumentary System, Colors, and Plural Endings, 51

LESSON 4   Respiratory System, 80

LESSON 5   Urinary System, 117

LESSON 6   Reproductive Systems, 148

LESSON 7   Cardiovascular and Lymphatic Systems, 182

LESSON 8   Digestive System, 218

LESSON 9   Eye and Ear, 257

LESSON 10   Musculoskeletal System, 287

LESSON 11   Nervous System and Behavioral Health, 329

LESSON 12   Endocrine System, 363

APPENDIX A   Word Parts Used in *Basic Medical Language,* 384

APPENDIX B   Abbreviations, 389; Error-Prone List, 395

APPENDIX C   Answers to Exercises, 399

Illustration Credits, 419

Index, 421

Evolve Appendices, Evolve Resources at *evolve.elsevier.com*

APPENDIX D   Pharmacology Terms

APPENDIX E   Health Information Technology Terms

Anatomy of a Lesson

Let's take a look at the structure of body systems lessons using Lesson 4 on the respiratory system as an example.

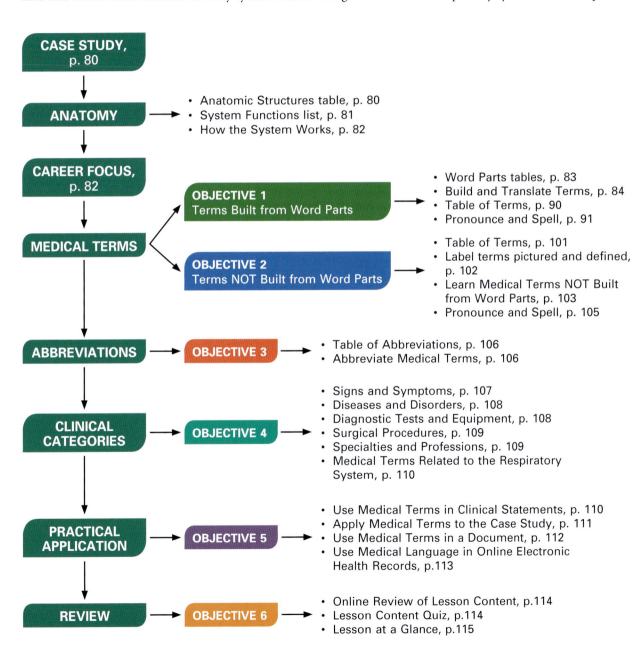

CASE STUDY, p. 80

ANATOMY
- Anatomic Structures table, p. 80
- System Functions list, p. 81
- How the System Works, p. 82

CAREER FOCUS, p. 82

MEDICAL TERMS

OBJECTIVE 1
Terms Built from Word Parts
- Word Parts tables, p. 83
- Build and Translate Terms, p. 84
- Table of Terms, p. 90
- Pronounce and Spell, p. 91

OBJECTIVE 2
Terms NOT Built from Word Parts
- Table of Terms, p. 101
- Label terms pictured and defined, p. 102
- Learn Medical Terms NOT Built from Word Parts, p. 103
- Pronounce and Spell, p. 105

ABBREVIATIONS

OBJECTIVE 3
- Table of Abbreviations, p. 106
- Abbreviate Medical Terms, p. 106

CLINICAL CATEGORIES

OBJECTIVE 4
- Signs and Symptoms, p. 107
- Diseases and Disorders, p. 108
- Diagnostic Tests and Equipment, p. 108
- Surgical Procedures, p. 109
- Specialties and Professions, p. 109
- Medical Terms Related to the Respiratory System, p. 110

PRACTICAL APPLICATION

OBJECTIVE 5
- Use Medical Terms in Clinical Statements, p. 110
- Apply Medical Terms to the Case Study, p. 111
- Use Medical Terms in a Document, p. 112
- Use Medical Language in Online Electronic Health Records, p.113

REVIEW

OBJECTIVE 6
- Online Review of Lesson Content, p.114
- Lesson Content Quiz, p.114
- Lesson at a Glance, p.115

Preface

WELCOME TO THE NEW EDITION OF *BASIC MEDICAL LANGUAGE*

The sixth edition offers a carefully-crafted learning system designed for quick and lasting acquisition of medical language needed for entry into the health professions. Word parts, medical terms, and abbreviations are introduced in manageable amounts, followed by immediate practice. Illustrations and narrative passages using medical terms in context weave between written exercises to reveal the medical concepts the terms represent. Bridging new learning with practical application remains a priority. In this new edition of the book, lesson content has been closely revised to focus on frequently used terms in clinical settings and in billing and coding. We have also included several **new features**:

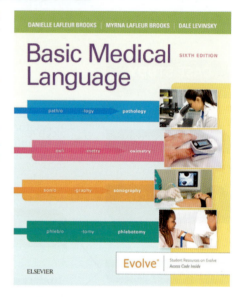

- End of lesson content quizzes
- Illustration exercises for Terms NOT Built from Word Parts
- Expanded abbreviation tables
- Online Resources: Tournament of Terminology Game, separate Practice Quizzes for word parts, terms, and abbreviations, and Gradable Exercises and Quizzes

Since 1994, we have dedicated ourselves to creating quality learning opportunities accessing the **multiple intelligences** and **learning styles** of our students. As such, the book and online resources continue to offer numerous and varied ways to interact with lesson content:

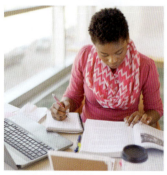

- Flashcards
- Interactive illustrations
- Career focus sections
- Pronunciation and spelling with audio
- Case studies with corresponding medical records
- Online EHR modules, games, and animations
- Lesson At a Glance review of word parts, terms, and abbreviations

Basic Medical Language offers a hybrid of print and electronic materials. Students have the opportunity to hold the book, pencil, and flashcards in their hands. They also have the opportunity to hear terms pronounced, practice spelling with immediate feedback, play games, view animations, and much more using the book's online resources. We believe we have reached an optimal balance of hands-on and virtual opportunities to support long-term learning.

We wish you the best as you begin your study of medical language and invite you to contact us at:

danielle.lafleurbrooks@ccv.edu   *myrnabrooks@comcast.net*   *dale.levinsky@gmail.com*

Warmly,
Danielle, Myrna, and *Dale*

FEATURES

Case Studies

Each lesson begins with a case study depicting a possible experience of a medical condition. Students apply medical terms presented in the lesson to the context of the case study.

CASE STUDY   Roberta Pawlaski

Roberta is experiencing difficulty breathing. She notices it gets worse when she tries to do chores around the house. This has been going on for about four days. She also has a cough and a runny nose. Today when she woke up she noticed that her throat was very sore. She also thinks that she might have a fever because she feels hot all over. She tried taking some over-the-counter cough medicine but this didn't seem to help. She notices when she coughs that a thick yellow mucus comes out. She hasn't had a cough like this since before she quit smoking about 10 years ago. She remembers that her grandson who stays with her after school has missed school because of a cold. She decides to call her doctor to schedule an appointment.

■ *Consider Roberta's situation as you work through the lesson on the respiratory system. At the end of the lesson, we will return to this case study and identify medical terms used to document Roberta's experience and the care she receives.*

Objectives

Lesson introductions list objectives and corresponding page numbers. Exercises, quizzes, and exams correlate directly with the objectives.

OBJECTIVES

1 ■ Build, translate, pronounce, and spell medical terms built from word parts (p. 86).
2 ■ Define, pronounce, and spell medical terms NOT built from word parts (p. 104).
3 ■ Write abbreviations (p. 109).
4 ■ Identify medical terms by clinical category (p. 110).
5 ■ Use medical language in clinical statements, the case study, and a medical record (p. 113).
6 ■ Recall and assess knowledge of word parts, medical terms, and abbreviations (p. 117).

Anatomy

Body system lessons briefly introduce related anatomy and physiology, including anatomic structure term tables with phonetic spelling, illustrations, and labeling exercises, which connect word parts with pictures of the anatomic structures they name.

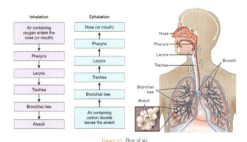

Figure 4.1 Flow of air.

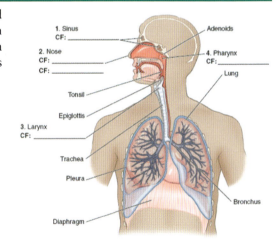

1. Sinus
   CF: _____
2. Nose
   CF: _____
   CF: _____
3. Larynx
   CF: _____

Adenoids
4. Pharynx
   CF: _____
Lung
Tonsil
Epiglottis
Trachea
Pleura
Bronchus
Diaphragm

Career Focus

Health professions related to the body system and lesson content are identified, along with tips on where to gather more information about specific fields.

CAREER FOCUS   Professionals Who Work with the Respiratory System

• **Respiratory Therapists (RTs)** treat, evaluate, and maintain function of the heart and lungs. RTs are highly skilled and perform pulmonary function tests, provide treatments (Figure 4.2), such as oxygen therapy and intermittent positive pressure breathing (IPPB), perform arterial blood gases (ABGs) to monitor carbon dioxide and oxygen in the blood, and assist with ventilation of seriously ill patients.
• **Respiratory Therapy Technicians** provide respiratory care under the supervision of respiratory therapists and physicians.
• **Sleep technologists**, also called **registered polysomnographic technologists (RPSGTs)**, perform polysomnography and other tests to diagnose and monitor sleep disorders. RPSGTs work under the guidance of a physician.

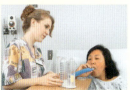

Figure 4.2 Respiratory therapist assisting a patient with incentive spirometry.

Word Parts

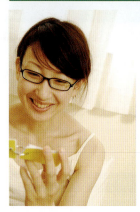

Word part tables present combining forms, suffixes, and prefixes related to lesson content as well as those introduced in previous lessons. Exercises, paper and electronic flashcards, and online activities reinforce learning.

5. **LABEL:** *Write word parts to complete Figure 4.7.*

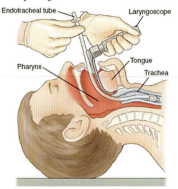

Endotracheal tube — Laryngoscope

Pharynx — Tongue — Trachea

Figure 4.7 The nurse anesthetist inserts a(n) _____/_____/_____ tube with a
within   trachea   pertaining to
_____/o/_____ to guide the tube into place.
larynx   instrument used for visual examination

Medical Terms Built from Word Parts

Students build, translate, and read medical terms in context. Learning may be extended through practice with online resources, including animations, games, exercises, and quizzes.

11. **READ: Pharyngitis** (far-in-JĪ-tis) is the medical term for sore throat. The larynx, commonly referred to as the voice box, contains the vocal cords. Frequently caused by a virus, **laryngitis** (lar-in-JĪ-tis) may be characterized by hoarseness or loss of voice.

12. **BUILD:** *Write word parts to build descriptive terms using the suffix –eal, meaning pertaining to.*

   a. pertaining to the pharynx (throat)   _____/_____
                                                              wr   s

   b. pertaining to the larynx (voice box)   _____/_____
                                                              wr   s

   c. pertaining to the larynx (voice box)   _____/o/_____/_____
      and pharynx (throat)   wr   cv   wr   s

   > **FYI**   The suffixes **-ic, -al, -ous, -ary,** and **-eal** all mean **pertaining to.** As you practice and use the medical terms, you will become more familiar with which suffix is used.

13. **TRANSLATE:** *Complete the definitions of the following terms built from the combining form **laryng/o**, meaning larynx. Use the meaning of word parts to fill in the blanks. Remember, the definition usually starts with the meaning of the suffix.*

   a. laryng/o/scope   _____ used for _____examination of the
                            larynx

   b. laryng/o/scopy   visual _____ of the _____

   c. laryng/ectomy   _____ (or surgical removal) of the _____

Medical Terms NOT Built from Word Parts

Lessons present tables of Medical Terms NOT Built from Word Parts with corresponding illustrations and exercises. Practice with online resources, including animations, games, exercises, and quizzes, reinforces learning.

MEDICAL TERMS NOT BUILT FROM WORD PARTS	
TERM	**DEFINITION**
asthma (AZ-ma)	respiratory disease characterized by coughing, wheezing, and shortness of breath; caused by constriction and inflammation of airways that is reversible between attacks
chronic obstructive pulmonary disease (COPD) (KRON-ik) (ob-STRUK-tive) (PUL-mŏ-nar-ē) (di ZEZ)	progressive lung disease blocking air flow, which makes breathing difficult. Chronic bronchitis and emphysema are two main components of COPD. Most COPD is a result of cigarette smoking.
computed tomography (CT) (kom-PU-ted) (tŏ-MOG-re-fē)	diagnostic imaging test producing scans composed from sectional radiographic images, which can be taken in any of the anatomic planes for a multidimensional view of internal structures. Chest computed tomography is often performed to follow up on abnormalities identified on previous chest radiographs. (Figure 4.14, *B*)
culture and sensitivity (C&S) (KUL-cher) (sen-si-TIV-i-tē)	laboratory test performed on a collected sample to determine the presence of pathogenic bacteria or fungi and to identify the most effective antimicrobial treatment. The test may be performed on sputum, throat cultures, blood, urine, and other fluids. Sputum culture and sensitivity tests are frequently used in the diagnosis of lower respiratory tract infections such as bronchitis and pneumonia.

EXERCISE E   Label

Write the medical terms pictured and defined using the previous table of Medical Terms NOT Built from Word Parts. Check your work with the Answer Key in Appendix C.

1. _____
diagnostic imaging test producing scans composed from sectional radiographic images, which can be taken in any of the anatomic planes for a multidimensional view of internal structures

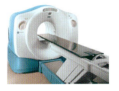

2. _____
image created by ionizing radiation

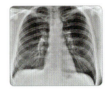

NEW—Label Exercise for Terms NOT Built from Word Parts to illustrate the medical concepts the terms represent.

Pronunciation & Spelling

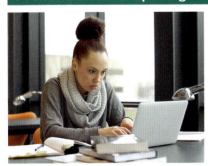

Pronunciation and spelling exercises may be completed on paper or online. Students may hear terms pronounced and practice spelling using online resources.

Abbreviations

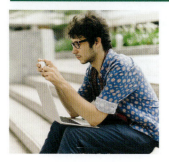

Tables introduce abbreviated medical terms related to lesson content. Exercises, electronic flashcards, and online activities provide practice for new learning. Appendix B provides additional abbreviations and a list of error-prone abbreviations.

NEW—Expanded tables listing more frequently used abbreviations.

ABBREVIATIONS RELATED TO THE RESPIRATORY SYSTEM			
Use the electronic **flashcards** to familiarize yourself with the following abbreviations.			
ABBREVIATION	**TERM**	**ABBREVIATION**	**TERM**
ABGs	arterial blood gases	O_2	oxygen
CO_2	carbon dioxide	OSA	obstructive sleep apnea
COPD	chronic obstructive pulmonary disease	PFT	pulmonary function tests
C&S	culture and sensitivity	PSG	polysomnography
CPAP	continuous positive airway pressure	RT	respiratory therapist

Clinical Categories

Students practice recall of all the terms, built from word parts and NOT built from word parts, presented in the lesson. Exercises group terms in clinical categories, such as signs and symptoms, to give a sense of how terms are used in the field.

NEW—The **clinical category lesson objective** provides an additional way to practice content and to understand the use of medical terms.

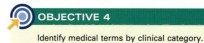

OBJECTIVE 4

Identify medical terms by clinical category.

Now that you have worked through the respiratory system lesson, review and practice medical terms grouped by clinical category. Categories include signs and symptoms, diseases and disorders, diagnostic tests and equipment, surgical procedures, specialties and professions, and other terms related to the respiratory system.

EXERCISE I | **Signs and Symptoms**

Write the medical terms for signs and symptoms next to their definitions.

1. _____ absence of breathing
2. _____ difficult breathing
3. _____ excessive breathing
4. _____ deficient breathing
5. _____ condition of excessive oxygen
6. _____ condition of deficient oxygen
7. _____ condition of deficient carbon dioxide
8. _____ condition of excessive carbon dioxide
9. _____ inflammation of the nose (nasal membranes)
10. _____ rapid flow of blood from the nose
11. _____ discharge from the nose

Practical Application

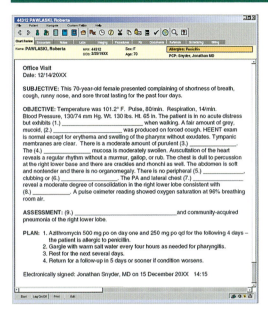

Students apply medical terms to case studies, corresponding medical records, clinical statements, and in electronic health records online.

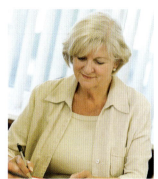

Electronic Health Record (EHR) Modules

Lessons 4-12 offer Electronic Health Record modules with three related medical records online. Students apply terms from the lesson within electronic medical records.

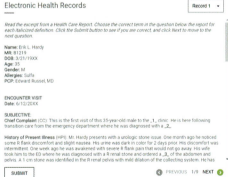

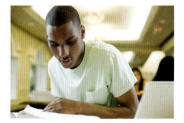

Lesson Content Quiz

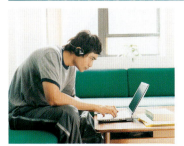

NEW—End of lesson content quizzes in the worktext and online in Gradable Student Resources allow students to quickly assess their understanding of medical terms and abbreviations.

EXERCISE T   Lesson Content Quiz

Test your knowledge of the terms and abbreviations introduced in this lesson. Circle the letter for the medical term or abbreviation related to the words in italics.

1. After weeks of experiencing a hoarse voice, the otolaryngologist performed a *visual examination of the larynx* on the patient to determine its cause.
   a. laryngoscope
   b. laryngoscopy
   c. laryngectomy

2. The term used to describe the *absence of spontaneous respiration* is a breathing disorder called:
   a. apnea
   b. hypopnea
   c. dyspnea

Lesson at a Glance

Lessons conclude with a concise review of word parts, terms, and abbreviations presented.

LESSON AT A GLANCE	RESPIRATORY SYSTEM WORD PARTS	

COMBINING FORMS
bronch/o
capn/o
laryng/o
muc/o
nas/o
ox/i
pharyng/o
pneum/o

pneumon/o
pulmon/o
rhin/o
sinus/o
somn/o
spir/o
thorac/o
trache/o

SUFFIXES
-ary
-centesis
-eal
-ectomy
-gram
-graphy
-ia
-meter

-pnea
-rrhagia
-rrhea
-scope
-scopic
-scopy
-stomy
-thorax

PREFIXES
a-, an-
dys-
endo-
hyper-
poly-

LESSON AT A GLANCE	RESPIRATORY SYSTEM MEDICAL TERMS AND ABBREVIATIONS

SIGNS AND SYMPTOMS
apnea
dyspnea
hypercapnia
hyperoxia
hyperpnea
hypocapnia
hypopnea
hypoxia
rhinitis
rhinorrhagia
rhinorrhea

DISEASES AND DISORDERS
asthma
bronchitis
bronchopneumonia
chronic obstructive pulmonary disease
   (COPD)

DIAGNOSTIC TESTS AND EQUIPMENT
bronchoscope
bronchoscopy
capnometer
computed tomography (CT)
culture and sensitivity (C&S)
endoscope
endoscopic
endoscopy
laryngoscope
laryngoscopy
oximeter
polysomnogram
polysomnography (PSG)
radiograph
spirometer
thoracoscope
thoracoscopic

tracheostomy
tracheotomy

SPECIALTIES AND PROFESSIONS
pulmonologist
pulmonology

RELATED TERMS
endotracheal (ET)
laryngeal
mucous
nasal
pharyngeal
pulmonary
sputum
thoracic

ABBREVIATIONS
| ABGs | CXR | PSG |
| CO_2 | ET | RT |

Online Learning Resources at evolve.elsevier.com

Evolve content online provides practice activities, gradable exercises and quizzes, and mobile resources that can be accessed from a portable device. Practice Student Resources are available to supplement your learning and scores are for student use only. Gradable Student Resources may populate your class' gradebook if your instructor has set it up to do so. Gradable Student Resources are available to all students whether or not your instructor chooses to record scores.

Practice Student Resources

- Word Part and Abbreviation Flashcards
- Pronunciation and Spelling
- Electronic Health Record Modules
- Games
- Practice Quizzes
- Career Videos
- Animations
- Additional Appendices on Pharmacology and Health Information Technology

Mobile Resources

- Word Part and Abbreviation Flashcards
- Practice Quizzes

Gradable Student Resources

- Exercises: Word Parts, Terms Built from Word Parts, Terms NOT Built from Word Parts, and Abbreviations
- Lesson Content Quiz

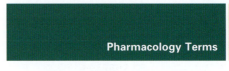

APPENDIX
D

Pharmacology Terms

Topics include:

General Drug Categories, p. e1.
General Pharmacy Terms, p. e2.
Routes of Administration, p. e4.

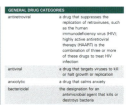

GENERAL DRUG CATEGORIES	
analgesic	an agent that reduces pain
anesthetic	an agent that reduces sensation locally or systemically and may cause loss of consciousness
antibacterial	a drug that targets bacteria to kill or halt growth or replication
antibiotic	a drug that targets bacteria, fungi, or protozoa to kill or halt growth or replication
anticholinergic agent	a drug that blocks the neurotransmitter acetylcholine to suppress the parasympathetic nervous system

GENERAL DRUG CATEGORIES	
antiretroviral	a drug that suppresses the replication of retroviruses, such as the human immunodeficiency virus (HIV); highly active antiretroviral therapy (HAART) is the combination of three or more of these drugs to treat HIV infection
antiviral	a drug that targets viruses to kill or halt growth or replication
anxiolytic	a drug that calms anxiety
bactericidal	the designation for an antimicrobial agent that kills or destroys bacteria

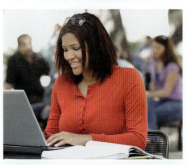

Create an Account and Register for Evolve Resources

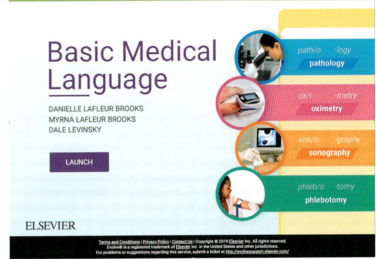

Use the following instructions to request Evolve Student Resources for *Basic Medical Language 6th Edition*. Technical help may be reached by calling 1-800-222-9570.

1. Go to the Evolve Education Portal at evolve.elsevier.com.
2. Click Login on the upper right corner of the screen.
3. Click Create account and select Student.
4. Enter your personal details and provide a new password of at least 7 characters.
5. Click Submit. After completing these steps: A pop-up appears with your automatically generated username and your provided password; an email with your login details will be sent to the email address you gave at registration, then you can log in to Evolve with your username and password.
6. Select the Catalog near the top of the screen. Use the search box and enter Basic Medical Language, 6th Edition.
7. Click on Evolve Resources for Basic Medical Language, 6th Edition.
8. Click Checkout/Redeem and follow the prompts to finish the process.
9. After completing these steps there are two ways to access Evolve Resources content:
   - My Evolve tab at evolve.elsevier.com. See the menu to the left of the screen; click on Resources, Student Resources, and then select Gradable Student Resources or Practice Student Resources as needed.
   - Evolve Links on your course site if your instructor has made them available. Links will take you to the activities, exercises, and quizzes your instructor has chosen.

Note: Gradable Student Resources will upload to the course gradebook if your instructor has set it up as such, otherwise the exercises and quizzes are for practice only.

FYI   Registration Steps may change as the Evolve website is updated. If difficulties arise, please:
- Call technical support at 1-800-222-9570.
- Type "evolve support center" in your browser and follow the links for help in accessing Evolve.

HOW WILL I LEARN?

The worktext and companion online resources hosted on the Evolve website offer a variety of ways to learn chapter content. The paper and online learning activities are coordinated and designed to cultivate long-term learning.

Word Parts

Worktext

- Read word parts and definitions
- Label anatomic diagrams
- Complete exercises and check responses
- Practice with paper flashcards

Online Resources

- Practice with online Flashcards using Activities
- Complete the Gradable Word Parts Exercise
- Take the Word Part Practice Quiz using Practice Activities

Medical Terms Built From Word Parts

Worktext

- Build terms
- Translate terms
- Label illustrations
- Read terms in context
- Pronounce and spell

Online Resources

- Listen to and repeat terms aloud using the Audio Glossary
- Spell terms using Practice Activities
- Build terms using Gradable Exercises
- Watch Animations

Medical Terms NOT Built From Word Parts

Worktext

- Read terms with definitions
- Label illustrations
- Complete in-context exercise
- Pronounce and spell

Online Resources

- Listen to and repeat terms aloud using the Audio Glossary
- Spell terms using Practice Activities
- Match terms with definitions using Gradable Exercises
- Watch Animations in Other Resources

Abbreviations

Worktext

- Read abbreviations with definitions
- Complete exercises grouped by clinical category
- Reference Appendix B with common abbreviations and an error-prone list

Online Resources

- Practice with online Flashcards using Practice Activities
- Complete the Gradable Abbreviations Exercise
- Take Abbreviation Practice Quiz using Practice Activities

Practical Application

Worktext

- Define terms grouped by clinical category
- Identify correct terms used in clinical statements
- Apply medical terms to the case study
- Write medical terms within a medical health record and answer related questions

Online Resources

- Apply medical terms to three related medical records in EHR modules

Review

Worktext

- Take lesson content quiz
- Practice recall with Lesson at a Glance

Online Resources

- Review word part and abbreviation flashcards using Practice Activities
- Play Games
- Take the Medical Term Practice Quiz using Practice Activities
- Take the Gradable Lesson Content Quiz

DEAR INSTRUCTOR

Thank you for choosing *Basic Medical Language*! We hope you find our learning system supportive of your teaching methods and effective for your students' learning styles. With the purchase of a new worktext, students receive paper flashcards for word parts and access to Evolve Resources for students. You may find the flashcards and online resources, such as pronunciation for term lists and games, useful for class activities and exam preparation.

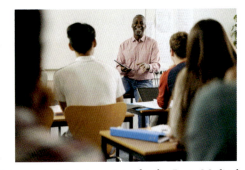

Additional teaching materials are available online at **evolve.elsevier. com** within Evolve Resources for Instructors. All resources are objective based, and we recommend beginning with the TEACH Lesson Plans for an overview of the various teaching tools. The first step in accessing teaching materials is to register for the *Basic Medical Language 6th Edition* Evolve Resources. Please visit evolve.elsevier.com or call **1-800-222-9570** to register.

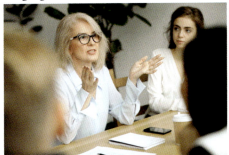

We welcome your comments and questions by email. Danielle, who currently teaches medical terminology in the traditional classroom, online, and in hybrid formats, is also happy to share ideas and materials. Contact us at Danielle.lafleurbrooks@ccv.edu, Myrnabrooks@comcast.net, and *dale.levinsky@gmail.com*. We also invite you to visit Myrna's educational blog MedTerm Topics at medtermtopics.com to keep up with trends in teaching medical terminology and emerging medical language.

Looking forward to hearing from you,

Danielle, Myrna, and Dale

Online Teaching Resources at evolve.elsevier.com

Instructor Resources

- Image Collection
- Sample Course Syllabus and Outline
- TEACH Handouts
- TEACH Lesson Plans
- TEACH PowerPoint Slides
- Test Bank

Assessment

- Formative and summative assessment plan for each lesson, TEACH Lesson Plans in Evolve Instructor Resources
- Pretest and Posttest, TEACH Lesson Plans in Evolve Instructor Resources
- Practice Quizzes, Evolve Practice Student Resources
- Quizzes, scores can upload to gradebook, Evolve Gradable Student Resources
- Test Bank to build quizzes and exams, Evolve Instructor Resources

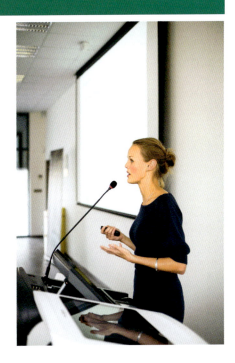

FYI For assistance in registering for Evolve Resources, call **1-800-222-9570** or visit **evolvesupport.elsevier.com**.

Also Available

Elsevier Adaptive Learning

Corresponding lesson-by-lesson to *Basic Medical Terminology*, sixth Edition, **Elsevier Adaptive Learning** combines the power of brain science with sophisticated, patented Cerego algorithms to help you learn faster and remember longer. It's fun, it's engaging, and it constantly tracks your performance and adapts to deliver content precisely when it's needed to ensure core information is transformed into lasting knowledge.

Reviewers and Advisors

REVIEWERS/ADVISORS

Cynthia A. Bjerklie, MEd
Medical Assisting Instructor
Community College of Vermont
Montpelier, Vermont

Richard K. Brooks, MD, FACP, FACG
Internal Medicine and Gastroenterology
Mayo Clinic (retired)
Scottsdale, Arizona

Erin Hayes, MS, MAT
Foundations of Medicine Instructor
Medicine & Healthcare Strand Leader
Blue Valley Center for Advanced Professional Studies
Overland Park, Kansas

Denise M. Hellman, RN, BN, MN
Nursing Instructor
Medicine Hat College
Division of Health Studies
Medicine Hat, Alberta

Charlene Thiessen, MEd
Program Director Emeritus, Medical Transcription
GateWay Community College
Phoenix, Arizona

PREVIOUS EDITION REVIEWERS

Ruth Buchner
Family and Consumer Science/Health Science
  Educator
Chippewa Falls Senior High School
Chippewa Falls, Wisconsin

Christine Costa, BS, GCM, HUC
Geriatric Care Manager
Tempe, Arizona

Heather Drake, RN, BSN
Instructor, Nursing
Southern West Virginia Community & Technical
  College
Mt. Gay, West Virginia

Melody Miller, LPN, VOC II
Medical Assistant Instructor
Lancaster County Career & Technology Center
Willow Street, Pennsylvania

Suezette Musick-Hicks, MEd, RRT, CPFT
Director, Respiratory Care Program
Black River Technical College
Pocahontas, Arkansas

Ann Vadala
Professor, Office Administration – Health Services
Coordinator, Health Care Administration
School of Business
St. Lawrence College
Kingston, Ontario

Tiffani Walker, MSRS, RT(R)
Clinical Coordinator, Radiology
North Central Texas College
Gainesville, Texas

Dokagari Woods, PhD, RN
Assistant Professor and Undergraduate Program
  Director, Nursing
Tarleton State University
Stephenville, Texas

Introduction to Medical Language, Body Structure, and Oncology

CASE STUDY **Tova Katz**

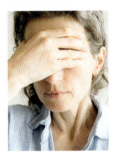

Tova has been having diarrhea. Even worse, she notices blood in it. She had this before when she was younger, and the disease process was identified, but she couldn't remember the name. She was put on medicine and got better. It looked like a positive outcome. Now it's been going on for 3 weeks. She has pain in her belly with cramps and feels kind of full all the time. She notices she is losing weight, even though she isn't trying. She also feels more tired than usual. Tova makes an appointment with her family doctor to see if she needs to go back on medicine.

■ *Consider Tova's situation as you work through the lesson on body structure and oncology. We will return to this case study and identify medical terms used to document Tova's experience and the care she receives.*

OBJECTIVES

1 ■ Identify the origins of medical language, the four word parts, and the combining form (p. 1).

2 ■ Build, translate, pronounce, and spell medical terms built from word parts (p. 6).

3 ■ Define, pronounce, and spell medical terms NOT built from word parts (p. 18).

4 ■ Write abbreviations (p. 21).

5 ■ Identify body structure and oncology terms (p. 22).

6 ■ Use medical language in clinical statements, the case study, and a medical record (p. 24).

7 ■ Recall and assess knowledge of word parts, medical terms, and abbreviations (p. 26).

OBJECTIVE 1

Identify the origins of medical language, the four word parts, and the combining form.

The vocabulary of medical language reflects its development over time, starting with the ancient Greeks who were among the first to study and write about medicine. The Romans continued this practice, adapting elements of the Greek language to use alongside Latin. Today, we can see the historical roots of medical language in the use of **terms built from Greek and Latin word parts**. As medical language evolved with scientific advancements, **eponyms**, **acronyms**, and terms from **modern language** have also come into use (Figure 1.1).

1

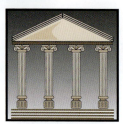

Greek and Latin
Terms built from Greek and Latin word parts such as ***arthritis***

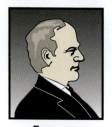

Eponyms
Terms named for a person or place; examples include **Alzheimer disease**, named after the first person to identify the disease, and **West Nile virus**, the first geographical location the virus was identified

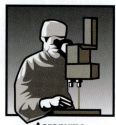

Acronyms
Terms formed from the first letters of the words in a phrase that can be spoken as a whole word and usually contain a vowel, such as ***laser*** (light amplification by stimulated emission of radiation)

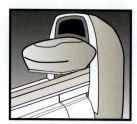

Modern language
Terms derived from the English language such as ***nuclear medicine scanner***

Figure 1.1 Origins of medical language.

FYI   **Alzheimer disease vs. Alzheimer's disease**

The need for clarity and consistency in medical language has resulted in the modern trend to eliminate the possessive form of eponyms and instead use the non-possessive form, which omits the apostrophe "s". The non-possessive form is observed by the Association for Healthcare Documentation Integrity, the American Medical Association's Manual of Style, in most medical dictionaries, and in this textbook. With either use, the noun that follows is not capitalized.

EXERCISE A   **Identify Origins of Medical Language**

For questions 1-4, write the letter of the origin of a medical term next to its description. Check responses using the Answer Key in Appendix C.

_____ **1.** Terms formed from the first letters of the words in a phrase that can be spoken as a whole word

_____ **2.** Terms derived from the English language reflecting scientific advancement and new technologies

_____ **3.** Terms built from word parts

_____ **4.** Terms named for a person or place

a. acronym
b. eponym
c. modern language
d. Greek and Latin

5. *Draw a line matching the origin of medical language with its example.*

   a. acronym   posttraumatic stress disorder
   b. eponym   MRSA
   c. modern language   arthritis
   d. Greek and Latin   Parkinson disease

Categories of Medical Terms and Learning Methods

For the purpose of our studies, medical terms are categorized as *built from word parts* and as *NOT built from word parts*. Specific learning methods will be used for each category.

CATEGORIES OF MEDICAL TERMS AND LEARNING METHODS

CATEGORY	ORIGIN	EXAMPLE	LEARNING METHODS
Terms Built from Word Parts (can be translated literally to find their meaning)	1. Word parts of Greek and Latin origin put together to form terms that can be translated to find their meanings	1. arthr/itis	1. Translating terms 2. Building terms
Terms NOT Built from Word Parts (cannot be easily translated literally to find their meaning)	1. Eponyms, terms named for a person or place	1. Alzheimer disease	1. Memorizing terms
	2. Acronyms, terms formed from the first letters of a phrase that can be spoken as a whole word and usually contain a vowel	2. MRSA (methicillin-resistant *Staphylococcus aureus*)	
	3. Modern Language, terms from the English language	3. complete blood count and differential	
	4. Terms of Greek and Latin word parts that cannot be easily translated to find their meanings	4. orthopedics	

Terms Built from Word Parts

Terms built from word parts may be easily understood by learning the meaning of the individual word parts. The four types of word parts that may be used in forming a medical term are **word root, suffix, prefix,** and **combining vowel.**

USING WORD PARTS TO BUILD MEDICAL TERMS

WORD PART	DESCRIPTION	ABBREVIATION
word root	core of the term; fundamental meaning. All medical terms have one or more word roots.	wr
suffix	attached to the end of the word root and provides additional information; modifies meaning. Not all medical terms have a suffix.	s
prefix	attached to the beginning of the word root and provides additional information; modifies meaning. Not all medical terms have a prefix.	p
combining vowel	vowel, usually an **o,** placed between two word roots and between a word root and a suffix (if the suffix does not begin with a vowel); eases pronunciation	cv

EXAMPLE 1: INTRAVENOUS

	WORD PART	MEANING
prefix	intra-	within
word root	ven	vein
suffix	-ous	pertaining to
term = p + wr + s	intra/ven/ous	pertaining to within a vein

> **FYI** Usually, the **meaning of the suffix** will initiate the definition of a medical term categorized as built from word parts.

EXAMPLE 2: OSTEOARTHRITIS

	WORD PART	MEANING
word root	oste	bone
combining vowel	o	none; eases pronunciation
word root	arthr	joint
suffix	-itis	inflammation
term = wr + cv + wr + s	oste/o/arthr/itis	inflammation of the bone and joint

Combining Form

A combining form is a word root with the combining vowel attached, separated by a slash. *For learning purposes, word roots are presented with their combining vowels as combining forms.*

EXAMPLES
arthr/o
oste/o
ven/o

> **FYI** **Word roots** are presented as **combining forms** throughout the text.

Terms NOT Built from Word Parts

Basic Medical Language would not be complete without including commonly used terms, such as **heart failure,** that are not built from word parts. Although there is less emphasis on these terms, they are important in the development of a medical vocabulary. While memorization is the primary method for learning terms not built from word parts, textbook exercises incorporate related information to help remember definitions and to develop a sense of how the terms are used in context.

Some terms containing recognizable word parts are categorized as *NOT Built from Word Parts* because they are difficult to translate. For example orth/o/ped/ic is made up of three word parts: **orth** meaning "straight," **ped** meaning "child" or "foot," and **-ic** meaning "pertaining to." Translated literally, orthopedic would seem to mean **pertaining to a straight child or foot**; however, the current use of the term orthopedic refers to the **branch of medicine dealing with the study and treatment of diseases and abnormalities of the musculoskeletal system.** Because the term *orthopedic* cannot be translated from word parts to understand its meaning, it is categorized as *NOT Built from Word Parts* in this textbook.

EXERCISE B Define Word Parts, Combining Form, and Categories of Medical Terms

Check your responses using the Answer Key in Appendix C.

A. *Match the phrases in the first column with the correct terms in the second column.*

_____ 1. Core of the term

_____ 2. Attached at the end of a word root

_____ 3. Definitions can be easily understood by knowing meanings of word parts.

_____ 4. Word root presented with its combining vowel

_____ 5. Used to ease pronunciation; usually an "o"

_____ 6. Definitions **cannot** be easily understood by knowing meanings of word parts.

_____ 7. Attached at the beginning of a word root

a. terms built from word parts
b. terms NOT built from word parts
c. word root
d. prefix
e. suffix
f. combining vowel
g. combining form

B. *Fill in the blanks to complete the following sentences.*

1. There are four types of word parts used to build medical terms. The fundamental meaning of a term may be understood by knowing the meaning of the core of the term or the _____ _____.

2. To modify the meaning of a term, a suffix may be added at the _____ of a word root or a prefix may be added at its _____.

3. Most often, when translating the meaning of a term built from word parts, begin with the definition of the word part attached to the end of the term, or the _____. The next step is to translate the word part attached to the beginning of the term, or the _____. Finally, add the definition of the word root to discern the full meaning of the term. For example, the term **intra/ven/ous** can be translated literally in this way to find its meaning, _____ to _____ a _____ (see Example 1 in the table on p. 4).

4. To ease pronunciation, a term may have a vowel placed between two word roots or between a word root and a suffix; use of a vowel in this way is known as a _____ _____. The term **oste/o/arthr/itis** has the combining vowel **o** inserted between the word roots **oste** and **arthr** to ease pronunciation. A combining vowel is not inserted between the word root **arthr** and the suffix **-itis** because the suffix begins with the vowel **i**. Osteoarthritis can be translated literally by defining the suffix and then word roots to mean _____ of the _____ and _____ (See Example 2 in the table on p. 4).

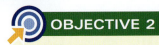

OBJECTIVE 2

Build, translate, pronounce, and spell medical terms built from word parts.

Body Structure and Oncology

The structure of the human body falls into four categories: cells, tissues, organs, and systems. Each structure is a highly organized unit of smaller structures (Figure 1.3). **Oncology** is the study of tumors. Tumors develop from excessive growth of cells. Oncology terms are introduced in this lesson because of their relationship to cells and cell abnormalities. Oncology terms naming tumors of specific organs and body systems are introduced in subsequent lessons.

BODY STRUCTURE

STRUCTURE	DESCRIPTION
cell	basic unit of all living things; the human body is composed of trillions of cells that vary in size and shape according to function
tissue	group of similar cells that perform a specific function
organ	two or more kinds of tissues that together perform special body functions
system	group of organs that work together to perform complex body functions

Body Tissues

Tissues can be grouped into four main categories, each having a specific function (Figure 1.4).

BODY TISSUES

TISSUE	DESCRIPTION
muscle tissue	composed of cells that have a special ability to contract, usually producing movement
nerve tissue	found in the nerves, spinal cord, and brain; coordinates and controls body activities
connective tissue	connects, supports, penetrates, and encases various body structures; forms bones, fat, cartilage, and blood
epithelial tissue	the major covering of the external surface of the body; forms membranes that line body cavities and organs and is the major tissue in glands; (also called **epithelium**)

Body Cavities and Organs

The body is not a solid structure, as it appears on the outside, but has cavities containing an orderly arrangement of the internal organs (Figure 1.6).

BODY CAVITIES AND ORGANS

CAVITY	ORGANS
cranial cavity	brain
spinal cavity	spinal cord
thoracic cavity	heart, aorta, lungs, esophagus, trachea, and bronchi
abdominal cavity	stomach, intestines, kidneys, liver, gallbladder, pancreas, spleen, and ureters
pelvic cavity	urinary bladder, certain reproductive organs, parts of the small and large intestines, and rectum

FYI   **Abdominopelvic cavity** refers to the abdominal cavity and the pelvic cavity. See Figure 1.6.

Body Systems

Each system is made up of organs that work together to perform specific tasks. Although body systems play individual roles, they are interrelated, working together to maintain life.

BODY SYSTEMS

BODY SYSTEM	ORGANS, GLANDS, AND TISSUES	BASIC FUNCTIONS
integumentary system	skin, hair, nails, and sweat and oil glands	covers and protects body, regulates body temperature, and helps manufacture vitamin D
respiratory system	nose, pharynx, larynx, trachea, bronchi, and lungs	exchanges oxygen and carbon dioxide between blood and external environment
urinary system	kidneys, ureters, urinary bladder, and urethra	removes waste material (urine), regulates fluid volume, and maintains electrolyte concentration
reproductive system	F: ovaries, uterus, uterine (fallopian) tubes, and vagina; M: testes, vas deferens, prostate gland, and penis	produces offspring, secretes hormones that produce feminine and masculine physical traits
cardiovascular system	heart and blood vessels	pumps and transports blood throughout the body
lymphatic system	lymph, lymph nodes, lymphatic vessels, spleen, and thymus	provides defense against infection and other diseases and drainage of extracellular fluid
digestive system	mouth, pharynx, esophagus, stomach, intestines, gallbladder, liver, and pancreas	prepares food for use by the body's cells and eliminates waste
musculoskeletal system	muscles, bones, cartilage, ligaments, and tendons	provides movement and framework for the body, protects vital organs, stores calcium, and produces blood cells
nervous system	brain, spinal cord, and nerves	regulates specific body activities by sending and receiving messages
endocrine system	pituitary, thyroid, thymus, adrenal glands, and pancreas	secretes hormones that regulate specific body activities

CAREER FOCUS   Professionals Who Work with Body Structure and Oncology Terms

- **Laboratory Technologists and Technicians** collect samples and perform tests to analyze body fluids such as blood and urine. Both technicians and technologists perform tests ordered by physicians; however, technologists perform more complex tests and laboratory procedures than technicians.

- **Pharmacy Technicians** work under the supervision of a licensed pharmacist to prepare and dispense prescriptions. Tech duties also include answering the phone, data entry, and customer service.

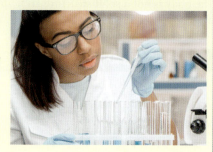

Figure 1.2 Laboratory technologist using a pipette to perform a lab test.

FOR MORE INFORMATION

- Access online resources at evolve.elsevier.com > Practice Student Resources > Other Resources > Career Videos to watch interviews with a **Medical Laboratory Technician** and a **Pharmacy Technician**.

WORD PARTS   Use the paper or online **flashcards** to familiarize yourself with the following word parts.

COMBINING FORM (WR + CV)	DEFINITION	COMBINING FORM (WR + CV)	DEFINITION
carcin/o	cancer	neur/o	nerve(s), nerve tissue
cyt/o	cell(s)	onc/o	tumor(s)
epitheli/o	epithelium, epithelial tissue	path/o	disease
hist/o	tissue(s)	radi/o	x-rays (ionizing radiation)
lip/o	fat, fat tissue	sarc/o	flesh, connective tissue
my/o	muscle(s), muscle tissue	viscer/o	internal organs

Word roots are the core of the word (fundamental meaning). Each medical term contains one or more word roots. *Combining forms* are word roots with their combining vowels.

SUFFIX (S)	DEFINITION	SUFFIX (S)	DEFINITION
-al	pertaining to	-oid	resembling
-genic	producing, originating, causing	-oma	tumor
-logist	one who studies and treats (specialist, physician)	-plasm	growth (substance or formation)
-logy	study of	-stasis	control, stop

Suffixes are attached to the end of the word root to modify its meaning. Not all medical terms have a suffix.

WORD PARTS	Use the paper or online **flashcards** to familiarize yourself with the following word parts—cont'd

PREFIX (P)	DEFINITION	PREFIX (P)	DEFINITION
meta-	beyond	**neo-**	new

Prefixes are attached to the beginning of the word root to modify its meaning. Not all medical terms have a prefix.

COMBINING VOWEL (CV)

A *combining vowel*, usually an o, is used to ease pronunciation:
- between two word roots
- between a word root and a suffix (if the suffix does not begin with a vowel)

Refer to Appendix A, for an alphabetized list of word parts and their meanings.

Pronunciation

Use the following Pronunciation Key to read the phonetic spellings of terms aloud. Phonetic spellings are provided with medical terms in the READ exercises and in term tables.

PRONUNCIATION KEY

GUIDELINES	EXAMPLES
1. Words are distorted minimally to indicate proper phonetic sound.	doctor (dok-tor), gastric (gas-trik)
2. Capital letters indicate the primary accent.	doctor (DOC-tor), gastric (GAS-trik)
3. The macron (ˉ) indicates the long vowel sound.	donate (dō-nāte)
	ā as in say **ō** as in no
	ē as in me **ū** as in cute
	ī as in spine
4. Vowels with no markings should have the short sound.	medical (med-i-cal)
	a as in sad **o** as in top
	e as in get **u** as in cut
	i as in sit

EXERCISE C   Build and Translate Terms Built from Word Parts

*Use the **Word Parts Table** to complete the following questions. Check your responses with the Answer Key in Appendix C.*

1. **MATCH:** Suffixes are attached to the end of word roots to provide additional information. *Draw a line to match the suffix with its definition.*

   a. -al   tumor
   b. -logy   pertaining to
   c. -oma   study of

2. **LABEL:** The word root is the core of a term. All medical terms built from word parts have one or more word roots. The combining form is the word root presented with its combining vowel. The structure of the human body falls into four categories: cells, tissues, organs, and systems.

   Write the combining forms for structures of the human body in Figure 1.3.

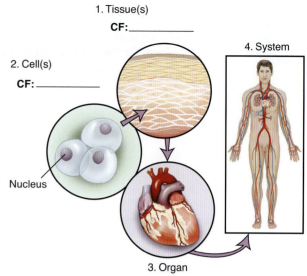

1. Tissue(s)
   CF:_____

2. Cell(s)
   CF:_____

4. System

Nucleus

3. Organ

Figure 1.3 Structure of the human body.

3. **TRANSLATE:** *Complete the definitions of the following terms by using the meaning of word parts to fill in the blanks. The definition of a term usually starts with the meaning of the suffix, and then moves to the beginning of the term.*

   Example: cyt/o/logy   *study* of *cell* (s)

   hist/o/logy   _____ of _____(s)

   > **FYI**   **Translate** exercises ask you to define medical terms using the meaning of combining forms and word parts. Begin the definition of the term with the meaning of the suffix, and then move to the beginning of the term and apply the meaning of the next word part (prefix) or combining form. **Check your answers using Appendix C.**

4. **READ:** Knowing the meaning of even a few combining forms and word parts will unlock the meaning of many medical terms. The term **cytology** (sī-TOL-o-jē) contains the combining form **cyt/o**, which means cell. The suffix **-logy** means study of. The medical term cyt/o/logy means study of cells. In the term **histology** (his-TOL-o-jē), **hist/o** means tissue(s). Hist/o/logy means study of tissues. Cytology and histology take place in a medical laboratory and involve microscopic examination of biopsied specimens.

   > **FYI**   The **o** in the terms cyt/o/logy and hist/o/logy is a **combining vowel**, which is used between word parts to ease pronunciation.

5. LABEL: Tissues are groups of cells that perform specific tasks. Four types of tissues are nerve, connective, muscle, and epithelium.

Write the combining forms for tissues of the human body to complete Figure 1.4.

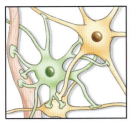

1. Nerve(s), nerve tissue
   CF: _____

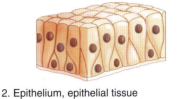

2. Epithelium, epithelial tissue
   CF: _____

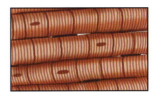

3. Flesh, connective tissue
   CF: _____

4. Muscle(s), muscle tissue.
   CF: _____

Figure 1.4 Types of tissue.

6. BUILD: Tumors may develop from tissues. Medical terms for specific types of tumors are often built with a combining form for the related anatomic structure and the suffix **–oma**.

Write the combining forms and word parts to build the terms defined. The definition of the term usually begins with the meaning of the suffix, followed by the meaning of the prefix or combining form at the beginning of the term.

> **FYI** **Build**
> exercises ask you to write the components of a medical term using its definition and the meanings of combining forms and word parts. Check your answers using Appendix C.

Example: tumor (composed of)   ____neur__ / __oma____
   nerve tissue   **wr**   **s**

a. tumor (composed of) muscle   _____/_____
   tissue   **wr**   **s**

b. tumor (composed of)   _____/_____
   epithelial tissue   **wr**   **s**

c. tumor (of) connective tissue   _____/_____
                                         wr   **s**

> **FYI** The definition of the medical term **sarcoma** does not contain the word "composed" because it grows in connective tissue rather than being made up of connective tissue.

7. **READ:** Definitions of medical terms built from Greek and Latin word parts may contain additional words that are not a part of the literal translation. For example, the definition of **neur/oma** is tumor (composed of) nerve tissue. You will become familiar with these variations as you learn the medical terms. Tumors may be considered benign (nonrecurring) or malignant (tending to become progressively worse). **Neuroma** (nū-RŌ-ma) and **myoma** (mī-Ō-ma) are benign tumors. An **epithelioma** (ep-i-thē-lē-Ō-ma) may be benign or malignant. **Sarcoma** (sar-KŌ-ma) usually indicates a highly malignant tumor arising from connective tissue, such as bone or cartilage.

> **FYI**   **Incidentaloma** refers to a mass or lesion discovered unexpectedly during a diagnostic imaging procedure and has nothing to do with the patient's symptoms or primary diagnosis.

8. **MATCH:** *Draw a line matching the word part with its definition.*

   a. lip/o   tumor
   b. cyt/o   fat, fat tissue
   c. -oma   resembling
   d. -oid   cell(s)

9. **TRANSLATE:** *Complete the definitions of the following terms by using the meaning of word parts to fill in the blanks. The definition of a term usually starts with the meaning of the suffix, and then moves to the beginning of the term.*

   a. lip/oma   _____ (composed of) _____ tissue
   b. lip/oid   _____ fat
   c. cyt/oid   resembling a _____

10. **READ:** **Lipoma** (li-PŌ-ma) refers to a benign tumor composed of fat tissue (a type of connective tissue). Lipomas are commonly found below the skin of the neck and trunk. **Lipoid** (LIP-oid) describes a fatlike substance. **Cytoid** (SĪ-toid) describes structures that resemble cells.

11. **LABEL:** *Write word parts to complete Figure 1.5.*

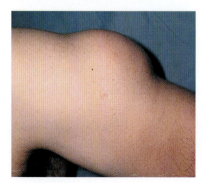

Figure 1.5 _____/_____.
                           fat   tumor

12. LABEL: The body is not a solid structure as it appears on the outside. It has five cavities: cranial, spinal, thoracic, abdominal, and pelvic. Sometimes the abdominal and pelvic cavities are referred to as the abdominopelvic cavity. Body cavities contain internal organs and other anatomical structures.

Write the combining form for internal organs in the space provided in Figure 1.6.

FYI The five body cavities may be grouped into more general categories known as the **dorsal cavity** and the **ventral cavity**. The ventral cavity, located in the anterior (front) portion of the body, is made up of the thoracic and abdominopelvic cavities. The dorsal cavity, located in the posterior (back) portion of the body, is made up of the cranial and spinal cavities.

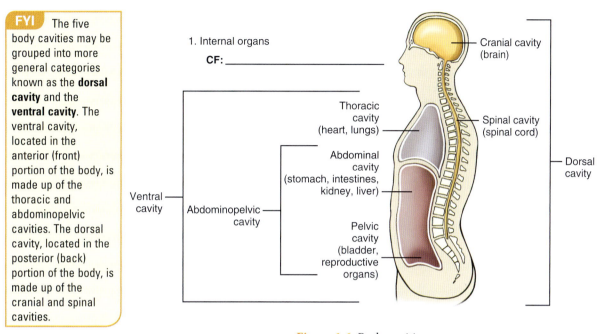

Figure 1.6 Body cavities.

13. BUILD: *Using the suffix -al meaning pertaining to, build the following descriptive terms.*

a. pertaining to internal organs   _____/_____
                                        wr   s

b. pertaining to epithelium   _____/_____
                                   wr   s

14. MATCH: *Draw a line matching the word part with its definition.*

a. path/o   study of
b. -genic   one who studies and treats (specialist, physician)
c. -logy   disease
d. -logist   producing, originating, causing

FYI   The suffix **-logist** may indicate a specialist such as a **psychologist, who is not a physician,** or a specialist such as an **oncologist, who is a physician.** For learning purposes in the text, if the specialist is a physician, it will be indicated in the definition, such as: **oncologist … a physician who studies and treats tumors.**

15. TRANSLATE: *Complete the definitions of the following terms by using the meaning of word parts to fill in the blanks. HINT: use* **producing** *for the definition of* **-genic.**

   a. path/o/logist   physician who studies _____

   b. path/o/genic   _____

   c. path/o/logy   _____ of disease

---

16. READ: A **pathologist** (pa-THOL-o-jist) studies cell, tissue, and organ specimens and performs autopsies to determine the presence and cause of disease. A pathologist is commonly employed in the **pathology** (pa-THOL-o-jē) department of a hospital or healthcare center and does not directly treat patients. Pathology, abbreviated as **PATH**, is a branch of medicine focused on the study of the causes of disease and death. **Pathogenic** (path-ō-JEN-ik), an adjective, describes a substance that produces disease.

---

17. BUILD: *Write the combining forms and word parts to build the following terms.*

   a. study of x-rays

                                               _____ / o / _____
                                                     wr   **cv**   **s**

   b. physician who studies and treats using x-rays

                                             _____ / o / _____
                                                     wr   **cv**   **s**

---

18. READ: Radiology (rā-dē-OL-o-jē) is the branch of medicine concerned with the use of radiation to diagnose and treat diseases. While literally translated as the study of x-rays, radiology includes other diagnostic imaging procedures, such as computed tomography, magnetic resonance imaging, sonography, and nuclear medicine. A **radiologist** (rā-dē-OL-o-jist) is a physician who interprets images generated by diagnostic imaging procedures and who performs treatments using imaging modalities.

---

19. MATCH: *Draw a line matching the word part with its definition.*

   a. carcin/o   beyond
   b. -oma   control, stop
   c. -genic   growth (substance or formation)
   d. meta-   cancer
   e. neo-   producing, originating, causing
   f. -plasm   new
   g. -stasis   tumor

> **FYI**   The suffixes **-plasm** and **-stasis** are considered to have embedded word roots, which means that they may appear in terms with a prefix and no other combining form. In these instances, suffixes with embedded word roots will be noted as **s(wr)**.

20. **BUILD:** *Write the combining forms and word parts to build the following terms related to cancer.*

    a. new growth

                                                  _____ / _____
                                                              p   **s(wr)**

    b. beyond control

                                                  _____ / _____
                                                              p   **s(wr)**

    c. producing cancer

                                                  _____ / o / _____
                                                     wr   **cv**   **s**

    d. cancerous tumor
        Hint: in this instance the definition of the term starts
        with the combining form rather than the suffix.

                                                  _____ / _____
                                                   wr   **s**

---

21. **READ:** A **neoplasm** (NĒ-ō-plazm) is a new growth, which may also be called a tumor. Tumors may be either malignant (cancerous) or may be benign (noncancerous). **Carcinoma** (kar-si-NŌ-ma), abbreviated as **CA**, is a term used to describe a malignant new growth. **Carcinogenic** (kar-sin-ō-JEN-ik), an adjective, describes a substance that produces cancer.

---

22. **LABEL:** *Write word parts to complete Figure 1.7.*

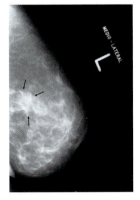

Figure 1.7 Mammogram demonstrating _____ / _____ of the breast.
                                          cancer   **tumor**

---

23. **READ:** **Metastasis** (me-TAS-ta-sis) abbreviated as **mets**, indicates the transfer of disease beyond the tissue or organ of origin. Metastasis often describes the spread of cancer from the place it developed to another site in the body. Variations of the term are **metastases** (me-TAS-ta-sēz), which is its plural form indicating more than one site of metastasis, and **metastatic** (MET-a-stat-ik), which is its adjective form used to describe a noun (e.g. metastatic cancer).

24. LABEL: *Write word parts to complete Figure 1.8, which illustrates the transfer of breast cancer cells from the tissue of origin to the brain.*

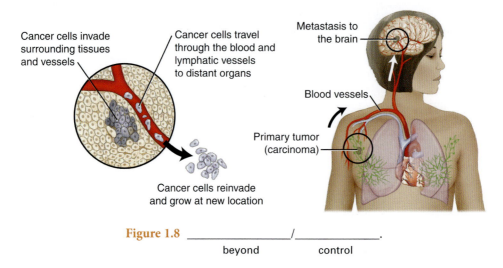

Cancer cells invade surrounding tissues and vessels

Cancer cells travel through the blood and lymphatic vessels to distant organs

Metastasis to the brain

Blood vessels

Primary tumor (carcinoma)

Cancer cells reinvade and grow at new location

Figure 1.8 _____/_____.
beyond   control

25. MATCH: *Draw a line to match the word part with its definition.*

    a. onc/o   one who studies and treats (specialist, physician)
    b. -logy   tumor(s)
    c. -logist   study of

26. TRANSLATE: *Complete the definitions of the following terms by using the meaning of word parts to fill in the blanks.*

    a. study of tumors   _____/ o /_____
                                        wr   cv   s

    b. physician who studies and treats tumors   _____/ o /_____
                                          wr   cv   s

27. READ: Oncology (ong-KOL-o-jē) is the medical specialty devoted to the treatment and care of cancer patients. An **oncologist** (ong-KOL-o-jist) is a physician who treats patients diagnosed with cancer.

28. REVIEW OF BODY STRUCTURE AND ONCOLOGY TERMS BUILT FROM WORD PARTS: the following is an alphabetical list of terms built and translated in the previous exercises.

MEDICAL TERMS BUILT FROM WORD PARTS			
TERM	**DEFINITION**	**TERM**	**DEFINITION**
1. carcinogenic (kar-sin-ō-JEN-ik)	producing cancer	**3. cytoid** (SĪ-toid)	resembling a cell
2. carcinoma (CA) (kar-si-NŌ-ma)	cancerous tumor (Figure 1.7)	**4. cytology** (sī-TOL-o-jē)	study of cells

MEDICAL TERMS BUILT FROM WORD PARTS—cont'd

TERM	DEFINITION	TERM	DEFINITION
5. **epithelial** (ep-i-THĒ-lē-al)	pertaining to epithelium	14. **oncologist** (ong-KOL-o-jist)	physician who studies and treats tumors
6. **epithelioma** (ep-i-thē-lē-Ō-ma)	tumor composed of epithelial tissue	15. **oncology** (ong-KOL-o-jē)	study of tumors
7. **histology** (his-TOL-o-jē)	study of tissues	16. **pathogenic** (path-ō-JEN-ik)	producing disease
8. **lipoid** (LIP-oid)	resembling fat	17. **pathologist** (pa-THOL-o-jist)	physician who studies disease
9. **lipoma** (li-PŌ-ma)	tumor composed of fat tissue (Figure 1.5)	18. **pathology (PATH)** (pa-THOL-o-jē)	study of disease
10. **metastasis (pl. metastases) (mets)** (me-TAS-ta-sis) (me-TAS-ta-sēz)	beyond control [transfer of disease beyond the tissue or organ of origin] (Figure 1.8)	19. **radiologist** (rā-dē-OL-o-jist)	physician who studies and treats using x-rays (and other diagnostic imaging procedures)
11. **myoma** (mī-Ō-ma)	tumor composed of muscle tissue	20. **radiology** (rā-dē-OL-o-jē)	study of x-rays (and other diagnostic imaging procedures)
12. **neoplasm** (NĒ-ō-plazm)	new growth	21. **sarcoma** (sar-KŌ-ma)	tumor of connective tissue
13. **neuroma** (nû-RŌ-ma)	tumor composed of nerve tissue	22. **visceral** (VIS-er-al)	pertaining to internal organs

EXERCISE D　Pronounce and Spell Terms Built from Word Parts

Practice pronunciation and spelling on paper and online.

1. `Practice on Paper`
    a. **Pronounce**: Read the phonetic spelling and say aloud the terms listed in the previous table, Review Terms Built from Word Parts. Refer to the pronunciation key on p. 9 as necessary.
    b. **Spell**: Have a study partner read the terms aloud. Write the spelling of the terms on a separate sheet of paper.

2. `Practice Online` ⊕
    a. **Access** online learning resources. Go to evolve.elsevier.com > Evolve Resources > Practice Student Resources.
    b. **Pronounce**: Select Audio Glossary > Lesson 1 > Exercise D. Select a term to hear its pronunciation and repeat aloud.
    c. **Spell**: Select Activities > Lesson 1 > Spell Terms > Exercise D. Select the audio icon and type the correct spelling of the term.

❑　Check the box when complete.

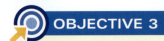

OBJECTIVE 3

Define, pronounce, and spell medical terms NOT built from word parts.

The terms listed below may contain word parts, but are difficult to translate literally.

MEDICAL TERMS **NOT** BUILT FROM WORD PARTS

TERM	DEFINITION
benign (be-NĪN)	not malignant, nonrecurring
biopsy (Bx) (BĪ-op-sē)	removal of living tissue to be viewed under a microscope for diagnostic purposes
chemotherapy (chemo) (kē-mō-THER-a-pē)	treatment of cancer by using pharmaceuticals
diagnosis (Dx) (dī-ag-NŌ-sis)	identification of a disease
infection (in-FEK-shun)	invasion of pathogens in body tissue
inflammation (in-fla-MĀ-shun)	localized, protective response to injury or tissue destruction characterized by redness, swelling, heat, and pain
malignant (ma-LIG-nant)	tending to become progressively worse, possibly resulting in death
prognosis (Px) (prog-NŌ-sis)	prediction of a possible outcome of a disease
radiation therapy (XRT) (rā-dē-Ā-shun THER-a-pē)	treatment of cancer with radioactive substances, x-rays, and other forms of radiation; types include external beam, internal placement, and systemic administration of pharmaceuticals; (also called **radiation oncology** and **radiotherapy**)
remission (rē-MISH-un)	lessening or absence of signs of disease
staphylococcus **(pl. staphylococci) (staph)** (staf-il-ō-KOK-us) (staf-il-ō-KOK-sī)	bacterium that grows in a pattern resembling grapelike clusters and can cause infections
streptococcus **(pl. streptococci) (strep)** (strep-tō-KOK-us) (strep-tō-KOK-sī)	bacterium that grows in a pattern resembling twisted chains and can cause infections

> **FYI**   **Inflammation** is a natural response that generally assists in the recovery from infection or injury, but it may also cause damage if it occurs inappropriately or is abnormally prolonged.

EXERCISE E   **Label**

Write the medical terms pictured and defined using the previous table of Medical Terms NOT Built from Word Parts. Check your work with the Answer Key in Appendix C.

1. _____(singular)

_____(plural)

bacterium that grows in a pattern resembling grapelike clusters and can cause infections

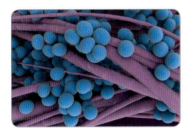

2. _____(singular)

_____(plural)

bacterium that grows in a pattern resembling twisted chains and can cause infections

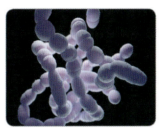

3. _____

invasion of pathogens in body tissue

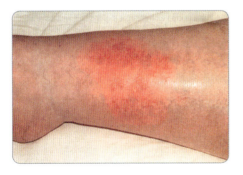

4. _____

removal of living tissue to be viewed under a microscope for diagnostic purposes

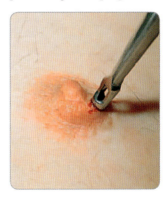

5. _____
treatment of cancer by using pharmaceuticals

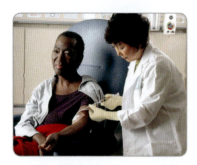

6. _____
treatment of cancer with a radioactive substances, x-rays, and other forms of radiation

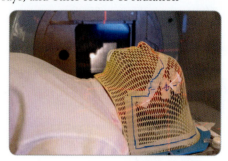

7. _____
tending to become progressively worse

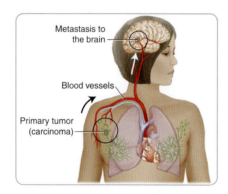

EXERCISE F **Learn Medical Terms NOT Built from Word Parts**

Fill in the blanks with medical terms defined in bold using the Medical Terms NOT Built from Word Parts table on the previous page. Check your work with the Answer key in Appendix C.

1. Neoplasms are classified as either **nonrecurring** _____ or **tending to become progressively worse** _____. A **removal of living tissue to be viewed under a microscope** _____ of a neoplasm may be performed and sent to the lab to make a diagnosis.

2. Once the **identification of disease** _____ of cancer has been made a **prediction of a possible outcome of a disease** _____ is considered.

3. A Px may be improved with treatments such as **treatment of cancer by using pharmaceuticals** _____ or **radioactive substances** _____. The course of the disease may improve, and the patient may have a **lessening or absence of signs of disease** _____.

4. **Localized, protective response to injury or tissue destruction characterized by redness, swelling, heat, and pain** _____ results from a wound or injury. After surgery, inflammation accompanied by a fever may be an indication of infection.

5. Many common bacterial **invasion of pathogens in body tissue** _____s are caused by **bacterium that grows in grapelike clusters (singular)** _____ and **bacterium that grows in twisted chains (singular)** _____.

EXERCISE G　**Pronounce and Spell Terms NOT Built from Word Parts**

Practice pronunciation and spelling on paper and online.

1. **Practice on Paper**
   a. **Pronounce**: Read the phonetic spelling and say aloud the terms listed in Medical Terms NOT Built from Word Parts table. Refer to the pronunciation key on p. 9 as necessary.
   b. **Spell**: Have a study partner read the terms aloud. Write the spelling of the terms on a separate sheet of paper.

2. **Practice Online** 🌐
   a. **Access** online learning resources. Go to evolve.elsevier.com > Evolve Resources > Practice Student Resources.
   b. **Pronounce**: Select Audio Glossary > Lesson 1 > Exercise G. Select a term to hear its pronunciation and repeat aloud.
   c. **Spell**: Select Activities > Lesson 1 > Spell Terms > Exercise G. Select the audio icon and type the correct spelling of the term.

❏　Check the box when complete.

OBJECTIVE 4

Write abbreviations.

ABBREVIATIONS RELATED TO ONCOLOGY

Use the online **flashcards** to familiarize yourself with the following abbreviations.

ABBREVIATION	TERM	ABBREVIATION	TERM
Bx	biopsy	PATH	pathology
CA	cancer, carcinoma	Px	prognosis
chemo	chemotherapy	staph	staphylococcus, staphylococci
Dx	diagnosis	strep	streptococcus, streptococci
lab	laboratory	XRT	radiation therapy
mets	metastasis, metastases		

EXERCISE H   Abbreviate Medical Terms

Write the correct abbreviation next to its medical term.

1. Diseases and disorders:

_____   cancer, carcinoma

2. Descriptive of the disease process:

   a. _____   metastasis, metastases

   b. _____   diagnosis

   c. _____   prognosis

3. Surgical procedures:

_____   biopsy

4. Treatments:

   a. _____   radiation therapy

   b. _____   chemotherapy

5. Specialties:

_____   pathology

6. Related Terms:

   a. _____   laboratory

   b. _____   staphylococcus, staphylococci

   c. _____   streptococcus, streptococci

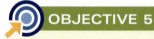

OBJECTIVE 5

Identify body structure and oncology terms.

Now that you have worked through the lesson, review and practice body structure and oncology terms. *Check your responses using the Answer Key in Appendix C.*

EXERCISE I   Body Structure Terms

Write the medical term next to its definition.

1. _____   resembling a cell

2. _____   resembling fat

3. _____   pertaining to epithelium

4. _____   pertaining to internal organs

EXERCISE J **Oncology Terms**

Write the medical term next to its definition.

Signs and Symptoms

1. _____ localized, protective response to injury or tissue destruction characterized by redness, swelling, heat, and pain

Diseases and Disorders

2. _____ new growth

3. _____ tumor composed of epithelial tissue

4. _____ tumor composed of nerve tissue

5. _____ tumor of connective tissue

6. _____ tumor composed of fat tissue

7. _____ tumor composed of muscle tissue

8. _____ cancerous tumor

9. _____ invasion of pathogens in body tissue

Descriptive of Disease and Disease Processes

10. _____ identification of a disease

11. _____ prediction of possible outcome of a disease

12. _____ tending to become progressively worse, possibly resulting in death

13. _____ not malignant, nonrecurring

14. _____ lessening or absence of signs of disease

15. _____ beyond control (transfer of the disease beyond the tissue or organ of origin); (singular)

Surgical Procedures

16. _____ removal of living tissue to be viewed under a microscope for diagnostic purposes

Treatments

17. _____ treatment of cancer with radioactive substances, x-rays, and other forms of radiation

18. _____ treatment of cancer using pharmaceuticals

Specialties and Professions

19. _____ physician who studies disease

20. _____ physician who studies and treats tumors

21. _____ study of tumors

22. _____ study of tissues

23. _____ study of disease

24. _____ study of cells

25. _____ study of x-rays (and other diagnostic imaging procedures)

26. _____ physician who studies and treats using x-rays (and other diagnostic imaging procedures)

Related Terms

27. _____ producing cancer

28. _____ producing disease

29. _____ bacterium that grows in a pattern resembling twisted chains and can cause infections (singular)

30. _____ bacterium that grows in a pattern resembling grapelike clusters and can cause infections (singular)

 OBJECTIVE 6

Use medical language in clinical statements, the case study, and a medical record.

EXERCISE K **Use Medical Terms in Clinical Statements**

Circle the medical term or abbreviation defined in the bolded phrases. Answers are listed in Appendix C. For pronunciation practice read the answers aloud.

1. **Producing disease** (Histology, Pathology, Pathogenic) bacteria may cause infection. A(n) **producing cancer** (carcinogenic, carcinoma, oncology) agent or substance may cause cancer.

2. A patient with a(n) **identification of a disease** (diagnosis, prognosis, remission) of **cancer** (chemo, CA, mets) may seek the services of a(n) **physician who studies and treats tumors** (histologist, pathologist, oncologist).

3. The **new growth** (neoplasm, myoma, epithelioma) was biopsied and sent to the laboratory for **study of cells** (pathology, cytology, histology) to determine if the tumor is **nonrecurring** (malignant, benign, inflammation) or **tending to become progressively worse** (malignant, benign, inflammation).

4. The **physician who studies disease** (oncologist, histologist, pathologist) described the tissue as **resembling fat** (lipoma, lipoid, cytoid).

5. Mrs. Gonzalez' **study of disease** (pathology, cytology, histology) report indicated the presence of **tumor of connective tissue** (carcinoma, sarcoma, lipoma) with **beyond control** (metastasis, remission, neoplasm). She will be transferred to the **study of tumors** (histology, oncology, epithelial) unit of the hospital. The **prediction of a possible outcome of a disease** (Dx, Bx, Px) is poor.

EXERCISE L   Apply Medical Terms to the Case Study

Think back to Tova, who was introduced in the case study at the beginning of the lesson. After working through Lesson 1 on body structure and oncology, consider the medical terms that might be used to describe her experience. List two terms relevant to the case study and their meanings. ■

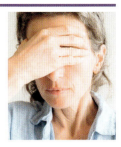

Medical Term   **Definition**

1. _____   _____

2. _____   _____

EXERCISE M   Use Medical Terms in a Document

Tova was able to see her primary care physician who referred her for further testing. The following medical document notes the care and treatment Tova received.

Use the definitions in numbers 1-12 to write medical terms within the following document.

1. removal of living tissue to be viewed under a microscope for diagnostic purpose

2. study of cells

3. physician who studies disease

4. identification of a disease

5. cancerous tumor

6. localized, protective response to injury or tissue destruction characterized by redness, swelling, heat, and pain

7. beyond control

8. tending to become progressively worse, possibly resulting in death

9. physician who studies and treats tumors

10. treatment of cancer using pharmaceuticals

11. prediction of possible outcome of a disease

12. treatment of cancer with radioactive substances, x-rays, and other forms of radiation

Refer to the medical record to answer questions 13-17. Mark T for true, and F for false.

13. _____ The cancer has spread from the colon to other surrounding organs.

14. _____ Ms. Katz's prognosis is carcinoma of the colon.

15. _____ Ms. Katz was referred to a pathologist for consideration of treatment of cancer using pharmaceuticals.

```
┌─────────────────────────────────────────────────────────────────────────┐
│ 04417 Katz, Tova                                              _ □ X       │
│ File    Patient    Navigate    Custom Fields    Help                      │
│ [« ] [» ] [👤][👥][▯][▮][▤][🏠][Rx][🕐][ℹ][✂][📋][🔒][▦][✔][🌐][🔍][?]      │
│ Chart Review  Encounters  Notes  Labs  Imaging  Procedures  Rx  Documents  Referrals  Scheduling  Billing │
│ Name: Katz, Tova          MR#: 04417       Sex: F      ┌ Allergies: None known ──┐ │
│                           DOB: 10/17/19XX  Age: 54     │ PCP: Patel, Aashish MD  │ │
│ ┌─────────────────────────────────────────────────────────────────────┐ ▲     │
│ │ CLINICAL NOTATION                                                     │       │
│ │                                                                       │       │
│ │ ENCOUNTER DATE: 02/21/20XX                                            │       │
│ │                                                                       │       │
│ │ A 54-year-old woman presented to the office with a 3-week history of  │       │
│ │ bloody diarrhea. She had been diagnosed with ulcerative colitis at    │       │
│ │ age 25 years. She was referred for a colonoscopy. The examination     │       │
│ │ revealed a suspicious lesion in the transverse colon.                 │       │
│ │ A (1.) _____ was performed and a (2.) _____ specimen │       │
│ │ was obtained. The (3.) _____ made a (4.) _____ of    │       │
│ │ (5.) _____ of the colon. Advanced dysplasia and (6.) _____ │       │
│ │ was present in the specimen. The patient underwent surgery and was    │       │
│ │ found to have no evidence of (7.) _____. Her entire     │       │
│ │ colon was removed because of a high risk for developing a (8.)         │       │
│ │ _____ lesion in the remaining colon.                       │       │
│ │ She made an uneventful recovery and was referred to an (9.) _____ │       │
│ │ for consideration of (10.) _____. Her (11.) _____ │       │
│ │ is generally positive. (12.) _____ is not indicated  │       │
│ │ in this case.                                                         │       │
│ │                                                                       │       │
│ │ Electronically signed: Aashish Patel, MD 02/21/20XX 14:43             │       │
│ └─────────────────────────────────────────────────────────────────────┘ ▼     │
│ ◀ ───────────────────────────────────────────────────────────────────── ▶     │
│    Start   Log On/Off   Print   Edit                          [🖥][🔊][⚡][🔒]  │
└─────────────────────────────────────────────────────────────────────────┘
```

16. Identify two abbreviations of medical terms used within the clinical notation.

Abbreviation _____   Term _____

Abbreviation _____   Term _____

17. Identify a new medical term in the medical record you would like to investigate. Use your medical dictionary or an online resource to look up the definition.

Medical Term	Definition
1. _____	_____
2. _____	_____

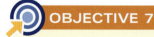

OBJECTIVE 7

Recall and assess knowledge of word parts, medical terms, and abbreviations.

EXERCISE N   **Online Review of Lesson Content**

🌐 *Recall and assess your learning from working through the lesson by completing online learning activities at evolve. elsevier.com > Evolve Resources > Practice Student Resources. Keep track of your progress by placing a check mark next to completed activities.*

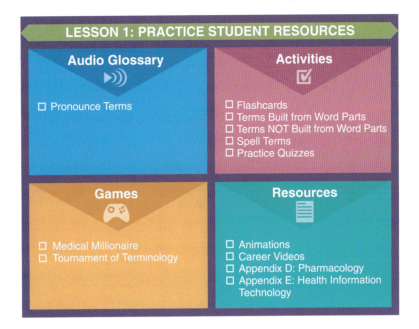

EXERCISE O **Lesson Content Quiz**

Test your knowledge of the terms and abbreviations introduced in this lesson. Circle the letter for the medical term or abbreviation related to the words in italics.

1. In the medical term cytology, *logy* is the:
   a. prefix
   b. suffix
   c. combining form

2. *Neuroma*, *myoma*, and *epithelioma* are all diagnoses which indicate the presence of a:
   a. tumor
   b. growth
   c. cancer

3. The oncologist ordered a *treatment using a radioactive substance.*
   a. chemo
   b. Dx
   c. XRT

4. *Pertaining to internal organs* leishmaniasis, also called black fever, is transmitted by sand flies.
   a. visceral
   b. epithelial
   c. lipoid

5. The skin biopsy was sent to the *study of tissues* department of the medical laboratory for analysis.
   a. cytology
   b. oncology
   c. histology

6. The respiratory *invasion of pathogens in body tissue* was caused by streptococcus bacteria.
   a. inflammation
   b. infection
   c. biopsy

7. The eye examination revealed no *resembling a cell* bodies.
   a. lipoid
   b. cytoid
   c. carcinogenic

8. The patient was transported to the *study of x-rays* department for her chest x-ray.
   a. radiology
   b. radiologist
   c. pathology

9. *Localized protective response to injury* was the first sign of an infection.
   a. carcinoma
   b. biopsy
   c. inflammation

10. The *physician who studies and treats using x-rays and other diagnostic procedures* interpreted the patient's CT scan of the abdomen and documented the findings.
    a. radiology
    b. radiologist
    c. oncologist

LESSON AT A GLANCE   **INTRODUCTION TO MEDICAL LANGUAGE, BODY STRUCTURE, AND ONCOLOGY WORD PARTS**

MEDICAL LANGUAGE ORIGINS
Greek and Latin word parts
acronyms
eponyms
modern language

WORD PARTS
word root
suffix
prefix
combining vowel

COMBINING FORMS
carcin/o
cyt/o
epitheli/o
hist/o
lip/o
my/o
neur/o
onc/o
path/o
radi/o
sarc/o
viscer/o

SUFFIXES
-al
-genic
-logist
-logy
-oid
-oma
-plasm
-stasis

PREFIXES
meta-
neo-

LESSON AT A GLANCE   **INTRODUCTION TO MEDICAL LANGUAGE, BODY STRUCTURE, AND ONCOLOGY MEDICAL TERMS AND ABBREVIATIONS**

SIGNS AND SYMPTOMS
inflammation

DISEASES AND DISORDERS
carcinoma (CA)
epithelioma
infection
lipoma
myoma
neoplasm
neuroma
sarcoma

DESCRIPTIVE OF DISEASE AND DISEASE PROCESSES
benign
diagnosis (Dx)
malignant
metastasis, metastases (mets)
prognosis (Px)
remission

SURGICAL PROCEDURES
biopsy

TREATMENTS
chemotherapy (chemo)
radiation therapy (XRT)

SPECIALTIES AND PROFESSIONS
cytology
histology
oncologist
oncology
pathologist
pathology (PATH)
radiologist
radiology

BODY STRUCTURE TERMS
cytoid
epithelial
lipoid
visceral

RELATED TERMS
carcinogenic
pathogenic
staphylococcus, staphylococci (staph)
streptococcus, streptococci (strep)

ABBREVIATIONS
Bx	lab	staph
CA	mets	strep
chemo	PATH	XRT
Dx	Px	

Directional Terms, Positions, and Imaging

A'idah Khalil

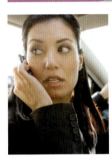

A'idah Khalil was just in a car accident, but luckily, she is awake and knows what is going on around her. The ambulance comes and the emergency team asks her where she is hurting. Her right foot hurts the most. She has pain in her upper right arm and notices some bleeding there. She also has some pain in her belly and back. The paramedics put her on a hard board, put some kind of collar around her neck, then load her into the ambulance and take her to the hospital.

■ *Consider A'idah's situation as you work through the lesson. We will return to this case study and identify medical terms used to document A'idah's experience and the care she receives.*

OBJECTIVES

1 ■ Build, translate, pronounce, and spell directional terms built from word parts (p. 29).

2 ■ Define, pronounce, and spell medical terms NOT built from word parts related to anatomic planes, abdominopelvic regions, and patient positions (p. 38).

3 ■ Write abbreviations (p. 42).

4 ■ Identify medical terms (p. 43).

5 ■ Use medical language in clinical statements, the case study, and a medical record (p. 45).

6 ■ Recall and assess knowledge of word parts, medical terms, and abbreviations (p. 48).

OBJECTIVE 1

Build, translate, pronounce, and spell directional terms built from word parts.

Directional terms communicate a specific location or direction of movement and often describe:

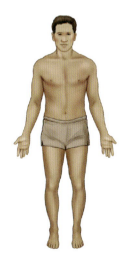

- Locations on or within the body, organs, and anatomic structures
- Direction of x-ray beams used in radiology
- Orientation of diagnostic images
- Surgical approaches

When using directional terms, the body is assumed to be in the standard, neutral position of reference called the **anatomic position.** In this position, the body is viewed as standing erect, arms at the side, palms of the hands facing forward, and feet side by side (Figure 2.1). The directional terms are the same whether the person is standing or supine (lying face up).

Figure 2.1 Anatomic position.

CAREER FOCUS   Professionals Who Use Directional Terms

Professionals working in radiology frequently use directional terms, anatomic planes, and patient positions. **Radiologic Technologists (RTs)** perform diagnostic imaging examinations and administer radiation therapy treatments. Types of radiologic technologists include:

- **Computed Tomography (CT) Technologists**, also called CT Technicians, operate CT equipment to produce cross-sectional or "sliced" images of internal structures.
- **Magnetic Resonance (MR) Technologists**, operate MR equipment to produce images using a strong magnetic field and radiofrequencies.
- **Radiographers** operate x-ray equipment using radiation to produce black and white images of bone structures and soft tissues.
- **Sonographers**, also called Ultrasound Technicians, operate sonography equipment to create images of internal organs using sound waves.
- **Radiation Therapists** administer high doses of radiation to treat cancer and other disease.

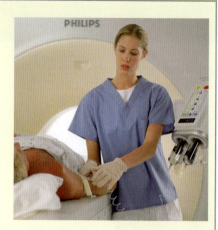

Figure 2.2 CT technologist preparing a patient for computed tomography.

FOR MORE INFORMATION

- Access online learning resources at evolve.elsevier.com > Practice Student Resources > Other Resources > Career Videos to watch interviews with a **CT Technologist**, a **Radiologic Technologist**, and an **Ultrasound Technologist**.

WORD PARTS   Use the paper or online **flashcards** to familiarize yourself with the following word parts.

COMBINING FORM (WR + CV)	DEFINITION	COMBINING FORM (WR + CV)	DEFINITION
anter/o	front	later/o	side
caud/o	tail (downward)	medi/o	middle
cephal/o	head (upward)	poster/o	back, behind
dist/o	away (from the point of attachment)	proxim/o	near (the point of attachment)
		super/o	above
dors/o	back	ventr/o	belly (front)
infer/o	below		
SUFFIX (S)	**DEFINITION**	**SUFFIX (S)**	**DEFINITION**
-ad	toward	-al, -ic, -ior	pertaining to

For definitions of word root, suffix, prefix, and combining vowel, see Using Word Parts to Build Medical Terms on p. 3.

EXERCISE A   **Build and Translate Directional Terms Built from Word Parts**

*Use the **Word Parts Table** to complete the following questions. Check your responses with the Answer Key in Appendix C.*

1. **MATCH:** *Draw a line to match the suffix with its definition. The following suffixes will be used to build and translate directional terms in the following exercises.*

   a. -al, -ic, -ior   toward
   b. -ad   pertaining to

2. **LABEL:** *Write the combining forms to complete Figure 2.3.*

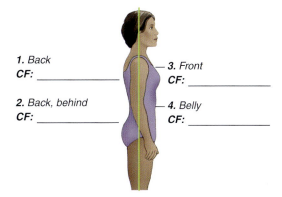

   1. Back
   CF: _____

   3. Front
   CF: _____

   2. Back, behind
   CF: _____

   4. Belly
   CF: _____

   Figure 2.3 Combining forms for front and back.

3. **TRANSLATE:** *Complete the definitions of the following terms by using the meaning of word parts to fill in the blanks. Remember, the definition usually starts with the meaning of the suffix.*

   a. ventr/al   _____ to the _____
   b. dors/al   pertaining _____ the _____
   c. anter/ior   _____ to the _____
   d. poster/ior   pertaining _____ the _____ (behind)

4. **READ: Ventral** (VEN-tral) and **anterior** (an-TĒR-ē-or) refer to the front of the body or anatomic structure described. The ventral cavity, located in the anterior portion of the body, is made up of the thoracic and abdominopelvic cavities. **Dorsal** (DOR-sal) and **posterior** (pos-TĒR-ē-or) refer to the back of the body or anatomic structure described. The dorsal cavity, located in the posterior portion of the body, is made up of the cranial and spinal cavities (See Figure 1-6, p. 13). Anterior and posterior are also used to describe the location of anatomical structures in relation to one another. For example, the sternum is anterior to the heart.

5. **LABEL:** *Write word parts to complete Figure 2.4.*

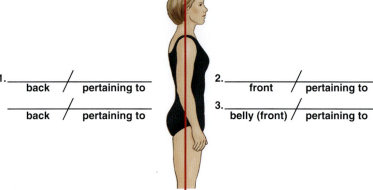

1. _____ / _____
   back   pertaining to

_____ / _____
   back   pertaining to

2. _____ / _____
   front   pertaining to

3. _____ / _____
   belly (front) / pertaining to

Figure 2.4 Directional terms describing the front and the back.

6. **TRANSLATE:** *Complete the definitions of the following terms by using the meaning of word parts to fill in the blanks.*

   a. poster/o/anter/ior (PA)   _____ to the _____ and to the _____

   b. anter/o/poster/ior (AP)   pertaining _____ the _____ and to the _____

7. **READ: Posteroanterior** (pos-ter-ō-an-TĒR-ē-or) and **anteroposterior** (an-ter-ō-pos-TĒR-ē-or) are used to describe the direction of the x-ray beam used in radiography. PA projection for a chest radiograph is used when the heart or other anterior structures are the focus of the diagnostic study. AP projection for a chest radiograph is used when the spine is the primary focus.

8. **LABEL:** *Write word parts to complete Figure 2.5.*

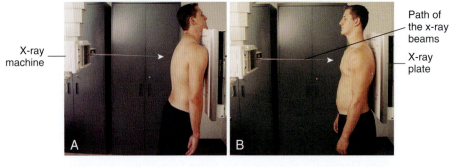

X-ray machine _____

Path of the x-ray beams

X-ray plate

A

B

Figure 2.5 A. _____ /o/_____ /_____ projection
       back   front   pertaining to

B. _____ /o/_____ /_____ projection
       front   back   pertaining to

Organs closest to the x-ray plate look the most accurate on a radiograph. In the PA projection (A), the x-ray beam moves from the back to the front of the body; in the AP projection (B), the x-ray beam moves through the front of the body to the back of the body.

9. LABEL: *Write combining forms to complete Figure 2.6.*

> **FYI Head and Trunk Only**
> Terms built from the combining forms **cephal/o** and **caud/o** are used to describe locations in the head and trunk of the body.

1. Above
CF: ____________

2. Head
CF: ____________

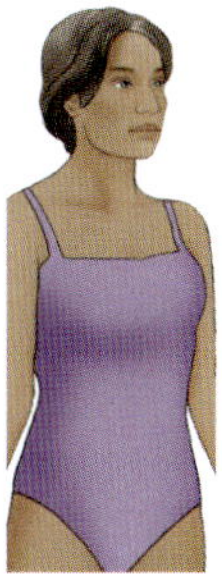

3. Tail
CF: ____________

4. Below
CF: ____________

Figure 2.6 Combining forms for above and below.

---

10. TRANSLATE: *Complete the definitions of the following terms by using the meaning of word parts to fill in the blanks.*

a. super/ior ____________________ to ____________________

b. infer/ior ____________________ to ____________________

c. anter/o/super/ior pertaining ________ the ______________ and ______________

---

11. READ: When considering the head and trunk of the body, **superior** (sū-PĒR-ē-or) indicates toward the head and **inferior** (in-FĒR-ē-or) indicates toward the pelvis (these terms do not apply to the limbs). The terms can also be used to describe the position of anatomical structures in relation to one another. For example, the eyes are superior to the mouth, and conversely, the mouth is inferior to the eyes. **Anterosuperior** (an-ter-ō-sū-PĒR-ē-or) indicates direction or location toward the front and above, as might be seen in describing a surgical approach, projection angle, or location within an anatomical structure.

---

12. TRANSLATE: *Complete the definitions of the following terms by using the meaning of word parts to fill in the blanks.*

a. cephal/ic ____________________ to the ____________________

b. caud/al pertaining ______________ the ____________________

c. cephal/ad ____________________ the ____________________

d. caud/ad ____________________ the ____________________

---

13. **READ:** **Cephalic** (se-FAL-ik) and **caudal** (KAW-dal) are used to describe locations within the head and trunk of the body and are not used to describe the limbs. Cephalic, literally translated as pertaining to the head, refers to a position above. Caudal, literally translated as pertaining to the tail, indicates a position below. It might be helpful to consider the final portion of the spine as the "tail" and the use of caudal as referring to the bottom portion of the trunk of the body. **Cephalad** (SEF-a-lad) and **caudad** (KAW-dad) indicate movement in a specific direction as might be seen describing a surgical approach or diagnostic projection angle. Cephalad indicates toward the head or upward. Caudad indicates toward the tail or downward.

14. **LABEL:** *Write word parts to complete Figure 2.7.*

> **FYI** **Terms Used Interchangeably**
> When describing anatomical structures in the head and trunk of the body, the following terms are used synonymously:
> **Anterior** and **ventral** describe the front.
> **Posterior** and **dorsal** describe the back.
> **Superior** and **cephalic** describe above.
> **Inferior** and **caudal** describe below.

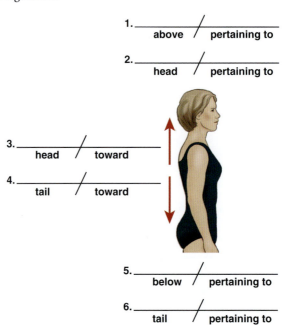

1. _____ / _____
   above / pertaining to

2. _____ / _____
   head / pertaining to

3. _____ / _____
   head / toward

4. _____ / _____
   tail / toward

5. _____ / _____
   below / pertaining to

6. _____ / _____
   tail / pertaining to

Figure 2.7 Directional terms describing above and below.

15. **LABEL:** *Write combining forms to complete Figure 2.8.*

> **FYI** **The midline** is a common reference point when describing anatomic locations. It is an imaginary line visualized in the middle of the body or anatomic structure, running from top to bottom and dividing the structure in half.

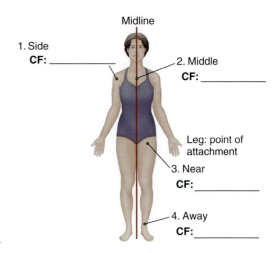

Midline

1. Side
   CF: _____

2. Middle
   CF: _____

Leg: point of attachment

3. Near
   CF: _____

4. Away
   CF: _____

Figure 2.8 Combining forms for middle, side, near, and away.

16. **BUILD:** *Write the word parts to build the following directional terms. Use the suffix –al.*

    a. pertaining to near [the point of attachment]   _____/_____

    　　　　　　　　　　　　　　　　　　　　　　　　　 wr 　　　　　　　 **s**

    b. pertaining to away [from the point of attachment]   _____/_____

    　　　　　　　　　　　　　　　　　　　　　　　　　 wr 　　　　　　　 **s**

17. **READ: Proximal** (PROK-si-mal) and **distal** (DIS-tal) are both used in reference to the point of attachment of the limb or anatomic structure described. When referring to a location on the arm, the shoulder is considered the point of attachment. Proximal indicates a location near the shoulder; distal indicates a position closer to the wrist (Figure 2.9).

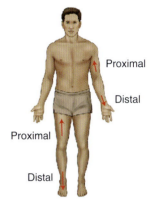

Figure 2.9 Proximal and distal.

18. **BUILD:** *Write the word parts to build the following directional terms. Use the suffix -al.*

    a. pertaining to the middle   _____/_____

    　　　　　　　　　　　　　　 wr 　　　　　　　 **s**

    b. pertaining to the side   _____/_____

    　　　　　　　　　　　　　 wr 　　　　　　　 **s**

19. **READ: Medial** (MĒ-dē-al) describes a location closer to the middle of the structure or the midline of the body. **Lateral** (LAT-e-ral) describes away from the middle of the structure or the midline of the body (Figure 2.10).

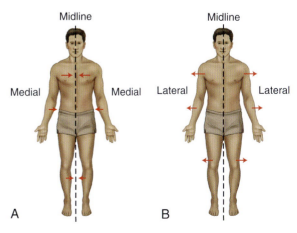

Figure 2.10 A. Medial, toward the midline. B. Lateral, toward the side.

20. LABEL: *Write word parts to complete Figure 2.11.*

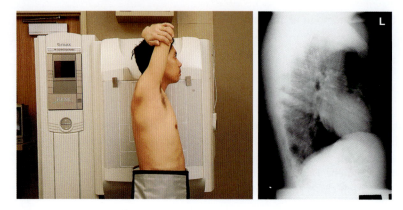

Figure 2.11 Chest radiograph, left _____/_____ position.
                                                     side   pertaining to

---

21. BUILD: *Write the word parts to build the following directional terms used to describe projection angles, surgical approaches, and specific locations within anatomical structures. Use the suffix -al.*

a. pertaining to the middle and to the side   _____/ o /_____/_____
                                                                      wr   cv   wr   s

b. pertaining to the front and to the middle   _____/ o /_____/_____
                                                                      wr   cv   wr   s

c. pertaining to the back and to the side   _____/ o /_____/_____
                                                                      wr   cv   wr   s

d. pertaining to above and to the side   _____/ o /_____/_____
                                                                      wr   cv   wr   s

e. pertain to below and to the side   _____/ o /_____/_____
                                                                      wr   cv   wr   s

f. pertaining to the front and to the side   _____/ o /_____/_____
                                                                      wr   cv   wr   s

---

22. REVIEW OF DIRECTIONAL TERMS BUILT FROM WORD PARTS: the following is an alphabetical list of terms built and translated in the previous exercises.

MEDICAL TERMS BUILT FROM WORD PARTS

TERM	DEFINITION	TERM	DEFINITION
1. anterior (ant) (an-TĒR-ē-or)	pertaining to the front (Figure 2.4)	**3. anteromedial** (an-ter-ō-MĒD-ē-al)	pertaining to the front and to the middle
2. anterolateral (an-ter-ō-LAT-er-al)	pertaining to the front and to the side	**4. anteroposterior (AP)** (an-ter-ō-pos-TĒR-ē-or)	pertaining to the front and to the back (Figure 2.5, B)

MEDICAL TERMS BUILT FROM WORD PARTS—cont'd

TERM	DEFINITION	TERM	DEFINITION
5. **anterosuperior** (an-ter-ō-sū-PĒR-ē-or)	pertaining to the front and above	15. **medial (med)** (MĒ-dē-al)	pertaining to the middle (Figure 2.10, A)
6. **caudad** (KAW-dad)	toward the tail (Figure 2.7)	16. **mediolateral** (mē-dē-ō-LAT-er-al)	pertaining to the middle and to the side
7. **caudal** (KAW-dal)	pertaining to the tail (Figure 2.7)	17. **posterior (post)** (pos-TĒR-ē-or)	pertaining to back, behind (Figure 2.4)
8. **cephalad** (SEF-a-lad)	toward the head (Figure 2.7)	18. **posteroanterior (PA)** (pos-ter-ō-an-TĒR-ē-or)	pertaining to the back and to the front (Figure 2.5, A)
9. **cephalic** (se-FAL-ik)	pertaining to the head (Figure 2.7)	19. **posterolateral** (pos-ter-ō-LAT-er-al)	pertaining to the back and to the side
10. **distal** (DIS-tal)	pertaining to away (from the point of attachment) (Figure 2.9)	20. **proximal** (PROK-si-mal)	pertaining to near (the point of attachment) (Figure 2.9)
11. **dorsal** (DOR-sal)	pertaining to the back (Figure 2.4)	21. **superior (sup)** (sū-PĒR-ē-or)	pertaining to above (Figure 2.7)
12. **inferior (inf)** (in-FĒR-ē-or)	pertaining to below (Figure 2.7)	22. **superolateral** (sū-per-ō-LAT-er-al)	pertaining to above and to the side
13. **inferolateral** (in-fer-ō-LAT-er-al)	pertaining to below and to the side	23. **ventral** (VEN-tral)	pertaining to the belly (Figure 2.4)
14. **lateral (lat)** (LAT-e-ral)	pertaining to the side (Figure 2.10, B; 2.11)		

EXERCISE B Pronounce and Spell Terms Built from Word Parts

Practice pronunciation and spelling on paper and online.

1. **Practice on Paper**
   a. **Pronounce**: Read the phonetic spelling and say aloud the terms listed in the previous table, Review Terms Built from Word Parts. Refer to the pronunciation key on p. 9 as necessary.
   b. **Spell**: Have a study partner read the terms aloud. Write the spelling of the terms on a separate sheet of paper.

2. **Practice Online** 🌐
   a. **Access** online learning resources. Go to evolve.elsevier.com > Evolve Resources > Practice Student Resources.
   b. **Pronounce**: Select Audio Glossary > Exercise B. Select a term to hear its pronunciation and repeat aloud.
   c. **Spell**: Select Activities > Spell Terms > Exercise B. Select the audio icon and type the correct spelling of the term.

❏ Check the box when complete.

OBJECTIVE 2

Define, pronounce, and spell medical terms NOT built from word parts related to anatomic planes, abdominopelvic regions, and patient positions.

Anatomic Planes and Imaging

Planes are imaginary, flat fields used as points of reference to identify or view the location of organs and anatomical structures (Figure 2.12). The body is assumed to be in the **anatomic position** (see Figure 2.1) unless specified otherwise. The terms identifying anatomic planes are categorized as NOT built from word parts. Though word parts may be present, the terms are difficult to translate. References to the anatomic planes are frequently used in diagnostic imaging to describe the angle from which images are captured; see the table following the list of anatomic planes for an overview of diagnostic imaging procedures.

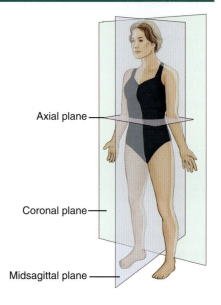

Figure 2.12 Anatomic Planes.

ANATOMIC PLANES

TERM	DEFINITION
axial plane (AK-see-uh-l) (plān)	horizontal field dividing the body into superior and inferior portions; (also called **transverse plane** and **horizontal plane**)
coronal plane (ko-RŌN-al) (plān)	vertical field passing through the body from side to side, dividing the body into anterior and posterior portions; (also called **frontal plane**)
sagittal plane (SAJ-i-tal) (plān)	vertical field running through the body from front to back, dividing the body into right and left sides. The midsagittal plane is the sagittal plane at the midline of the body.

OVERVIEW OF DIAGNOSTIC IMAGING PROCEDURES

PROCEDURE	DESCRIPTION
radiography	produces an image of internal structures using ionizing radiation; the resulting images are called radiographs. Radiography, the procedure, and radiograph, the resulting image, are both also called **x-ray**.
computed tomography (CT)	produces a series of sectional images of internal structures using ionizing radiation; computer software assembles data into images called scans
magnetic resonance (MR)	produces images of internal structures using high strength magnetic fields; computer software assembles data into images called scans
nuclear medicine (NM)	produces images of internal structures using gamma rays emitted from radioactive material introduced to the bloodstream; computer software assembles data into images called scans
sonography	produces images of internal structures using high frequency sound waves; computer software assembles data into images called scans; (also called **ultrasonography** abbreviated as **US**)

Abdominopelvic Regions

To assist in communication of location, the abdomen and pelvis are divided into nine regions (Figure 2.13). Abdominopelvic regions are often used in the physical examination and medical history to describe signs and symptoms. The terms identifying regions are categorized as NOT built from word parts. Though word parts may be present, the terms are difficult to translate.

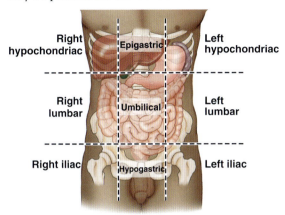

ABDOMINOPELVIC REGIONS (NUMBER OF REGIONS INDICATED IN PARENTHESES)	
TERM	**DEFINITION**
umbilical region (1) (um-BIL-i-kal) (RĒ-jun)	around the navel (umbilicus)
lumbar regions (2) (LUM-bar) (RĒ-junz)	to the right and left of the umbilical region, near the waist
epigastric region (1) (ep-i-GAS-trik) (RĒ-jun)	superior to the umbilical region
hypochondriac regions (2) (hī-pō-KON-drē-ak) (RĒ-junz)	to the right and left of the epigastric region
hypogastric region (1) (hī-pō-GAS-trik) (RĒ-jun)	inferior to the umbilical region
iliac regions (2) (IL-ē-ak) (RĒ-junz)	to the right and left of the hypogastric region, near the groin (also called **inguinal regions**)

Figure 2.13 Abdominopelvic regions.

Patient Positions

Position terms are used in healthcare settings to communicate how the patient's body is placed for physical examination, diagnostic procedures, surgery, treatment, and recovery (Figure 2.17).

TERM	**DEFINITION**
Fowler position (FOW-ler) (pe-ZISH-en)	semi-sitting position with slight elevation of the knees
orthopnea position (or-THOP-nē-a) (pe-ZISH-en)	sitting upright in a chair or in bed supported by pillows behind the back. Sometimes the patient tilts forward resting on a pillow supported by an overbed table. (also called **orthopneic position**)
prone position (prōn) (pe-ZISH-en)	lying on abdomen, facing downward (head may be turned to one side)
Sims position (simz) (pe-ZISH-en)	lying on side in a semi-prone position with the knee drawn up toward the chest and with the arm drawn behind, parallel to the back. "Right" and "left" precede the term to indicate the patient's right or left side. Originally, the term specifically indicated the patient's left side; therefore, if the Sims position is used without a description of right or left, it is assumed the patient is to be placed on the left side.
supine position (SOO-pīn) (pe-ZISH-en)	lying on back, facing upward
Trendelenburg position (tren-DEL-en-berg) (pe-ZISH-en)	lying on back with body tilted so that the head is lower than the feet

FYI **Fowler position** indicates the patient is in a sitting position with the head of the bed raised between 30° and 90°. Variations in the angle are denoted by **high Fowler**, indicating an upright position at approximately 90°, **Fowler** indicating an angle between 45° and 60°, **semi-Fowler**, 30° to 45°, and **low Fowler**, where the head is slightly elevated.

FYI **Orthopnea** is built from the combining form **orth/o** meaning straight, and the suffix **-pnea** meaning breathing. Patients who need to sit up straight to breathe are placed in the **orthopnea** position.

EXERCISE C   **Learn Anatomic Planes, Abdominopelvic Regions, and Patient Positions**

Fill in the blanks with medical terms defined using the previous tables. Check your responses with the Answer Key in Appendix C.

1. *Label Figure 2.14 by filling in the blanks.*

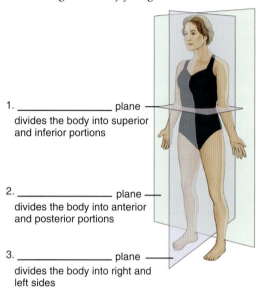

1. _____ plane divides the body into superior and inferior portions

2. _____ plane divides the body into anterior and posterior portions

3. _____ plane divides the body into right and left sides

Figure 2.14 Label anatomic planes.

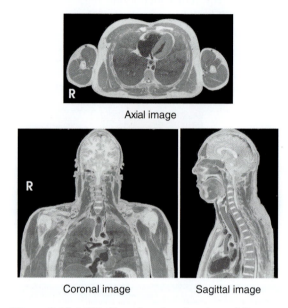

Axial image

Coronal image   Sagittal image

Figure 2.15 MRI slices showing the view of diagnostic images taken in the axial, coronal, and sagittal planes.

2. *Label Figure 2.16 by filling in the blanks.*

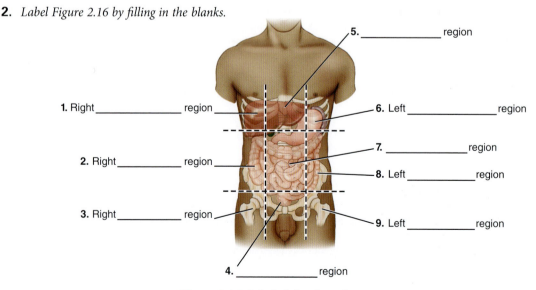

5. _____ region

1. Right _____ region

2. Right _____ region

3. Right _____ region

4. _____ region

6. Left _____ region

7. _____ region

8. Left _____ region

9. Left _____ region

Figure 2.16 Label abdominopelvic regions.

3. *Label Figure 2.17 by filling in the blanks.*

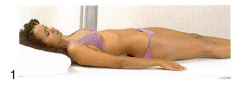

1

_____ position,
lying on back, facing upward

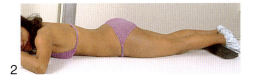

2

_____ position,
lying on abdomen, facing downward

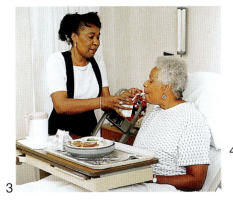

3

_____position,
semi-sitting position with slight
elevation of the knees

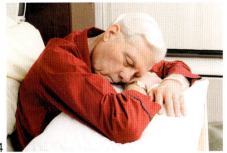

4

_____position,
sitting upright and tilted forward resting
on a pillow supported by an overbed
table

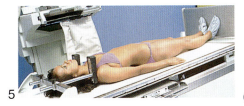

5

_____position,
lying on back with body tilted so that
the head is lower than the feet

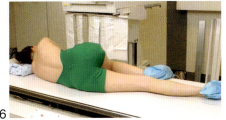

6

Modified _____position,
lying on left side with right knee
drawn up (notice the arm is placed in
front, rather than behind the body)

Figure 2.17 Label patient positions.

EXERCISE D | **Pronounce and Spell Anatomic Planes, Abdominopelvic Regions, and Patient Positions**

1. **Practice on Paper**
    a. **Pronounce:** Read the phonetic spelling and say aloud the terms for anatomic planes, abdominopelvic regions, and patient positions. Refer to the pronunciation key on p. 9 as necessary.
    b. **Spell:** Have a study partner read the terms aloud. Write the spelling of terms on a separate sheet of paper.

2. **Practice Online** ⊕
    a. **Access** online learning resources. Go to evolve.elsevier.com > Evolve Resources > Practice Student Resources.
    b. **Pronounce:** Select Audio Glossary > Exercise D. Select a term to hear its pronunciation and repeat aloud.
    c. **Spell:** Select Activities > Spell Terms > Exercise D. Select the audio icon and type the correct spelling of the term.

❑ Check the box when complete.

OBJECTIVE 3

Write abbreviations.

Abdominopelvic Quadrants

The abdominopelvic area also can be divided into four quadrants by using imaginary vertical and horizontal lines that intersect at the umbilicus. These divisions are used to communicate the location of pain, incisions, markings, and so forth (Figure 2.18). The four divisions are:

1. right upper quadrant (RUQ)
2. left upper quadrant (LUQ)
3. right lower quadrant (RLQ)
4. left lower quadrant (LLQ)

> **FYI**   The **abdominopelvic quadrants** provide a more general denotation than **abdominopelvic regions.** The quadrants are often used to describe signs and symptoms.

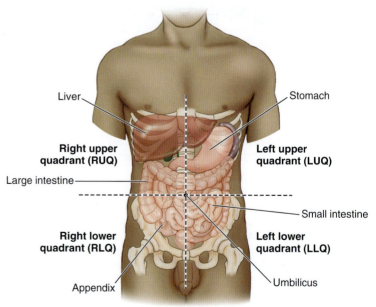

Figure 2.18 Abdominopelvic quadrants.

ABBREVIATIONS FOR ABDOMINOPELVIC QUADRANTS AND DIRECTIONAL TERMS

Use the online **flashcards** to familiarize yourself with the following abbreviations.

ABBREVIATION	TERM	ABBREVIATION	TERM
ant	anterior	med	medial
AP	anteroposterior	PA	posteroanterior
inf	inferior	post	posterior
lat	lateral	RLQ	right lower quadrant
LLQ	left lower quadrant	RUQ	right upper quadrant
LUQ	left upper quadrant	sup	superior

EXERCISE E Abbreviate Medical Terms

Write the correct abbreviation next to its medical term.

1. Directional Terms:

   a. _____ superior
   b. _____ inferior
   c. _____ medial
   d. _____ lateral
   e. _____ posteroanterior
   f. _____ anteroposterior
   g. _____ posterior
   h. _____ anterior

2. Abdominopelvic Quadrants:

   a. _____ right upper quadrant
   b. _____ right lower quadrant
   c. _____ left upper quadrant
   d. _____ left lower quadrant

OBJECTIVE 4

Identify medical terms.

Now that you have worked through the lesson, review and practice directional terms, anatomic planes, abdominopelvic regions, and patient positions.

EXERCISE F Directional Terms

Write directional term next to its definition.

1. _____ pertaining to the head
2. _____ pertaining to above
3. _____ pertaining to above and to the side
4. _____ pertaining to the back and to the side

5. _____ pertaining to the back and to the front

6. _____ pertaining to back, behind (starts with "p")

7. _____ pertaining to the back (starts with "d")

8. _____ pertaining to the middle and to the side

9. _____ pertaining to the front and to the middle

10. _____ pertaining to the middle

11. _____ pertaining to the side

12. _____ pertaining to below and to the side

13. _____ pertaining to below

14. _____ pertaining to near (the point of attachment)

15. _____ pertaining to away (from the point of attachment)

16. _____ toward the tail

17. _____ toward the head

18. _____ pertaining to the tail

19. _____ pertaining to the belly

20. _____ pertaining to the front

21. _____ pertaining to the front and above

22. _____ pertaining to the front and to the back

23. _____ pertaining to the front and to the side

EXERCISE G   Anatomic Planes

Write the anatomic plane next to its definition.

1. _____ plane   horizontal field dividing the body into superior and inferior portions

2. _____ plane   vertical field passing through the body from side to side, dividing the body into anterior and posterior portions

3. _____ plane   vertical field running through the body from front to back, dividing the body into right and left sides

EXERCISE H   Abdominopelvic Regions

Write the abdominopelvic region(s) next to its definition.

1. _____ region   around the navel

2. _____ region   superior to the umbilical region

3. _____ region   inferior to the umbilical region

4. _____ regions   to the right and left of the epigastric region

5. _____ regions   to the right and left of the umbilical region

6. _____ regions   to the right and left of the hypogastric region

| **EXERCISE I** | **Patient Positions** |

Write patient position next to its definition.

1. _____ position lying on back, facing upward

2. _____ position lying on abdomen, facing downward

3. _____ position sitting upright in a chair or in a bed supported by pillows behind the back; sometimes the patient tilts forward resting on a pillow supported by an overbed table

4. _____ position lying on back with body tilted so that the head is lower than the feet

5. _____ position lying on side in a semi-prone position with the knee drawn up toward the chest and with the arm drawn behind, parallel to the back

6. _____ position semi-sitting position with slight elevation of the knees

OBJECTIVE 5

Use medical language in clinical statements, the case study, and a medical record.

| **EXERCISE J** | **Use Medical Terms in Clinical Statements** |

Read the Procedure for Palpating Arterial Pulses and answer questions 1-4.

Procedure for Palpating Arterial Pulses

Palpate arteries with the distal pads of the first two fingers. The fingertips are used because they are the most sensitive parts of the hand. Unless contraindicated, simultaneous palpation is preferred.

Temporal: Palpate over the temporal bone on each side of the head, lateral to each eyebrow.

Carotid: Palpate the anterior edge of the sternocleidomastoid muscle, just medial and inferior to the angle of the jaw. To avoid reduction of blood flow, do not palpate right and left carotid pulses simultaneously.

Radial: Palpate anterolateral side of wrist, proximal to the first carpal-metacarpal junction.

Femoral: This pulse is inferior to the medial inguinal ligament; the pulse is found midway between anterosuperior iliac spine and pubic tubercle.

Posterior tibial: This pulse is found posterior and slightly inferior to the medial malleolus of the ankle.

Dorsalis pedis: With the foot slightly dorsiflexed, lightly palpate the dorsal surface of the foot, just lateral to the first metatarsal.

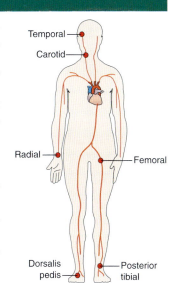

> **FYI**   **Dorsal:** When used with the foot, the directional term **dorsal** describes the upper surface of the foot opposite the sole.

Answer the following questions. For questions 2 to 4, circle the letter that correctly completes the sentence. Check answers in Appendix C.

1. Underline the directional terms used in the Procedure for Palpating Arterial Pulses.

2. The temporal pulse is palpated
   a. just above the eyebrow.
   b. to the side of the eyebrow.
   c. below the eyebrow.
   d. to the middle of the eyebrow.

3. The radial pulse is palpated on the
   a. front and side of the wrist.
   b. back and side of the wrist.
   c. back and middle of the wrist.
   d. front and middle of the wrist.

4. The femoral pulse is located
   a. below the inguinal ligament.
   b. above the inguinal ligament.
   c. to the front of the inguinal ligament.
   d. medial to the inguinal ligament.

For the following questions, circle the medical term defined in the bolded phrases. Medical terms from Lesson 1 may be included. Answers are listed in Appendix C. For pronunciation practice read the answers aloud.

5. The gastroenterologist found a polyp in the colon **pertaining to away from the point of attachment** (proximal, medial, distal) to the splenic flexure.

6. The primary care physician ordered a(n) **pertaining to the front and to the back** (AP, PA, lat) radiographic image of the chest.

7. A(n) **pertaining to the side** (lateral, medial, anterior) chest radiograph displays the anatomy in the **plane that divides the body into right and left sides** (sagittal, coronal, axial) plane.

8. Mr. Hernandez visited a dermatologist because of changes in a nevus located in the **pertaining to the middle** (proximal, medial, distal) aspect of his left eyelid.

9. The incision was made at the **pertaining to above** (superior, inferior, caudal) pole of the lesion.

10. The patient presented to her physician with pain in the right **regions to the right and left of the umbilical region** (hypochondriac, lumbar, iliac) region.

11. The electrocardiogram showed no ST changes in the **pertaining to the front** (anterior, posterior, dorsal) leads.

12. Images for computed tomography (CT) scanning can be produced from the sagittal plane, the **dividing the body into anterior and posterior portions** (coronal, axial, sagittal) plane, and the **dividing the body into superior and inferior portions** (coronal, axial, sagittal) plane.

13. The drainage catheter is placed over the right **pertaining to the front** (superior, inferior, anterior) pelvis.

14. The doctor's order indicated that the patient with dyspnea was to be placed in the **sitting upright** (Fowler, Sims, orthopnea) position to facilitate breathing.

15. The patient being treated for cardiovascular shock was placed in the **lying on back with the head lower than the feet** (prone, Trendelenburg, Fowler) position.

16. **Pertaining to the back** (Dorsal, Ventral, Medial) is often used to describe the back of the hand or upper surface of the foot.

17. Just before birth, the fetus shifted to a **pertaining to the head** (cephalic, caudal, anterior) presentation.

18. A **pertaining to the tail** (cephalic, caudal, dorsal) epidural steroid injection may be performed to relieve chronic low back pain.

EXERCISE K   **Apply Medical Terms to the Case Study**

Think back to A'idah who was introduced in the case study at the beginning of the lesson. After working through Lesson 2, consider the directional terms and abdominopelvic regions that might be used to describe the location of the pain she experienced. List three terms and their meanings. ■

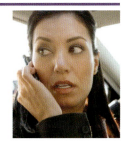

Medical Term	**Definition**
1. _____	_____
2. _____	_____
3. _____	_____

EXERCISE L   **Use Medical Terms in a Document**

Paramedics transported A'idah to the emergency department (ED) of the nearest hospital. The following medical record documents the encounter.

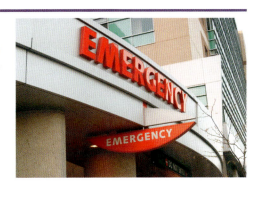

Use the definitions in 1-6 to write medical terms in the blanks on the following ED note.

1. to the right and left of the hypogastric region

2. to the right and left of the umbilical region

3. pertaining to away

4. pertaining to the middle

5. pertaining to the side

6. pertaining to near

Refer to the medical record to answer questions 7-8.

7. In the Physical Exam section of the document, identify and define the directional term ending in **ly.** The addition of **ly** transforms the term from adjective to adverb. Adjectives describe nouns, whereas adverbs describe verbs.

   Term: _____ Definition: _____

8. Identify and define the directional term abbreviated in the Diagnostic Studies section of the note.

   Term: _____ Definition: _____

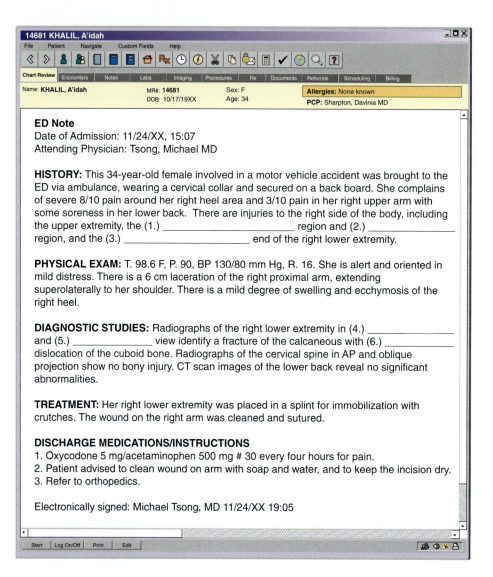

14681 KHALIL, A'idah

File   Patient   Navigate   Custom Fields   Help

Chart Review   Encounters   Notes   Labs   Imaging   Procedures   Rx   Documents   Referrals   Scheduling   Billing

Name: **KHALIL, A'idah**   MR#: **14681**   Sex: F   **Allergies:** None known
DOB: 10/17/19XX   Age: 34   **PCP:** Sharpton, Davinia MD

ED Note
Date of Admission: 11/24/XX, 15:07
Attending Physician: Tsong, Michael MD

HISTORY: This 34-year-old female involved in a motor vehicle accident was brought to the ED via ambulance, wearing a cervical collar and secured on a back board. She complains of severe 8/10 pain around her right heel area and 3/10 pain in her right upper arm with some soreness in her lower back. There are injuries to the right side of the body, including the upper extremity, the (1.) _____ region and (2.) _____ region, and the (3.) _____ end of the right lower extremity.

PHYSICAL EXAM: T. 98.6 F, P. 90, BP 130/80 mm Hg, R. 16. She is alert and oriented in mild distress. There is a 6 cm laceration of the right proximal arm, extending superolaterally to her shoulder. There is a mild degree of swelling and ecchymosis of the right heel.

DIAGNOSTIC STUDIES: Radiographs of the right lower extremity in (4.) _____ and (5.) _____ view identify a fracture of the calcaneous with (6.) _____ dislocation of the cuboid bone. Radiographs of the cervical spine in AP and oblique projection show no bony injury. CT scan images of the lower back reveal no significant abnormalities.

TREATMENT: Her right lower extremity was placed in a splint for immobilization with crutches. The wound on the right arm was cleaned and sutured.

DISCHARGE MEDICATIONS/INSTRUCTIONS
1. Oxycodone 5 mg/acetaminophen 500 mg # 30 every four hours for pain.
2. Patient advised to clean wound on arm with soap and water, and to keep the incision dry.
3. Refer to orthopedics.

Electronically signed: Michael Tsong, MD 11/24/XX 19:05

Start   Log On/Off   Print   Edit

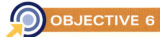

OBJECTIVE 6

Recall and assess knowledge of word parts, medical terms, and abbreviations.

EXERCISE M   **Online Review of Lesson Content**

🌐 *Recall and assess your learning from working through the lesson by completing online learning activities at evolve. elsevier.com > Evolve Resources > Practice Student Resources. Keep track of your progress by placing a check mark next to completed activities.*

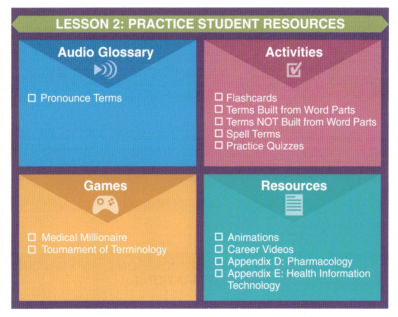

LESSON 2: PRACTICE STUDENT RESOURCES

Audio Glossary ▶))
- ☐ Pronounce Terms

Activities ☑
- ☐ Flashcards
- ☐ Terms Built from Word Parts
- ☐ Terms NOT Built from Word Parts
- ☐ Spell Terms
- ☐ Practice Quizzes

Games 🎮
- ☐ Medical Millionaire
- ☐ Tournament of Terminology

Resources 📄
- ☐ Animations
- ☐ Career Videos
- ☐ Appendix D: Pharmacology
- ☐ Appendix E: Health Information Technology

EXERCISE N   **Lesson Content Quiz**

Test your knowledge of the terms and abbreviations introduced in this lesson. Circle the letter for the medical term or abbreviation related to the words in italics.

1. A patient with pancreatitis presents with severe pain and tenderness in the *superior to the umbilical* region.
   a. lumbar
   b. hypogastric
   c. epigastric

2. The patient was placed in a *semi-sitting position with a slight elevation of the knees* on the examining table in preparation for his physical exam.
   a. Fowler position
   b. Sims position
   c. supine position

3. The MRI scan showed images of the brain from the perspective of the *vertical field passing through the body from side to side, dividing the body into anterior and posterior portions.*
   a. axial plane
   b. coronal plane
   c. sagittal plane

4. A 74-year-old male presented with pain in the *LLQ* consistent with diverticulitis.
   a. left leg quadrant
   b. lower left quadrant
   c. left lower quadrant

5. A patient with heart failure may experience shortness of breath when *in the position of lying on the back, facing upward.*
    a. prone position
    b. supine position
    c. Trendelenburg position

6. The thyroid gland is *pertaining to above* to the sternum.
    a. anterior
    b. inferior
    c. superior

7. The computed tomography scan of the chest showed images from *the perspective of the horizontal field dividing the body into superior and inferior portions.*
    a. axial plane
    b. coronal plane
    c. sagittal plane

8. The patient presented with a mass in the *pertaining to above and to the side* portion of the left breast.
    a. anteroposterior
    b. superolateral
    c. mediolateral

LESSON AT A GLANCE   **DIRECTIONAL TERMS, POSITIONS, AND IMAGING WORD PARTS**

COMBINING FORMS

anter/o	later/o
caud/o	medi/o
cephal/o	poster/o
dist/o	proxim/o
dors/o	super/o
infer/o	ventr/o

SUFFIXES

-ad
-al
-ic
-ior

LESSON AT A GLANCE   **DIRECTIONAL TERMS, POSITIONS, AND IMAGING MEDICAL TERMS AND ABBREVIATIONS**

DIRECTIONAL TERMS
anterior (ant)
anterolateral
anteromedial
anteroposterior (AP)
anterosuperior
caudad
caudal
cephalad
cephalic
distal
dorsal
inferior (inf)
inferolateral
lateral (lat)
medial (med)
mediolateral
posterior (post)
posteroanterior (PA)
posterolateral
proximal
superior (sup)
superolateral
ventral

ANATOMIC PLANES
axial plane
coronal plane
sagittal plane

ABDOMINOPELVIC REGIONS
epigastric region
hypochondriac regions
hypogastric region
iliac regions
lumbar regions
umbilical region

PATIENT POSITIONS
Fowler position
orthopnea position
prone position
Sims position
supine position
Trendelenburg position

ABDOMINOPELVIC QUADRANTS
left lower quadrant (LLQ)
left upper quadrant (LUQ)
right lower quadrant (RLQ)
right upper quadrant (RUQ)

ABBREVIATIONS

ant	LLQ	post
AP	LUQ	RLQ
inf	med	RUQ
lat	PA	sup

Amanda Sheehan

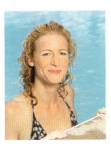

Amanda has a dark spot on her arm that worries her. She noticed it for the first time this morning as she put lotion on after her shower. It is fairly smooth and brown, but it isn't round like her other moles. When she runs her finger over it, the new spot feels more bumpy. Her other moles and freckles are flat. A few years ago she had a mole with what looked like small, black bubbles removed and looked at. It turned out to be skin cancer. She had another small, minor skin cancer removed from her ear a year later. The specialist that Amanda saw told her to come back right away if she noticed any changes in her moles or any new spots on her skin.

■ *Consider Amanda's situation as you work through the lesson on the integumentary system. At the end of the lesson, we will return to this case study and identify related medical terms.*

OBJECTIVES

1 ■ Build, translate, pronounce, and spell medical terms built from word parts (p. 53).

2 ■ Define, pronounce, and spell medical terms NOT built from word parts (p. 65).

3 ■ Write abbreviations (p. 69).

4 ■ Distinguish plural endings from singular endings (p. 70).

5 ■ Identify medical terms by clinical category (p. 72).

6 ■ Use medical language in clinical statements, the case study, and a medical record (p. 74).

7 ■ Recall and assess knowledge of word parts, medical terms, and abbreviations (p. 77).

INTRODUCTION TO THE INTEGUMENTARY SYSTEM

Anatomic Structures of the Integumentary System

skin (skin)	organ covering the body; made up of layers
epidermis (ep-i-DUR-mis)	outer layer of skin
dermis (DUR-mis)	inner layer of skin; also called **true skin**
hair (hār)	compressed, keratinized cells that arise from hair follicles

Anatomic Structures of the Integumentary System—cont'd

nails (nālz)	horny plates made from flattened epithelial cells, found on the dorsal surface of the ends of fingers and toes
sweat glands (swet) (glandz)	tiny, coiled, tubular structures that emerge through pores on the skin's surface and secrete sweat
sebaceous glands (se-BĀ-shas) (glandz)	special oil glands that secrete sebum (oil) into the hair follicles
appendages of the skin (a-PEN-da-jez) (of) (the) (skin)	common reference to hair, nails, sweat glands, and sebaceous glands
nerve endings (nurv) (EN-dingz)	provide sensory information, such as heat, cold, pain, and vibration

Functions of the Integumentary System

- Protects against harmful environmental elements
- Protects against fluid loss
- Produces vitamin D
- Regulates body temperature
- Excretes waste
- Provides sensory information

How the Integumentary System Works

The medical term integumentary originates from the Latin word *tegere*, meaning to cover. The integumentary system literally covers the body, providing a barrier to the external environment. The skin (also called the cutaneous membrane) is the largest organ in the human body and is made up of two layers: the epidermis and the dermis (Figure 3.2). The dermis is thicker, made of connective tissue, and contains blood vessels and nerve endings. Hair, nails, sweat glands, and sebaceous glands are referred to as the appendages of the skin. The skin and its appendages make up the integumentary system.

Colors

In addition to introducing word parts and medical terms relating to the integumentary system, this lesson includes combining forms indicating color. Medical terms built from word parts conveying color are often used to describe signs of a disease process or condition.

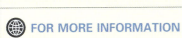
CAREER FOCUS   **Professionals Who Work with the Integumentary System**

- **Nursing Assistants** provide daily care for hospital and long-term care patients, including skin care and observation of changes in the skin (Figure 3.1).

- **Medical Estheticians** perform procedures such as skin evaluation, facial massages, and hair removal. They support dermatologists and plastic surgeons with patients' preoperative and postoperative exams.

FOR MORE INFORMATION

- Access online resources at evolve.elsevier.com > Practice Student Resources > Other Resources > Career Videos to watch interviews with **Certified Nursing Assistants** working in orthopedics and in a rehabilitation center.

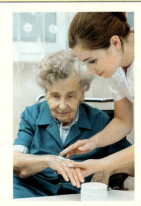
Figure 3.1 Nursing assistant providing skin care for a resident.

OBJECTIVE 1

Build, translate, pronounce, and spell medical terms built from word parts.

WORD PARTS   Presented with the Integumentary System and Colors

Use the paper or online **flashcards** to familiarize yourself with the following word parts.

COMBINING FORM (WR + CV)	DEFINITION	COMBINING FORM (WR + CV)	DEFINITION
Integumentary System		**Colors**	
acr/o	extremities	cyan/o	blue
cutane/o	skin	erythr/o	red
derm/o	skin	leuk/o	white
dermat/o	skin	melan/o	black
myc/o	fungus	xanth/o	yellow
onych/o	nail		

WORD PARTS — Presented with the Integumentary System and Colors—cont'd

SUFFIX (S)	DEFINITION	SUFFIX (S)	DEFINITION
-a, -e, -y	no meaning	-lysis	dissolution, separating
-itis	inflammation	-ous	pertaining to
-osis	abnormal condition		

PREFIX (P)	DEFINITION	PREFIX (P)	DEFINITION
epi-	on, upon, over	per-	through
hypo-	below, deficient, under	sub-	below, under
intra-	within	trans-	through, across, beyond

WORD PARTS PRESENTED IN PREVIOUS LESSONS — Used to Build Integumentary System and Color Terms

COMBINING FORM (WR +CV)	DEFINITION	COMBINING FORM (WR + CV)	DEFINITION
cyt/o	cell(s)	path/o	disease

SUFFIX (S)	DEFINITION	SUFFIX (S)	DEFINITION
-al, -ic	pertaining to	-logy	study of
-logist	one who studies and treats (specialist, physician)	-oma	tumor

Refer to Appendix A, Word Parts Used in *Basic Medical Language*, for alphabetical lists of word parts and their meanings.

EXERCISE A   **Build and Translate Terms Built from Word Parts**

*Use the **Word Parts Tables** to complete the following questions. Check your responses with the Answer Key in Appendix C.*

1. **LABEL:** *Write the combining forms for anatomical structures of the integumentary system on Figure 3.2. The combining forms will be used to build and translate medical terms in Exercise A.*

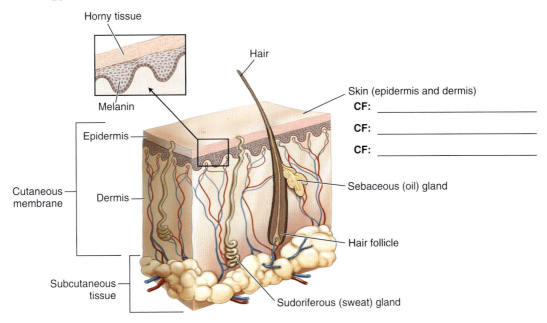

Figure 3.2 Cross section of the skin and combining forms for skin.

FYI   **Cutane/o** is of Latin origin; **derm/o** and **dermat/o** are of Greek origin.

---

2. **MATCH:** *Draw a line to match the word part with its definition.*

   a. -logist   study of
   b. -logy   inflammation
   c. path/o   one who studies and treats (specialist, physician)
   d. -itis   no meaning
   e. -y   disease

---

3. **TRANSLATE:** *Complete the definitions of the following terms by using the meaning of word parts to fill in the blanks. Remember, the definition usually starts with the meaning of the suffix.*

   a. dermat/o/logy   _____ of the _____
   b. dermat/o/logist   physician who _____ and _____ diseases of the _____
   c. dermat/o/path/y   (any) _____ of the _____
   d. dermat/itis   _____ of the _____
   e. dermat/o/path/o/logist   _____ who (microscopically) studies _____ of the skin

4. **READ:** **Dermatology** (der-ma-TOL-o-jē) is the medical specialty dedicated to the study of the skin, hair, nails, and mucous membranes of the eyelids, nose, and mouth. A **dermatologist** (der-ma-TOL-o-jist) diagnoses and treats pediatric and adult patients presenting with various forms of **dermatopathy** (der-ma-TOP-a-thē), including skin cancer, **dermatitis** (der-ma-TĪ-tis), and other skin conditions. A **dermatopathologist** (der-ma-tō-pat-THOL-o-jist) is trained in dermatology and pathology. A dermatopathologist works in the lab and makes diagnoses based on microscopic examination of tissue samples of skin, hair, and nails.

5. **LABEL:** *Write word parts to complete Figure 3.3.*

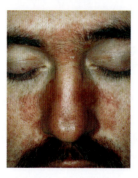

Figure 3.3 _____/_____ may be caused by an allergen, infection, or other disease.
                        skin   inflammation

6. **MATCH:** *Draw a line to match the word part with its definition.*

   a. epi–   below, deficient, under
   b. hypo–   within
   c. intra–   pertaining to
   d. trans–   on, upon, over
   e. -al, -ic   through, across, beyond

7. **BUILD:** *Using the combining form **derm/o** and the word parts reviewed in the previous exercise, build the following descriptive terms. Remember, the definition usually starts with the meaning of the suffix. Hint: use the suffix **-al** for all but the last term.*

a. pertaining to the skin   _____/_____
                                              wr   s

b. pertaining to upon the skin   _____/_____/_____
                                          p   wr   s

c. pertaining to within the skin   _____/_____/_____
                                          p   wr   s

d. pertaining to through the skin _____/_____/_____
                                          p   wr   s

e. pertaining to under the skin   _____/_____/_____
                                          p   wr   s

> **FYI** A combining vowel is not placed between a prefix and a word root, as seen in the medical terms **trans/derm/al** and other terms built in the previous exercise.

8. READ: Dermal (DER-mal) is a general term denoting relationship to the skin, specifically the dermis. The term **epidermal** (ep-i-DER-mal) refers to the uppermost layer of skin or the epidermis. The adjectives **hypodermic** (hī-pō-DER-mik), **intradermal** (in-tra-DER-mal), and **transdermal** (trans-DER-mel) are used to describe administration of medications. Injections may be given with a syringe and hypodermic needle, which penetrates the skin. An intradermal injection places a small amount of liquid within the dermis. Transdermal administration, using a patch, cream, or ointment, slowly introduces medication as it absorbs through the skin.

9. LABEL: *Write word parts to complete Figure 3.4.*

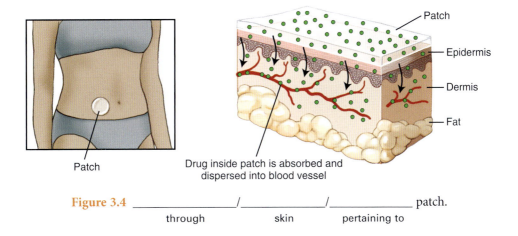

Patch

Drug inside patch is absorbed and dispersed into blood vessel

Patch

Epidermis

Dermis

Fat

Figure 3.4 _____/_____/_____ patch.
                    through   skin   pertaining to

10. MATCH: *Draw a line to match the word part with its definition.*

a. per-   below, under
b. -ous   pertaining to
c. sub-   through

11. TRANSLATE: *Use the meaning of word parts to complete the definitions of the following terms built from the combining form* **cutane/o,** *meaning skin. Remember, the definition usually starts with the meaning of the suffix.*

a. cutane/ous   _____ to the _____

b. sub/cutane/ous   pertaining to _____ the _____

c. per/cutane/ous   _____ to _____ the skin

FYI   **Terms with the Same Definition, But Used Differently**

Transdermal and **percutaneous** both mean through the skin. Transdermal is used to describe a route of administration introducing medicine into the bloodstream by absorption through the skin. Percutaneous is used to describe surgical procedures performed through the skin.

Hypodermic and **subcutaneous** both mean under the skin. Hypodermic describes the needle and/or syringe frequently used to inject substances into the body. Subcutaneous describes the injection itself. For example, a hypodermic needle is used to administer a subcutaneous injection.

---

12. READ: Cutaneous (kū-TĀ-nē-us) membrane refers to the epidermis and the dermis. **Subcutaneous** (sub-kū-TĀ-nē-us) tissue lies beneath the dermis and contains fat, connective tissue, larger blood vessels and nerves. A subcutaneous injection delivers fluid to the tissue below the dermis. **Percutaneous** (per-kū-TĀ-nē-us) is used to describe procedures performed through the skin of the patient by the physician, such as a percutaneous endoscopic gastrostomy (PEG) and percutaneous coronary intervention (PCI).

---

13. LABEL: *Write word parts to complete Figure 3.5.*

FYI

MEMORY TIP
Hypodermic explains **h**ow.
Subcutaneous **s**hows where.

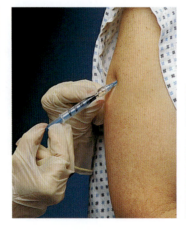

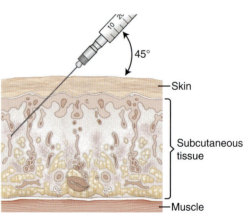

Skin

Subcutaneous tissue

Muscle

45°

Figure 3.5 Insertion of a _____/_____/_____ needle into the
                             under   skin   pertaining to

_____/_____/_____ tissue.
      under   skin   pertaining to

14. LABEL: *Write the combining form for nail to complete Figure 3.6.*

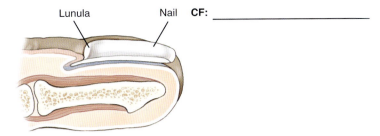

Lunula   Nail   **CF:** _____

Figure 3.6 Cross section of the finger with nail and the combining form for nail.

15. MATCH: *Draw a line to match the word part with its definition.*

a. -osis   separation
b. -lysis   abnormal condition
c. myc/o   fungus

16. BUILD: *Using the combining form **onych/o**, write the word parts to build terms related to the nail.*

a. abnormal condition of the nail   _____ / _____
                                                   wr   s

b. abnormal condition of fungus in the nail   _____ / o / _____ / _____
   Hint: the combining form for nail appears first.   wr   cv   wr   s

c. separation of the nail   _____ / o / _____
                                                   wr   cv   s

17. READ: Onychosis (on-i-KŌ-sis) describes any disease or disorder of the nail. **Onychomycosis** (on-i-kō-mī-KŌ-sis), the most common nail disorder, encompasses all fungal infections of the toenails and fingernails. **Onycholysis** (on-ē-KOL-i-sis) is another common disorder that may be caused by psoriasis, fungal infections, or traumatic injury.

18. LABEL: *Write word parts to complete Figure 3.7.*

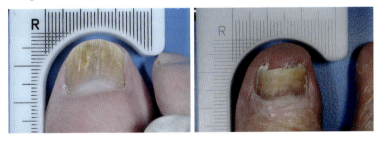

Figure 3.7 Examples of _____ / o / _____ / _____.
                                    nail   fungus   abnormal condition

19. REVIEW OF INTEGUMENTARY SYSTEM TERMS BUILT FROM WORD PARTS: the following is an alphabetical list of terms built and translated in the previous exercises.

MEDICAL TERMS BUILT FROM WORD PARTS

TERM	DEFINITION	TERM	DEFINITION
1. cutaneous (kū-TĀ-nē-us)	pertaining to the skin	9. hypodermic (hypo) (hī-pō-DER-mik)	pertaining to under the skin (Figure 3.5)
2. dermal (DER-mal)	pertaining to the skin	10. intradermal (ID) (in-tra-DER-mal)	pertaining to within the skin
3. dermatitis (der-ma-TĪ-tis)	inflammation of the skin (Figure 3.3)	11. onychomycosis (on-i-kō-mī-KŌ-sis)	abnormal condition of fungus in the nail (Figure 3.7)
4. dermatologist (der-ma-TOL-o-jist)	physician who studies and treats diseases of the skin	12. onychosis (on-i-KŌ-sis)	abnormal condition of the nail
5. dermatology (DERM) (der-ma-TOL-o-jē)	study of the skin	13. onycholysis (on-ē-KOL-i-sis)	separation of the nail
6. dermatopathologist (der-ma-tō-pat-THOL-o-jist)	physician who (microscopically) studies diseases of the skin	14. percutaneous (per-kū-TĀ-nē-us)	pertaining to through the skin
7. dermatopathy (der-ma-TOP-a-thē)	(any) disease of the skin	15. subcutaneous (subcut) (sub-kū-TĀ-nē-us)	pertaining to under the skin (Figure 3.5)
8. epidermal (ep-i-DER-mal)	pertaining to upon the skin	16. transdermal (TD) (trans-DER-mel)	pertaining to through the skin (Figure 3.4)

EXERCISE B   Pronounce and Spell Terms Built from Word Parts

Practice pronunciation and spelling on paper and online.

1. **Practice on Paper**
   a. **Pronounce:** Read the phonetic spelling and say aloud the terms listed in the previous table, Review Terms Built from Word Parts. Refer to the pronunciation key on p. 9 as necessary.
   b. **Spell:** Have a study partner read the terms aloud. Write the spelling of the terms on a separate sheet of paper.

2. **Practice Online** 🌐
   a. **Access** online learning resources. Go to evolve.elsevier.com > Evolve Resources > Practice Student Resources.
   b. **Pronounce:** Select Audio Glossary > Exercise B. Select a term to hear its pronunciation and repeat aloud.
   c. **Spell:** Select Activities > Spell Terms > Exercise B. Select the audio icon and type the correct spelling of the term.

❏ Check the box when complete.

EXERCISE C Build and Translate MORE Terms Built from Word Parts

*Use the **Word Parts Tables** near the beginning of the lesson to complete the following questions. Check your responses with the Answer Key in Appendix C.*

1. **LABEL:** *Write the combining forms for colors in Figure 3.8. The combining forms will be used to build and translate medical terms in Exercise C.*

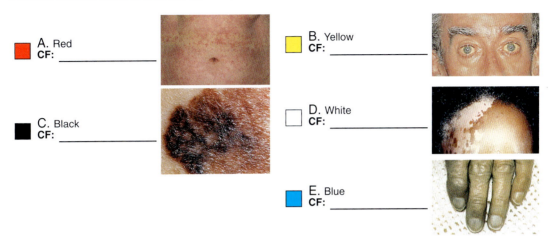

A. Red
CF: _____

B. Yellow
CF: _____

C. Black
CF: _____

D. White
CF: _____

E. Blue
CF: _____

Figure 3.8 Combining forms for color matched with examples of color as seen in the skin.

2. **MATCH:** *Draw a line to match the word part with its definition.*

   a. derm/o   skin
   b. -a   no meaning

3. **TRANSLATE:** *Use the meaning of word parts to complete the definitions of terms built from the combining form **derm/o**.*

   a. leuk/o/derm/a   _____ _____
   b. melan/o/derm/a   _____ _____
   c. erythr/o/derm/a   _____ _____
   d. xanth/o/derm/a   _____ _____

4. **READ: Leukoderma** (lū-kō-DER-ma) describes white patches of skin resulting from a disease process or reaction to a chemical substance. In leukoderma, there is an abnormal lack of pigmentation in the skin. Conversely, **melanoderma** (mel-a-nō-DER-ma) describes an abnormal increase in pigmentation, resulting in darkening of the skin. **Xanthoderma** (zan-thō-DER-ma) is a general term describing any yellow discoloration of the skin, such as seen in jaundice. **Erythroderma** (e-rith-rō-DER-ma) indicates abnormal redness of large areas of the skin. Inflammatory skin disease and adverse drug reactions may cause erythroderma, though in some cases no cause is identified (idiopathic erythroderma). If peeling of skin accompanies erythroderma, it may also be called exfoliative dermatitis.

5. LABEL: *Write word parts to complete Figure 3.9.*

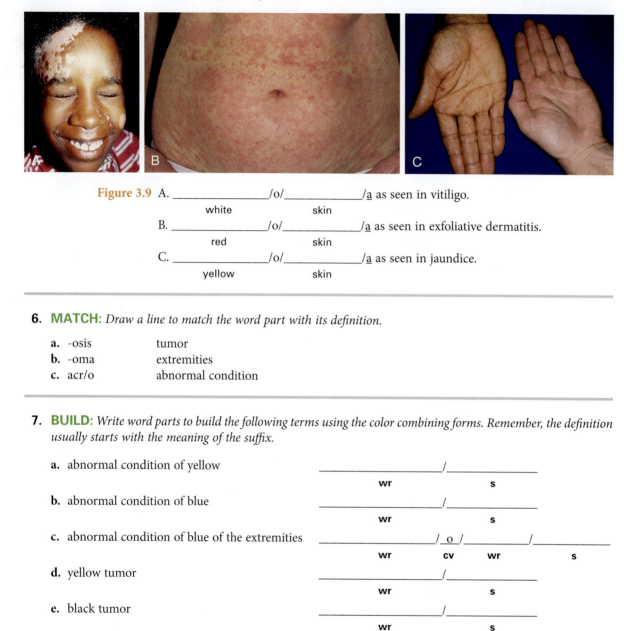

Figure 3.9 A. _____/o/_____/a as seen in vitiligo.
                         white   skin

             B. _____/o/_____/a as seen in exfoliative dermatitis.
                         red   skin

             C. _____/o/_____/a as seen in jaundice.
                         yellow   skin

---

6. MATCH: *Draw a line to match the word part with its definition.*

    a. -osis   tumor

    b. -oma   extremities

    c. acr/o   abnormal condition

---

7. BUILD: *Write word parts to build the following terms using the color combining forms. Remember, the definition usually starts with the meaning of the suffix.*

    a. abnormal condition of yellow   _____/_____
                                                             wr   s

    b. abnormal condition of blue   _____/_____
                                                             wr   s

    c. abnormal condition of blue of the extremities   _____/_o_/_____/_____
                                                             wr   cv   wr   s

    d. yellow tumor   _____/_____
                                                             wr   s

    e. black tumor   _____/_____
                                                             wr   s

8. **READ:** **Melanoma** (mel-a-NŌ-ma) is a malignant tumor that occurs primarily on the skin. **Xanthoma** (zan-THŌ-ma) is a benign tumor usually occurring in the subcutaneous tissue and creating a raised skin lesion yellowish in color. **Cyanosis** (sī-a-NŌ-sis) describes a bluish discoloration of the skin or mucous membranes caused by an inadequate supply of oxygen in the blood. **Acrocyanosis** (ak-rō-sī-a-NŌ-sis) refers to an abnormal bluish discoloration of the skin limited to the extremities, usually the hands and feet, which may be caused by narrowing of the arteries in distal portions of the arms and legs. **Xanthosis** (zan-THŌ-sis) is an abnormal condition of yellowing, sometimes associated with cancer.

9. **LABEL:** *Write word parts to complete Figure 3.10.*

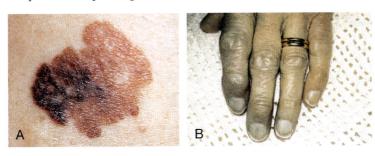

Figure 3.10   A._____/_____.
                        black   tumor
              B._____/_____ of the nail beds.
                        blue   abnormal condition

10. **MATCH:** *Draw a line to match the word part with its definition.*

   a. cyt/o   no meaning
   b. -e   cell(s)

11. **TRANSLATE:** *Using the meaning of word parts, complete the definitions of the following terms referring to types of blood cells.*

   a. leuk/o/cyt/e   _____ (blood) _____
   b. erythr/o/cyt/e   _____ (blood) _____

> **FYI**   The final **e** in **erythr/o/cyt/e** and **leuk/o/cyt/e** is a noun suffix that has no meaning and does not alter the meaning of the medical term.

12. **READ:** **Erythrocyte** (e-RITH-rō-sīt) and **leukocyte** (LŪ-kō-sīt) refer to cells contained in the blood. They are often referred to as red blood cells (**RBC**) and white blood cells (**WBC**), although the word root for blood does not appear in the definition of each medical term. Erythrocytes carry oxygen and carbon dioxide. Leukocytes help fight infection.

13. **LABEL:** *Write word parts to complete Figure 3.11.*

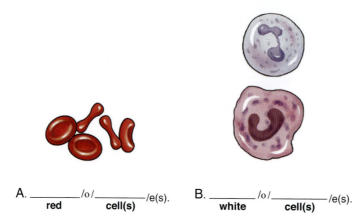

A. _____ /o/ _____ /e(s).
     red   cell(s)

B. _____ /o/ _____ /e(s).
     white   cell(s)

Figure 3.11 Blood cells.

14. **REVIEW OF MORE INTEGUMENTARY SYSTEM TERMS BUILT FROM WORD PARTS:** the following is an alphabetical list of terms built and translated in the previous exercises.

MEDICAL TERMS BUILT FROM WORD PARTS

TERM	DEFINITION	TERM	DEFINITION
1. **acrocyanosis** (ak-rō-sī-a-NŌ-sis)	abnormal condition of blue of the extremities	7. **melanoderma** (mel-a-nō-DER-ma)	black skin
2. **cyanosis** (sī-a-NŌ-sis)	abnormal condition of blue (Figure 3.10, *B*)	8. **melanoma** (mel-a-NŌ-ma)	black tumor (malignant, primarily of the skin) (Figure 3.10, *A*)
3. **erythrocyte** (e-RITH-rō-sīt)	red (blood) cell (Figure 3.11, *A*)	9. **xanthoderma** (zan-thō-DER-ma)	yellow skin (Figure 3.9, *C*)
4. **erythroderma** (e-rith-rō-DER-ma)	red skin (Figure 3.9, *B*)	10. **xanthoma** (zan-THŌ-ma)	yellow tumor (benign, primarily in the skin)
5. **leukocyte** (LŪ-kō-sīt)	white (blood) cell (Figure 3.11, *B*)	11. **xanthosis** (zan-THŌ-sis)	abnormal condition of yellow
6. **leukoderma** (lū-kō-DER-ma)	white skin (Figure 3.9, *A*)		

> **FYI**   Additional combining forms describing color are **chlor/o,** meaning green, and **glauc/o** and **poli/o,** both meaning gray. **Chrom/o** is the combining form for color. See your medical dictionary or online resource for more information on how they are used.

EXERCISE D   **Pronounce and Spell MORE Terms Built from Word Parts**

Practice pronunciation and spelling on paper and online.

1. **Practice on Paper**
   a. **Pronounce**: Read the phonetic spelling and say aloud the terms listed in the previous table, Review of MORE Terms Built from Word Parts. Refer to the pronunciation key on p. 9 as necessary.
   b. **Spell**: Have a study partner read the terms aloud. Write the spelling of the terms on a separate sheet of paper.

2. **Practice Online** 🌐
   a. **Access** online learning resources. Go to evolve.elsevier.com > Evolve Resources > Practice Student Resources.
   b. **Pronounce:** Select Audio Glossary > Exercise D. Select a term to hear its pronunciation and repeat aloud.
   c. **Spell:** Select Activities > Spell Terms > Exercise D. Select the audio icon and type the correct spelling of the term.

❑ Check the box when complete.

 OBJECTIVE 2

Define, pronounce, and spell medical terms NOT built from word parts.

The terms listed below may contain word parts, but are difficult to translate literally.

MEDICAL TERMS NOT BUILT FROM WORD PARTS

TERM	DEFINITION
abscess (AB-ses)	localized collection of pus accompanied by swelling and inflammation; abscesses can occur in tissues, organs (e.g., skin abscess), and contained spaces (e.g., abdominal abscess)
basal cell carcinoma (BCC) (BĀ-sal) (sel) (kar-si-NŌ-ma)	malignant epithelial tumor arising from the bottom layer of the epidermis called the basal layer; it seldom metastasizes, but invades local tissue and often recurs in the same location
cellulitis (sel-ū-LĪ-tis)	inflammation of the skin and subcutaneous tissue caused by infection; characterized by redness, pain, heat, and swelling
edema (e-DĒ-ma)	puffy swelling of tissue from the accumulation of fluid
erythema (er-i-THĒ-ma)	redness
herpes (HER-pēz)	inflammatory skin disease caused by herpes virus characterized by small blisters in clusters
impetigo (im-pe-TĪ-gō)	superficial skin infection characterized by red lesions which progress to blisters and then honey-colored crusts; most commonly caused by either staphylococcus or streptococcus bacteria.
jaundice (JAWN-dis)	condition characterized by a yellow tinge to the skin, mucous membranes, and sclera (whites of the eyes)

MEDICAL TERMS NOT BUILT FROM WORD PARTS—cont'd

TERM	DEFINITION
laceration (lac) (las-er-Ā-shun)	torn, ragged-edged wound
lesion (LĒ-zhun)	any visible change in tissue resulting from injury or disease
methicillin-resistant *Staphylococcus aureus* (MRSA) (meth-i-SIL-in) (rē-ZIS-tent) (staf-uh-lō-KOK-us) (OR-ē-us)	strain of common bacteria that has developed resistance to methicillin and other antibiotics. It can produce skin and soft tissue infections, and sometimes bloodstream infections and pneumonia, which can be fatal if not treated.
nevus (pl. nevi) (NĒ-vus), (NĒ-vī)	malformation of the skin, usually brown, black, or flesh colored (also called a **mole** or a **birthmark**)
pallor (PAL-or)	paleness
pressure injury (PRESH-ur) (IN-ju-rē)	damage of the skin and the subcutaneous tissue caused by prolonged pressure, often occurring in bedridden patients (also called **pressure ulcer** and **bedsore**; formerly called decubitus ulcer)
squamous cell carcinoma (SCC) (SQWĀ-mus) (sel) (kar-si-NO-ma)	malignant growth developing from scalelike epithelial tissue of the surface layer of the epidermis; it invades local tissue and may metastasize. While most commonly appearing on the skin, SCC can occur in other parts of the body including mouth, lips, and genitals.

EXERCISE E   Label

Write the medical terms pictured and defined using the previous table of Medical Terms NOT Built from Word Parts. Check your work with the Answer Key in Appendix C.

1. _____

malignant epithelial tumor arising from the bottom layer of the epidermis called the basal layer

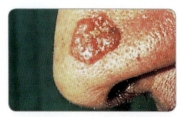

2. _____

malignant growth developing from scalelike epithelial tissue of the surface layer of the epidermis

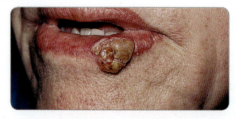

3. _____

damage of the skin and the subcutaneous tissue caused by prolonged pressure

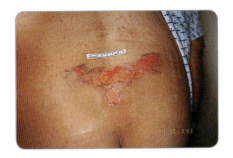

4. _____

inflammation of the skin and subcutaneous tissue caused by infection; characterized by redness, pain, heat, and swelling

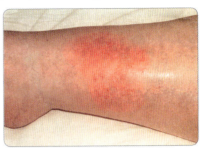

5. _____

inflammatory skin disease caused by a virus characterized by small blisters in clusters

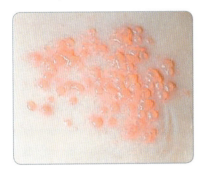

6. _____

malformation of the skin, usually brown, black, or flesh colored

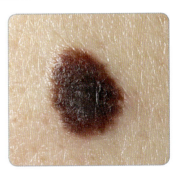

7. _____

bacterial skin infection characterized by red lesions which progress to blisters and then honey-colored crusts

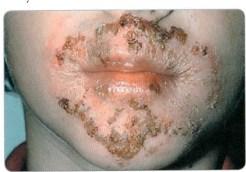

8. _____

torn, ragged-edged wound

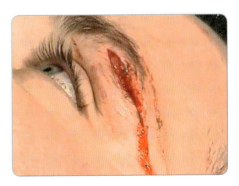

EXERCISE F   Learn Medical Terms NOT Built from Word Parts

Fill in the blanks with medical terms defined in **bold** *using the Medical Terms NOT Built from Word Parts table. Check your responses with the Answer Key in Appendix C.*

1. **Any visible change in tissue resulting from injury or disease** _____ is a broad term that includes sores, wounds, ulcers, and tumors.

2. **Damage of the skin and the subcutaneous tissue caused by prolonged pressure** _____ (*plural form*) often occur in bedridden patients.

3. A boil is a(n) **localized collection of pus** _____ involving the hair follicle and subcutaneous tissue.

4. **Torn, ragged-edged wounds** _____(s) may be caused by sharp objects cutting the skin and result in pain and bleeding.

5. **Puffy swelling of tissue from the accumulation of fluid** _____ of the ankles and feet often makes it difficult to wear shoes.

6. The dermatologist performed a biopsy of the patient's **malformation of the skin** _____, which recently showed changes in shape and color.

7. Unlike malignant **tumor arising from the bottom layer of the epidermis** _____ _____, a **malignant growth developing from scalelike epithelial tissue** _____ _____ has the potential to metastasize.

8. Many types of **inflammatory skin disease caused by a virus and characterized by small blisters in clusters** _____ exist. *Herpes simplex*, for example, causes fever blisters; *herpes zoster*, also called shingles, is characterized by painful skin eruptions that follow nerves inflamed by the virus.

9. **Superficial skin infection characterized by red lesions which progress to blisters and then honey-colored crusts** _____ is highly contagious and most commonly occurs in infants and young children.

10. Strep and staph may also cause a more serious infection called **inflammation of the skin and subcutaneous tissue** _____. This bacterial skin infection, which can spread rapidly, is characterized by **redness** _____, pain, heat, and swelling.

11. **Paleness** _____, an abnormal loss of color in skin and mucous membranes, can be widespread or localized and is caused by a reduction in blood flow.

12. **Yellow tinge to the skin, mucous membranes, and sclera** _____ occurs in adults and infants and results from an excess of bilirubin, a yellow-colored pigment of erythrocytes. Infant jaundice is common and usually resolves without treatment. Adult jaundice may indicate a more serious disease process affecting liver function.

13. **Strain of common bacteria that has developed resistance to methicillin and other antibiotics** _____ is quite common in hospitals and long-term care facilities but is increasingly emerging as an important infection in the general population.

EXERCISE G   Pronounce and Spell Medical Terms NOT Built from Word Parts

Practice pronunciation and spelling with the textbook and online.

1. **Practice on Paper**
   a. **Pronounce:** Read the phonetic spelling and say aloud the terms listed in the previous Medical Terms NOT Built from Word Parts table. Refer to pronunciation key on p. 9 as necessary.
   b. **Spell:** Have a study partner read the terms aloud. Write the spelling of the terms on a separate sheet of paper.

2. **Practice Online** ⊚
   a. **Access** online learning resources. Go to evolve.elsevier.com > Evolve Resources > Practice Student Resources.
   b. **Pronounce:** Select Audio Glossary > Exercise G. Select a term to hear its pronunciation and repeat aloud.
   c. **Spell:** Select Activities > Spell Terms > Exercise G. Select the audio icon and type the correct spelling of the term.

❏ Check the box when complete.

OBJECTIVE 3

Write abbreviations.

ABBREVIATIONS RELATED TO THE INTEGUMENTARY SYSTEM

Use the online **flashcards** to familiarize yourself with the following abbreviations.

ABBREVIATION	TERM	ABBREVIATION	TERM
BCC	basal cell carcinoma	RBC	erythrocyte
DERM	dermatology	SCC	squamous cell carcinoma
hypo	hypodermic	TD	transdermal
ID	intradermal	subcut	subcutaneous
lac	laceration	WBC	leukocyte
MRSA	methicillin-resistant *Staphylococcus aureus*		

EXERCISE H   Abbreviate medical terms

Write the correct abbreviation next to its medical term. Check your responses with the Answer Key in Appendix C.

1. Diseases and disorders:

   a. _____   laceration

   b. _____   squamous cell carcinoma

   c. _____   basal cell carcinoma

2. Related Terms

a. _____ dermatology

b. _____ hypodermic

c. _____ methicillin-resistant *Staphylococcus aureus*

d. _____ leukocyte

e. _____ erythrocyte

f. _____ transdermal

g. _____ intradermal

h. _____ subcutaneous

 OBJECTIVE 4

Distinguish plural endings from singular endings.

In the English language, plurals are formed by simply adding an **s** or **es** to the end of a word. For example, hand becomes plural by adding an **s** to form hands. Likewise, box becomes plural by adding **es** to become boxes. In the language of medicine, many terms have Latin or Greek suffixes, and forming plurals for these terms is not quite as easy. Listed below are singular and plural endings used in medical language.

SINGULAR AND PLURAL ENDINGS

LATIN ENDINGS		GREEK ENDINGS	
SINGULAR	PLURAL	SINGULAR	PLURAL
-a	-ae	-ma	-mata
-ax	-aces	-nx	-nges
-ex	-ices	-on	-a
-is	-es	-sis	-ses
-ix	-ices		
-um	-a		
-us	-i		

EXERCISE I   Learn Plural Endings

Using the Singular and Plural Endings box, convert the following terms from singular form to plural form and identify the plural ending. Check your answers with the answer key in Appendix C.

SINGULAR TERM	ENDING	PLURAL TERM	ENDING
Example: vertebra	*-a*	*vertebrae*	*-ae*
1. thorax	-ax	_____	_____
2. appendix	-ix	_____	_____
3. cervix	-ix	_____	_____
4. diagnosis	-sis	_____	_____
5. prognosis	-sis	_____	_____
6. metastasis	-sis	_____	_____
7. pelvis	-is	_____	_____
8. testis	-is	_____	_____
9. bronchus	-us	_____	_____
10. nevus	-us	_____	_____
11. streptococcus	-us	_____	_____
12. fungus	-us	_____	_____
13. bacterium	-um	_____	_____
14. ovum	-um	_____	_____
15. sarcoma	-ma	_____	_____
16. fibroma	-ma	_____	_____
17. pharynx	-nx	_____	_____
18. larynx	-nx	_____	_____
19. apex	-ex	_____	_____
20. cortex	-ex	_____	_____
21. ganglion	-on	_____	_____
22. spermatozoon	-on	_____	_____
23. pleura	-a	_____	_____
24. sclera	-a	_____	_____
25. bursa	-a	_____	_____

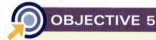 OBJECTIVE 5

Identify medical terms by clinical category.

Now that you have worked through the integumentary system lesson, review and practice medical terms grouped by clinical category. Categories include signs and symptoms, diseases and disorders, surgical procedures, specialties and professions, and other terms related to the integumentary system. Check your responses with the Answer Key in Appendix C.

EXERCISE J   Signs and Symptoms

Write the medical terms for signs and symptoms next to their definitions.

1. _____ puffy swelling of tissue from the accumulation of fluid

2. _____ any visible change in tissue resulting from injury or disease

3. _____ paleness

4. _____ condition characterized by a yellow tinge to the skin, mucous membranes, and whites of the eyes

5. _____ redness

6. _____ abnormal condition of blue of the extremities

7. _____ abnormal condition of blue

8. _____ black skin

9. _____ white skin

10. _____ yellow skin

11. _____ abnormal condition of yellow

EXERCISE K   Diseases and Disorders

Write the medical terms for diseases and disorders next to their definitions.

1. _____ localized collection of pus accompanied by swelling and inflammation

2. _____ inflammation of the skin and subcutaneous tissue caused by infection, characterized by redness, pain, heat, and swelling

3. _____ damage of the skin and the subcutaneous tissue caused by prolonged pressure

4. _____ torn, ragged-edged wound

5. _____ abnormal condition of the nail

6. _____ (any) disease of the skin

7. _____ inflammation of the skin

8. _____   red skin

9. _____   abnormal condition of fungus in the nail

10. _____   superficial skin infection characterized by red lesions which progress to blisters and then honey-colored crusts

11. _____   inflammatory skin disease caused by herpes virus characterized by small blisters in clusters

12. _____   yellow tumor (benign, primarily in the skin)

13. _____   black tumor (primarily of the skin)

14. _____   malignant growth developing from scalelike epithelial tissue of the surface layer of the epidermis

15. _____   malignant epithelial tumor arising from the bottom layer of the epidermis called the basal layer

16. _____   strain of common bacteria that has developed resistance to methicillin and other antibiotics

17. _____   separation of the nail

EXERCISE L   Specialties and Professions

Write the medical terms for specialties and professions next to their definitions.

1. _____   study of the skin

2. _____   physician who studies and treats diseases of the skin

3. _____   physician who (microscopically) studies diseases of the skin

EXERCISE M   Medical Terms Related to the Integumentary System and Colors

Write the medical terms related to the integumentary system and color next to their definitions.

1. _____   red (blood) cell

2. _____   white (blood) cell

3. a._____   pertaining to the skin

   b._____

4. _____   pertaining to upon the skin

5. _____   pertaining to within the skin

6. a._____   pertaining to under the skin

   b._____

7. a._____   pertaining to through the skin

   b._____

8. _____   malformation of the skin, usually brown, black, or flesh colored (also called a mole or birthmark)

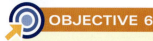

OBJECTIVE 6

Use medical language in clinical statements, the case study, and a medical record.

Check your responses for the following exercises with the Answer Key in Appendix C.

EXERCISE N   Use Medical Terms in Clinical Statements

Circle the medical term defined in the bolded phrases. Medical terms from previous lessons are included. For pronunciation practice read the answers aloud.

1. As the patient became more immobile, she was at increased risk of developing a(n) **damage of the skin and the subcutaneous tissue caused by prolonged pressure** (abscess, laceration, pressure injury). The nursing assistant took preventative measures, including changing the patient's position, keeping her skin dry, and looking for **redness** (erythema, jaundice, pallor).

2. The two-year-old patient who presented with several pimplelike **visible change in tissue resulting from injury or disease** (lesions, lacerations, pressure ulcers) accompanied by erythema was diagnosed with **superficial skin infection characterized by red lesions which progress to blisters and then honey-colored crusts** (herpes, impetigo, jaundice).

3. After clearing out a weedy patch in his front yard, Mr. Pisaniello noticed unusual **redness** (jaundice, pallor, erythema) on his forearm that itched quite a bit. He sought treatment from a **physician who studies and treats diseases of the skin** (dermatopathy, dermatologist, dermatopathologist). He was diagnosed as having contact **inflammation of the skin** (dermatitis, erythroderma, dermatopathy) thought to be caused by poison ivy.

4. Fungal infections can occur in various area of the body, including the skin, hair, and nails. **Abnormal condition of fungus in the nail(s)** (onychomycosis, onychosis, onycholysis) occurs more frequently in toenails and may lead to discoloration, thickening, crumbling, and/or splitting of the nail.

5. The skin test for tuberculosis is administered by a(n) **within the skin** (hypodermic, intradermal, percutaneous) injection.

6. The hospice patient had **black tumor** (melanoma, melanoderma, xanthoma), a form of skin cancer, with **beyond control** (benign, malignant, metastasis) to the brain. To relieve her pain, the nurse used a **pertaining to under the skin** (percutaneous, transdermal, hypodermic) needle to administer morphine into the **pertaining to under the skin** (intradermal, epidermal, subcutaneous) tissue.

7. The most common form of skin cancer is **malignant epithelial tumor arising from the bottom layer of the epidermis** (basal cell carcinoma, squamous cell carcinoma, melanoma), and it most often occurs on sun-exposed skin. **Malignant growth developing from scalelike epithelial tissue of the surface layer of the epidermis** (basal cell carcinoma, squamous cell carcinoma, melanoma) is also a common form of skin cancer. BCC and SCC are both linked to long-term sun exposure and are likely to occur on the head, neck, and backs of the hands.

8. **Strain of common bacteria that has developed resistance to many antibiotics** (SCC, BCC, MRSA) is common in hospitals, but is also occurring more frequently in the general population. First symptoms often include **inflammation of the skin and subcutaneous tissue characterized by redness, heat, pain, and swelling** (edema, dermatitis, cellulitis) and **localized collection of pus accompanied by swelling and inflammation** (abscess, laceration, lesion).

9. Plural and Singular Endings: for the following statements, circle the correct form of term in the parentheses.
   a. The patient had (metastasis, metastases) from the primary site of cancer of the breast to her lymph glands and bone.
   b. Several pulmonary (embolus, emboli) were identified on the CT scan.
   c. An (ova, ovum) is a female egg cell.
   d. Two (testis, testes) are enclosed in the scrotum.
   e. The patient had two small (lipoma, lipomata) removed from his upper back.

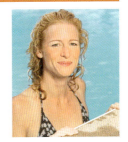

EXERCISE O   Apply Medical Terms to the Case Study

Think back to Amanda who was introduced in the case study at the beginning of the lesson. After working through Lesson 3 on the integumentary system, consider the medical terms that might be used to describe her experience. List three terms relevant to the case study and their meanings. ▪

	Medical Term	Definition
1.	_____	_____
2.	_____	_____
3.	_____	_____

EXERCISE P   Use Medical Terms in a Document

Amanda was able to see her dermatologist, who surgically removed the lesion for examination. The following medical record documents the biopsy results.

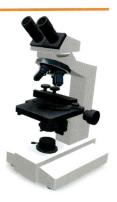

Use the definitions in numbers 1-10 to write medical terms within the following document.

1. study of disease
2. black tumor (primarily skin cancer)
3. malignant epithelial tumor arising from the bottom layer of the epidermis called the basal layer
4. malformation of the skin, usually brown, black, or flesh colored
5. removal of living tissue to be viewed under a microscope for diagnostic purposes
6. pertaining to near the point of attachment
7. pertaining to upon the skin
8. pertaining to the front
9. not malignant, not recurring
10. physician who (microscopically) studies diseases of the skin

```
┌──────────────────────────────────────────────────────────────────────┐
│ 49785 Sheehan, Amanda                                          _ □ ✕  │
│ File    Patient    Navigate    Custom Fields    Help                   │
│ [toolbar icons]                                                        │
│ Chart Review  Encounters  Notes  Labs  Imaging  Procedures  Rx  Documents  Referrals  Scheduling  Billing │
│ Name: Sheehan, Amanda      MR#: 49785        Sex: F     Allergies: None known   │
│                            DOB: 6/15/19XX    Age: 29    PCP: Papas, Aenea MD     │
```

(1.) _____ REPORT

DATE/TIME COLL: Jun 12 20XX, 12:00

DATE RECEIVED: Jun 12 20XX, 16:00

DATE REPORTED: Jun 15 20XX

REPORT STATUS: FINAL REPORT

HISTORY: Previous incidence of (2.) _____ and
(3.) _____, no metastases

PRE-OP DIAGNOSIS: Melanoma vs. compound (4.) _____

PROCEDURE: Tissue (5.) _____

SPECIMEN: Skin biopsy, anterior, (6.) _____ right arm

GROSS DESCRIPTION: One container is received. Specimen in formalin labeled with the
patient's name is a shave biopsy of gray-white hair bearing skin measuring 0.4 × 0.3 cm in
surface dimension and averaging 0.1 cm in thickness. The (7.) _____ surface
contains a symmetric, smooth, ordered, pigmented lesion measuring 0.3 cm in greatest
diameter. The specimen is bisected and totally submitted.

MICROSCOPIC EXAMINATION: A microscopic examination has been performed.

DIAGNOSIS: Lesion, (8.) _____, proximal right arm;
(9.) _____compound nevus.

Electronically signed: J. Alvarez, MD, (10.) _____,
6/15/20XX 10:48

```
│ Start │ Log On/Off │ Print │ Edit │                                    │
└──────────────────────────────────────────────────────────────────────┘
```

Refer to the medical record as needed to answer questions 11-13.

11. The skin biopsy was obtained from:
   a. near the shoulder on the back of the right arm
   b. near the shoulder on the front of the right arm
   c. near the wrist on the back of the right arm
   d. near the wrist on the front of the right arm

12. Identify singular and plural forms of medical terms used in the pathology report. Write "P" for plural and "S" for singular next to the terms. Refer to the Singular and Plural Endings table.
   a. melanoma _____
   b. melanomata _____
   c. nevi _____
   d. nevus _____
   e. metastasis _____
   f. metastases _____
   g. biopsy _____
   h. biopsies _____

13. Using a medical dictionary or an online source, write the meanings of the following terms used in the pathology report:

    a. compound _____

    b. pigmented _____

    c. bisected _____

    d. microscopic _____

OBJECTIVE 7

Recall and assess knowledge of word parts, medical terms, and abbreviations.

EXERCISE Q **Online Review of Lesson Content**

🌐 *Recall and assess your learning from working through the lesson by completing online learning activities at evolve.elsevier.com > Evolve Resources > Practice Student Resources. Keep track of your progress by placing a check mark next to completed activities.*

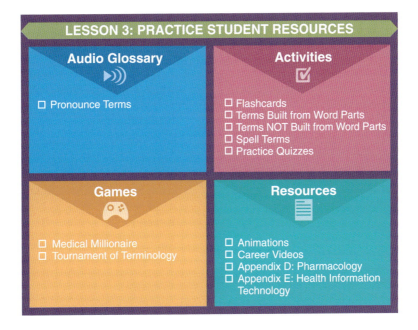

EXERCISE R   **Lesson Content Quiz**

Test your knowledge of the terms and abbreviations introduced in this lesson. Circle the letter for the medical term or abbreviation related to the words in italics.

1. Vitiligo is a progressive skin condition that is a form of *white skin.*
   a. melanoderma
   b. leukoderma
   c. erythroderma

2. A *physician who (microscopically) studies diseases of the skin* may examine deep samples of tissue to evaluate skin cancer.
   a. dermatologist
   b. pathologist
   c. dermatopathologist

3. A *malignant epithelial tumor arising from the bottom layer of the epidermis called the basal layer* may occur on the tip of the nose, the ears, or other sun-exposed areas.
   a. BCC
   b. SCC
   c. RBC

4. *Yellow skin* refers to any yellowish discoloration of the skin, while jaundice is an indicator of disease, and is usually caused by obstruction in the gastrointestinal system.
   a. xanthoma
   b. xanthosis
   c. xanthoderma

5. A *malformation of the skin, usually brown, black, or flesh colored* that changes significantly should be examined by a physician to rule out melanoma.
   a. nevus
   b. laceration
   c. abscess

6. *Inflammation of the skin and subcutaneous tissue caused by infection* can become very serious and should be treated immediately with antibiotics and supportive measures.
   a. dermatitis
   b. cellulitis
   c. cyanosis

7. A tuberculosis (TB) skin test, is a(n) *pertaining to within the skin* injection that must be interpreted 48-72 hours later.
   a. hypodermic
   b. transdermal
   c. intradermal

8. *Abnormal condition of fungus in the nail* is often caused by *T. rubrum* and may be preceded by "athlete's foot," a fungal dermatopathy.
   a. onychomycosis
   b. onycholysis
   c. onychosis

9. Pallor may sometimes be caused by anemia, which is a(n) *red (blood) cell* deficiency.
   a. leukocyte
   b. erythrocyte
   c. cyanosis

10. *Inflammatory skin disease caused by a virus characterized by small blisters in clusters* is one of many infections that affect that skin.
    a. impetigo
    b. herpes
    c. acrocyanosis

LESSON AT A GLANCE | INTEGUMENTARY SYSTEM, COLORS, AND PLURAL ENDINGS WORD PARTS

COMBINING FORMS

Integumentary System
acr/o
cutane/o
derm/o
dermat/o
myc/o
onych/o

Colors
cyan/o
erythr/o
leuk/o
melan/o
xanth/o

SUFFIXES
-a, -e, -y
-itis
-osis
-ous
-lysis

PREFIXES
epi-
hypo-
intra-
per-
sub-
trans-

LESSON AT A GLANCE | INTEGUMENTARY SYSTEM, COLORS, AND PLURAL ENDINGS MEDICAL TERMS AND ABBREVIATIONS

SIGNS AND SYMPTOMS
acrocyanosis
cyanosis
edema
erythema
jaundice
lesion
leukoderma
melanoderma
pallor
xanthoderma
xanthosis

DISEASES AND DISORDERS
abscess
basal cell carcinoma (BCC)
cellulitis
dermatitis
dermatopathy
erythroderma
herpes
impetigo
laceration (lac)
melanoma
methicillin-resistant *staphyloccus aureus* (MRSA)

onycholysis
onychomycosis
onychosis
pressure injury
squamous cell carcinoma (SCC)
xanthoma

SPECIALITIES AND PROFESSIONS
dermatologist
dermatology (DERM)
dermatopathologist

RELATED TERMS
cutaneous
dermal
epidermal
erythrocyte (RBC)
hypodermic (hypo)
intradermal (ID)
leukocyte (WBC)
nevus
percutaneous
subcutaneous (subcut)
transdermal (TD)

ABBREVIATIONS

BCC	RBC
DERM	SCC
hypo	TD
ID	subcut
lac	WBC
MRSA	

SINGULAR AND PLURAL ENDINGS

-a	-ae
-ax	-aces
-ex	-ices
-is	-es
-ix	-ices
-ma	-mata
-nx	-nges
-on	-a
-sis	-ses
-um	-a
-us	-i

Respiratory System

Roberta Pawlaski

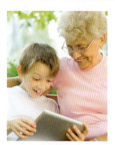

Roberta is experiencing difficulty breathing. She notices it gets worse when she tries to do chores around the house. This has been going on for about four days. She also has a cough and a runny nose. Today when she woke up she noticed that her throat was very sore. She also thinks that she might have a fever because she feels hot all over. She tried taking some over-the-counter cough medicine but this didn't seem to help. She notices when she coughs that a thick yellow mucus comes out. She hasn't had a cough like this since before she quit smoking about 10 years ago. She remembers that her grandson who stays with her after school has missed school because of a cold. She decides to call her doctor to schedule an appointment.

■ *Consider Roberta's situation as you work through the lesson on the respiratory system. At the end of the lesson, we will return to this case study and identify medical terms used to document Roberta's experience and the care she receives.*

OBJECTIVES

1	■	Build, translate, pronounce, and spell medical terms built from word parts (p. 83).
2	■	Define, pronounce, and spell medical terms NOT built from word parts (p. 101).
3	■	Write abbreviations (p. 106).
4	■	Identify medical terms by clinical category (p. 107).
5	■	Use medical language in clinical statements, the case study, and a medical record (p. 110).
6	■	Recall and assess knowledge of word parts, medical terms, and abbreviations (p. 114).

INTRODUCTION TO THE RESPIRATORY SYSTEM

Anatomic Structures of the Respiratory System

alveoli (*s.* alveolus) (al-VĒ-ō-lī), (al-VĒ-o-lus)	air sacs at the smallest subdivision of the bronchial tree; oxygen and carbon dioxide are exchanged through the alveolar walls and the capillaries that surround them
bronchus (*pl.* bronchi) (BRONG-kus), (BRONG-kī)	one of two branches from the trachea that conducts air into the lungs, where it divides and subdivides. The branchings resemble a tree; therefore, they are referred to as a **bronchial tree**.
larynx (LAR-inks)	location of vocal cords; air enters from the pharynx; (also called **voice box**)
lungs (lungs)	two spongelike organs in the thoracic cavity. The right lung has three lobes, and the left lung has two lobes.

Anatomic Structures of the Respiratory System—cont'd

nose (nōz)	lined with mucous membranes and fine hairs; acts as a filter to moisten and warm air
pharynx (FAR-inks)	serves as food and air passageway; air enters from the nasal cavities and/or mouth and passes through the pharynx to the larynx. Food enters the pharynx from the mouth and passes into the esophagus. (also called **throat**)
sinuses (SĪ-nus-es)	air cavities within the cranial bones; membrane lining the air cavities produces mucus, which drains into the nasal passages; (also called **paranasal sinuses**)
thorax (THOR-aks)	chest; the part of the body between the neck and the diaphragm encased by the ribs. The **thoracic cavity** is the hollow space between the neck and diaphragm.
trachea (TRĀ-kē-a)	passageway for air to the bronchi from the larynx; (also called **windpipe**)

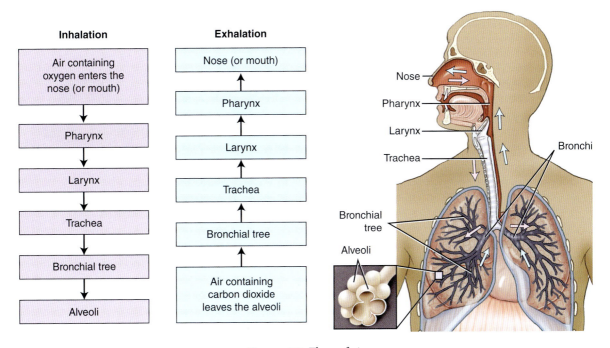

Figure 4.1 Flow of air.

Functions of the Respiratory System

- Moves air in and out of lungs
- Provides for intake of oxygen and release of carbon dioxide
- Provides air flow for speech
- Enables sense of smell

How the Respiratory System Works

The respiratory system is divided into two parts: the upper respiratory tract and the lower respiratory tract. **The upper respiratory tract** includes the nose, pharynx, and larynx. **The lower respiratory tract** includes the trachea, bronchi, and lungs. The thoracic cavity, or chest cavity, encases the lower respiratory tract. The function of the respiratory system is the exchange of oxygen (O_2) and carbon dioxide (CO_2) between the atmosphere and the body's cells. The process is called respiration or breathing. **Inhalation** occurs as air passes through the **nose** or mouth into the **pharynx, larynx,** and **trachea** before entering the **lungs** through the **bronchi.** There, oxygen passes from the sacs in the lungs, called **alveoli,** to the blood in tiny vessels called **capillaries. Exhalation** occurs as carbon dioxide passes back from the capillaries to the alveoli and is expelled through the respiratory tract (see Figure 4.1).

CAREER FOCUS | **Professionals Who Work with the Respiratory System**

- **Respiratory Therapists (RTs)** treat, evaluate, and maintain function of the heart and lungs. RTs are highly skilled and perform pulmonary function tests, provide treatments, such as oxygen therapy and intermittent positive pressure breathing (IPPB), perform arterial blood gases (ABGs) to monitor carbon dioxide and oxygen in the blood, and assist with ventilation of seriously ill patients.

- **Respiratory Therapy Technicians** provide respiratory care under the supervision of respiratory therapists and physicians.

- **Sleep technologists,** also called **registered polysomnographic technologists (RPSGTs),** perform polysomnography and other tests to diagnose and monitor sleep disorders. RPSGTs work under the guidance of a physician.

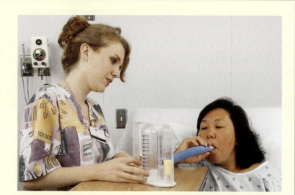

Figure 4.2 Respiratory therapist assisting a patient with incentive spirometry.

- **Sleep technicians** also called **certified polysomnographic technicians (CPSGTs),** prepare sleep testing equipment, gather patient information, and provide explanations of procedures. CPSGTs work under the guidance of a sleep technologist or respiratory therapist.

🌐 **FOR MORE INFORMATION**

- To view a video on careers in **respiratory therapy**, go to the American Association of Respiratory Care's website and search for the video *Life and Breath.*

- Access online resources at evolve.elsevier.com > Practice Student Resources > Other Resources > Career Videos to watch an interview with a **Sleep Technologist**.

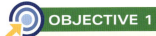

OBJECTIVE 1

Build, translate, pronounce, and spell medical terms built from word parts.

WORD PARTS   Presented with the Respiratory System

Use paper or online **flashcards** to familiarize yourself with the following word parts.

COMBINING FORM (WR + CV)	DEFINITION	COMBINING FORM (WR + CV)	DEFINITION
bronch/o	bronchus (s.), bronchi (pl.)	pneumon/o	lung, air
capn/o	carbon dioxide	pulmon/o	lung
laryng/o	larynx (voice box)	rhin/o	nose
muc/o	mucus	sinus/o	sinus (s.), sinuses (pl.)
nas/o	nose	somn/o	sleep
ox/i	oxygen	spir/o	breathe, breathing
pharyng/o	pharynx (throat)	thorac/o	chest, chest cavity
pneum/o	lung, air	trache/o	trachea (windpipe)

SUFFIX (S)	DEFINITION	SUFFIX (S)	DEFINITION
-ary, -eal	pertaining to	-pnea	breathing
-centesis	surgical puncture to remove fluid (with a sterile needle)	-rrhagia	rapid flow of blood, excessive bleeding
		-rrhea	flow, discharge
-ectomy	surgical removal, excision	-scope	instrument used for visual examination
-gram	record, radiographic image		
-graphy	process of recording, radiographic imaging	-scopic	pertaining to visual examination
		-scopy	visual examination
-ia	diseased state, condition of	-stomy	creation of an artificial opening
		-thorax	chest, chest cavity
-meter	instrument used to measure	-tomy	cut into, incision

PREFIX (P)	DEFINITION	PREFIX (P)	DEFINITION
a-, an-	absence of, without	hyper-	above, excessive
dys-	difficult, painful, abnormal	poly-	many, much
endo-	within		

WORD PARTS PRESENTED IN PREVIOUS LESSONS   Used to Build Terms for the Respiratory System

SUFFIX (S)	DEFINITION	SUFFIX (S)	DEFINITION
-al, -ous	pertaining to	-logist	one who studies and treats (specialist, physician)
-itis	inflammation		
		-logy	study of

PREFIX (P)	DEFINITION		
hypo-	below, deficient, under		

Refer to Appendix A, Word Parts Used in *Basic Medical Language,* for alphabetical lists of word parts and their meanings.

EXERCISE A | **Build and Translate Terms Built from Word Parts**

Use the **Word Parts Tables** *to complete the following questions. Check your responses with the Answer Key in Appendix C*

1. **LABEL:** *Write the combining forms for anatomical structures of the respiratory system on Figure 4.3. These anatomical combining forms will be used to build and translate medical terms in Exercise A.*

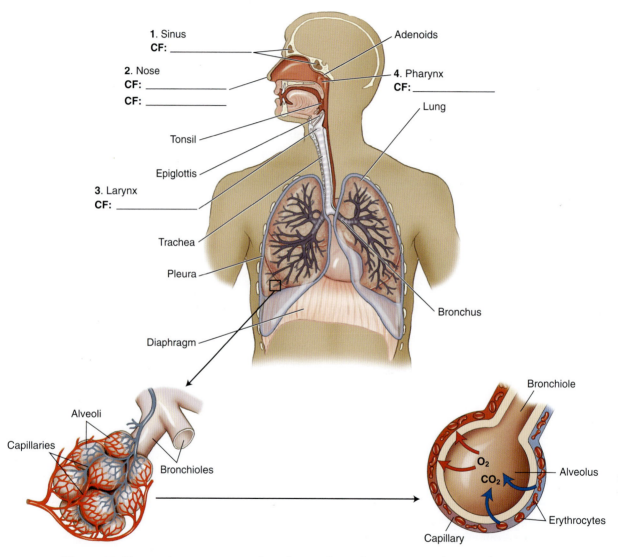

1. Sinus
CF: _____

2. Nose
CF: _____
CF: _____

Tonsil

Epiglottis

3. Larynx
CF: _____

Trachea

Pleura

Diaphragm

Adenoids

4. Pharynx
CF: _____

Lung

Bronchus

Alveoli

Capillaries

Bronchioles

Bronchiole

O₂
CO₂

Alveolus

Erythrocytes

Capillary

Figure 4.3 The respiratory system and combining forms for sinus, nose, larynx, and pharynx.

2. **MATCH:** *Draw a line to match the suffix with its definition.*

    a. -rrhea   inflammation
    b. -rrhagia   rapid flow of blood
    c. -itis   flow, discharge

> **FYI**   **-rrhagia** and **-rrhea** are two of four **rrh** suffixes you will learn in medical terminology. Note the **h** in **rrh**. The **h** is often missing in misspelled words.

3. **BUILD:** *Using the combining form **rhin/o** and the suffixes reviewed in the previous exercise, build the following terms describing conditions related to the nose and nasal membranes:*

    a. inflammation of the nose (nasal membranes)   _____/_____
                                                              wr   s

    b. discharge from the nose   _____/_o_/_____
                                                              wr   cv   s

    c. rapid flow of blood from the nose   _____/_o_/_____
                                                              wr   cv   s

4. **READ: Rhinorrhagia** (rī-nō-RĀ-ja), the medical term for "nosebleed," describes rapid flow of blood from the nose. **Rhinorrhea** (rī-nō-RĒ-a), the medical term for "runny nose," describes discharge from the nose as seen in the common cold and in **rhinitis** (rī-NĬ-tis), a symptom of allergies.

5. **MATCH:** *Draw a line to match the combining form or suffix with its definition.*

    a. -tomy   mucus
    b. -al, -ous   inflammation
    c. muc/o   pertaining to
    d. -itis   cut into, incision

6. **TRANSLATE:** *Complete the definitions of the following terms by using the meaning of word parts to fill in the blanks. Remember, the definition usually starts with the meaning of the suffix.*

    a. nas/al   _____ to the _____
    b. muc/ous   _____ to _____
    c. sinus/itis   _____ of the _____ (membranes)
    d. sinus/o/tomy   (cut into or)_____ of a _____

7. **READ:** Paranasal sinuses are hollow spaces located near the **nasal** (NĀ-zal) cavity and drain into it. The paranasal sinuses produce mucus, a slimy fluid that lubricates and protects the **mucous** (MŪ-kus) membranes. **Sinusitis** (sī-nū-SĪ-tis), which presents with nasal congestion, headache, and fever, often extends into the nasal passageways. A **sinusotomy** (sī-nū-SOT-o-mē) may be performed to relieve symptoms in more severe cases. An otolaryngologist, often referred to as an ENT, is a specialist trained to treat problems of the ear, nose, and throat. ENTs also perform surgeries of the head and neck, including sinusotomy.

> **FYI**   **Mucus** and **mucous** are pronounced the same. **Mucus** is a noun, the substance, whereas **mucous** is an adjective describing a noun, as in mucous membrane.

8. **LABEL:** *Write word parts to complete Figure 4.4.*

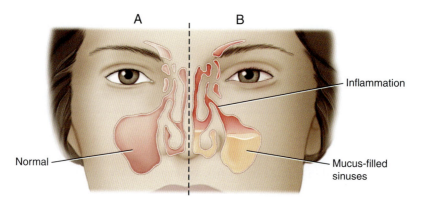

Figure 4.4 A) Normal sinuses. B) _____/_____.
                                         sinus   inflammation

9. **MATCH:** *Draw a line to match the suffix with its definition.*

a. -itis   pertaining to
b. -eal   inflammation
c. -ectomy   visual examination
d. -scope   surgical removal, excision
e. -scopy   instrument used for visual examination

10. **BUILD:** *Write word parts to build terms describing inflammation (hint: use **nas/o** for the combining form meaning nose):*

a. inflammation of the pharynx (throat)   _____/_____
                                                              wr   s

b. inflammation of the nose (nasal membranes) and   _____/_o_/_____/_____
   pharynx (throat)   wr   cv   wr   s

c. inflammation of the larynx (voice box)   _____/_____
                                                              wr   s

11. **READ:** **Pharyngitis** (far-in-JĪ-tis) is the medical term for sore throat. The larynx, commonly referred to as the voice box, contains the vocal cords. Frequently caused by a virus, **laryngitis** (lar-in-JĪ-tis) may be characterized by hoarseness or loss of voice.

12. **BUILD:** *Write word parts to build descriptive terms using the suffix* **–eal**, *meaning pertaining to.*

    a. pertaining to the pharynx (throat)   _____/_____
    wr   s

    b. pertaining to the larynx (voice box)   _____/_____
    wr   s

    c. pertaining to the larynx (voice box)   _____/ o /_____/_____
       and pharynx (throat)
    wr   cv   wr   s

    > **FYI**   The suffixes **-ic, -al, -ous, -ary,** and **-eal** all mean **pertaining to.** As you practice and use the medical terms, you will become more familiar with which suffix is used.

13. **TRANSLATE:** *Complete the definitions of the following terms built from the combining form* **laryng/o**, *meaning larynx. Use the meaning of word parts to fill in the blanks. Remember, the definition usually starts with the meaning of the suffix.*

    a. laryng/o/scope   _____ used for _____ examination of the larynx
    b. laryng/o/scopy   visual _____ of the _____
    c. laryng/ectomy   _____ (or surgical removal) of the _____

14. **READ:** A **laryngoscope** (lar-RING-gō-skōp) is used to perform **laryngoscopy** (lar-in-GOS-ko-pē). Treatment of **laryngeal** (lar-IN-jē-al) cancer may include a **laryngectomy** (lar-in-JEK-to-mē).

    > **FYI**   Manuel Garcia, a Spanish singing teacher, invented the modern **laryngoscope** in 1854. The first successful **laryngectomy** was performed in 1873 by the famous Viennese surgeon Christian Albert Theodor Billroth.

15. **MATCH:** *Draw a line to match the prefix or suffix with its definition.*

    a. a-, an-   breathing
    b. dys-   absence of, without
    c. hyper-   difficult, painful, abnormal
    d. hypo-   below, deficient, under
    e. -pnea   above, excessive

    > **FYI**   **Tips for Use of Word Parts**
    > - The prefix **a-** is used when the following word root begins with a consonant. **An-** is used when the following word root begins with a vowel.
    > - For translating the meaning of respiratory system terms, use "excessive" for the definition of **hyper-** and use "deficient" for the definition of **hypo-**.
    > - The suffix **–pnea** is used with a prefix only. The word root **pne** means breathing and is embedded in the suffix **-pnea**.

16. TRANSLATE: *Complete the definitions of the following terms by using the meaning of word parts to fill in the blanks. Remember, the definition usually starts with the meaning of the suffix.*
*Terms built using the suffix -**pnea**:*

a. a/pnea _____ of _____

b. dys/pnea _____ breathing

c. hypo/pnea   deficient _____

d. hyper/pnea _____ breathing

---

17. READ: **Apnea** (AP-nē-a) refers to absence of spontaneous respiration. **Dyspnea** (DISP-nē-a), a symptom, describes shortness of breath or any other breathing difficulty outside of a person's normal experience. **Hypopnea** (hī-POP-nē-a) and **hyperpnea** (hī-perp-NĒ-a) describe airflow in terms of rate and quantity. Hypopnea represents a deficient or decreased rate and depth of breathing. Hyperpnea represents an excessive or increased rate and depth of breathing. The medical terms apnea and hypopnea are key findings in obstructive sleep apnea.

---

18. MATCH: *Draw a line to match the combining form, prefix, or suffix with its definition.*

a. -ia   above, excessive
b. -meter   instrument used to measure
c. hyper-   condition of
d. hypo-   below, deficient, under
e. capn/o   oxygen
f. ox/i   breathing
g. spir/o   carbon dioxide

---

19. BUILD: *Write word parts to build terms describing excessive or deficient amounts of oxygen and carbon dioxide in the body:*

a. condition of excessive oxygen (in the tissues)   _____/_____/_____
                                                          p   wr   s

b. condition of excessive carbon dioxide (in the blood)   _____/_____/_____
                                                               p   wr   s

c. condition of deficient carbon dioxide (in the blood)   _____/_____/_____
                                                               p   wr   s

d. condition of deficient oxygen (in the tissues)   _____/_____/_____
                                                          p   wr   s

FYI   The **o** from **hypo** has been dropped in the medical term **hypoxia**. The final vowel of a prefix may be dropped when the word to which it is added begins with a vowel.

20. READ: Condition of deficient oxygen in the tissues, or **hypoxia** (hī-POK-sē-a), may be caused by the inability of erythrocytes to transport oxygen to the tissues or from being at high altitude. Condition of excessive oxygen, **hyperoxia** (hī-per-OK-sē-a), usually results from an increase in the concentration of oxygen given to a patient. Condition of excessive carbon dioxide, or **hypercapnia** (hī-per-KAP-nē-a), can result from disorders such as emphysema or chronic obstructive pulmonary disease; whereas condition of deficient carbon dioxide, or **hypocapnia** (hī-pō-KAP-nē-a), usually results from hyperventilation, which is ventilation of the lungs beyond normal body needs.

21. TRANSLATE: *Complete the definitions of the following terms by using the meaning of word parts to fill in the blanks. Remember, the definition usually starts with the meaning of the suffix. Terms built using the suffix -**meter**:*

a. capn/o/meter   _____ used to measure _____ _____

b. ox/i/meter   instrument used to _____ _____

c. spir/o/meter   _____ used to measure _____ (or lung volumes)

22. READ: A **capnometer** (kap-NOM-e-ter) measures carbon dioxide concentration in exhaled air. A pulse **oximeter** (ok-SIM-e-ter) is placed on a figure tip and measures the oxygen level in the blood. A **spirometer** (spī-ROM-e-ter) measures the amount of air that can be inhaled and exhaled.

23. LABEL: *Write word parts to complete Figure 4.5.*

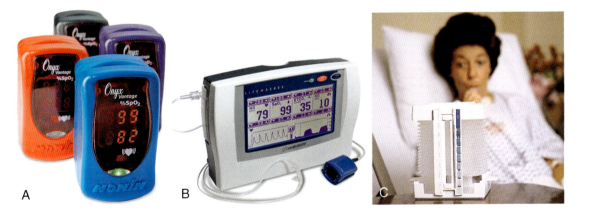

Figure 4.5 A) Pulse _____/i/_____.
oxygen   instrument used to measure
B) _____/o/_____.
carbon dioxide   instrument used to measure
C) _____/o/_____.
breathing   instrument used to measure

24. **REVIEW OF RESPIRATORY SYSTEM TERMS BUILT FROM WORD PARTS:** the following is an alphabetical list of terms built and translated in the previous exercises.

MEDICAL TERMS BUILT FROM WORD PARTS

TERM	DEFINITION	TERM	DEFINITION
1. apnea (AP-nē-a)	absence of breathing	14. laryngoscopy (lar-in-GOS-ko-pē)	visual examination of the larynx
2. capnometer (kap-NOM-e-ter)	instrument used to measure carbon dioxide (Figure 4.5, *B*)	15. mucous (MŪ-kus)	pertaining to mucus
3. dyspnea (DISP-nē-a)	difficult breathing	16. nasal (NĀ-zal)	pertaining to the nose
4. hypercapnia (hī-per-KAP-nē-a)	condition of excessive carbon dioxide	17. nasopharyngitis (nā-zō-far-in-JĪ-tis)	inflammation of the nose and pharynx
5. hyperoxia (hī-per-OK-sē-a)	condition of excessive oxygen	18. oximeter (ok-SIM-e-ter)	instrument used to measure oxygen (Figure 4.5, *A*)
6. hyperpnea (hī-perp-NĒ-a)	excessive breathing	19. pharyngeal (fa-RIN-jē-al)	pertaining to the pharynx
7. hypocapnia (hī-pō-KAP-nē-a)	condition of deficient carbon dioxide	20. pharyngitis (far-in-JĪ-tis)	inflammation of the pharynx
8. hypopnea (hī-POP-nē-a)	deficient breathing	21. rhinitis (rī-NĪ-tis)	inflammation of the nose (nasal membranes)
9. hypoxia (hī-POK-sē-a)	condition of deficient oxygen	22. rhinorrhagia (rī-nō-RĀ-ja)	rapid flow of blood from the nose
10. laryngeal (lar-IN-jē-al)	pertaining to the larynx	23. rhinorrhea (rī-nō-RĒ-a)	discharge from the nose
11. laryngectomy (lar-in-JEK-to-mē)	excision of the larynx	24. sinusitis (sī-nū-SĪ-tis)	inflammation of the sinus (membranes) (Figure 4.4, *B*)
12. laryngitis (lar-in-JĪ-tis)	inflammation of the larynx	25. sinusotomy (sī-nū-SOT-o-mē)	incision of a sinus
13. laryngoscope (lar-RING-gō -skōp)	instrument used for visual examination of the larynx (Figure 4.7)	26. spirometer (spī-ROM-e-ter)	instrument used to measure breathing (lung volume) (Figure 4.5, *C*)

EXERCISE B Pronounce and Spell Terms Built from Word Parts

Practice pronunciation and spelling on paper and online.

1. **Practice on Paper**
   a. **Pronounce:** Read the phonetic spelling and say aloud the terms listed in the previous table, Review Terms Built from Word Parts. Refer to the pronunciation key on p. 9 as necessary.
   b. **Spell:** Have a study partner read the terms aloud. Write the spelling of the terms on a separate sheet of paper.

2. **Practice Online** 🌐
   a. **Access** online learning resources. Go to evolve.elsevier.com > Evolve Resources > Practice Student Resources.
   b. **Pronounce:** Select Audio Glossary > Exercise B. Select a term to hear its pronunciation and repeat aloud.
   c. **Spell:** Select Activities > Spell Terms > Exercise B. Select the audio icon and type the correct spelling of the term.

❏ Check the box when complete.

EXERCISE C Build and Translate MORE Medical Terms Built from Word Parts

1. **LABEL:** *Write the word parts for anatomical structures of the respiratory system on Figure 4.6. These anatomical combining forms and suffix will be used to build and translate medical terms in Exercise C.*

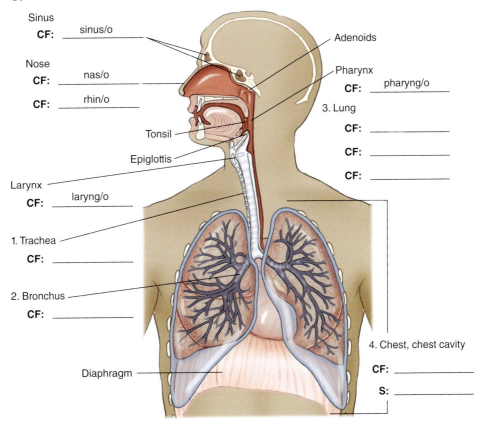

Sinus
  CF: ___sinus/o___

Nose
  CF: ___nas/o___
  CF: ___rhin/o___

Tonsil

Epiglottis

Larynx
  CF: ___laryng/o___

1. Trachea
   CF: _____

2. Bronchus
   CF: _____

Diaphragm

Adenoids

Pharynx
  CF: ___pharyng/o___

3. Lung
   CF: _____
   CF: _____
   CF: _____

4. Chest, chest cavity
   CF: _____
   S: _____

Figure 4.6 The respiratory system and word parts for trachea, bronchus, lung, and chest cavity.

2. MATCH: *Draw a line to match the prefix or suffix with its definition.*

a. -stomy   instrument used for visual examination
b. -tomy   creation of an artificial opening
c. endo-   pertaining to
d. -al   within
e. -scope   cut into, incision

---

3. TRANSLATE: *Complete the definitions of terms built from the combining form **trache/o** by using the meaning of word parts to fill in the blanks. Remember, the definition usually starts with the meaning of the suffix.*

a. trache/o/tomy   (cut into or) _____ of the _____

b. trache/o/stomy   creation of an _____ _____ into the _____

c. endo/trache/al   _____ to _____ the _____

---

4. READ: An **endotracheal** (en-dō-TRĀ-kē-al) tube, or **ET** tube, is inserted through the mouth or nose into the trachea to maintain an open airway, the passageway for the movement of the air to and from the lungs. This tube remains in place for a limited amount of time, such as during a surgical procedure. A **laryngoscope** (lar-RING-gō-skōp) is used to place the tube. Insertion of the tube is called endotracheal intubation.

---

5. LABEL: *Write word parts to complete Figure 4.7.*

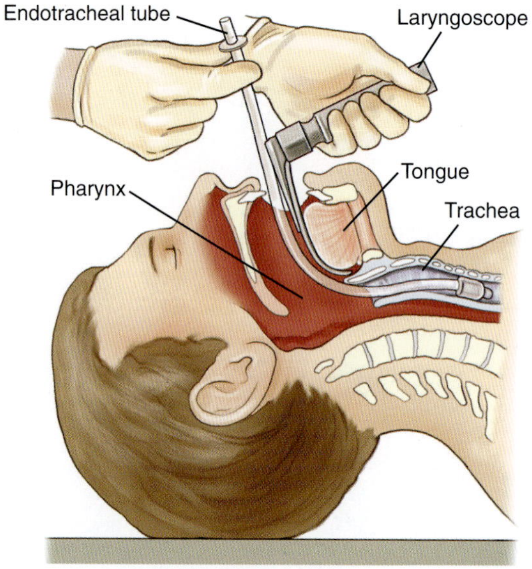

Figure 4.7 The nurse anesthetist inserts a(n) _____/_____/_____ tube with a
                                                        within   trachea   pertaining to

_____/o/_____ to guide the tube into place.
         larynx   instrument used for visual examination

6. **READ:** A **tracheotomy** (trā-kē-OT-o-mē) establishes an open airway when normal breathing is obstructed. An emergency tracheotomy may be performed, for instance, when a person's upper airway is blocked. If the opening needs to be maintained, a tube is inserted, creating a **tracheostomy** (trā-kē-OS-to-mē). A tracheostomy may be temporary, as for prolonged mechanical ventilation to support breathing, or it may be permanent, as in airway reconstruction after a **laryngectomy** (lar-in-JEK-to-mē) to treat **laryngeal** (lar-IN-jē-al) cancer.

> **FYI** The terms **tracheotomy** and **tracheostomy** are used interchangeably, though tracheotomy names the procedure entailing an incision into the trachea and tracheostomy names the resulting opening.

7. **LABEL:** *Write word parts to complete Figure 4.8.*

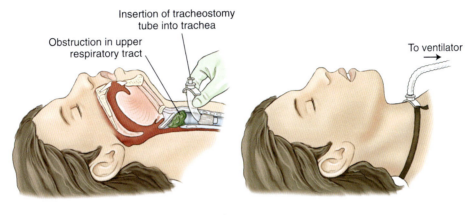

Insertion of tracheostomy tube into trachea

Obstruction in upper respiratory tract

To ventilator

Figure 4.8 _____ /o/ _____.
trachea   creation of an artificial opening

8. **MATCH:** *Draw a line to match the suffix with its definition.*

a. -scope   instrument used for visual examination
b. -scopy   inflammation
c. -itis   visual examination

9. **BUILD:** *Write word parts to build the following terms using the combining form **bronch/o**, meaning bronchi.*

a. inflammation of the bronchi

_____/_____
                wr   s

b. instrument used for visual examination of the bronchi

_____/ o /_____
                wr   cv   s

c. visual examination of the bronchi

_____/ o /_____
                wr   cv   s

> **FYI** The medical term **bronchus** is singular; the plural form, **bronchi**, refers to the multiple branches within the lung. See Lesson 3 for plural endings.

10. READ: **Bronchoscopy** (bron-KOS-ko-pē) is performed by using a **bronchoscope** (BRON-kō-skōp) inserted through the nostril or mouth and passed through the pharynx, larynx, and trachea into the bronchus.

11. LABEL: *Write word parts to complete Figure 4.9.*

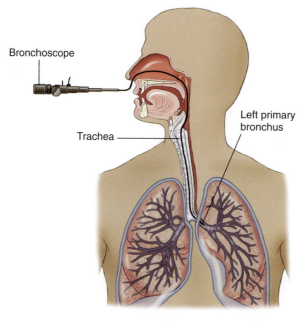

Bronchoscope

Left primary bronchus

Trachea

Figure 4.9 _____/o/_____.

                  bronchi   visual examination

12. MATCH: *Draw a line to match the suffix with its definition.*

a. -ia   pertaining to
b. -ectomy   study of
c. -ary   one who studies and treats (specialist, physician)
d. -logy   diseased state, condition of
e. -logist   surgical removal, excision

13. TRANSLATE: *Complete the definitions of the following terms by using the meaning of word parts to fill in the blanks. Remember, the definition usually starts with the meaning of the suffix. Terms built from the combining form **pulmon/o**, meaning lung:*

a. pulmon/ary   _____ to the _____

b. pulmon/o/logy   _____ of the _____

c. pulmon/o/logist   physician who _____ and _____ diseases of the lung

14. READ: The medical term **pulmonary** (PUL-mō-nar-ē), an adjective, describes anatomic location, as in pulmonary artery, or the location of a disease, as in pulmonary tuberculosis. **Pulmonology** (pul-mon-OL-o-jē), a subspecialty of internal medicine, focuses on treating diseases and disorders of the lungs and bronchial tubes. The pulmonology department of a hospital provides evaluation, diagnosis, and treatment of patients with conditions affecting the lungs. **Pulmonologists** (pul-mon-OL-o-jists) may be involved with the care of hospitalized patients who are critically ill. They also care for lung transplant candidates and patients with pulmonary diseases including severe asthma, pneumonia, emphysema, chronic obstructive pulmonary disease (COPD), cystic fibrosis (CF), and tuberculosis (TB).

15. BUILD: *Write word parts to build terms using the combining form* **pneumon/o**, *meaning lung, air.*

a. diseased state of the lungs

                                      _____/_____
                                            wr   s

b. diseased state of the bronchi and lungs

               _____/_o_/_____/_____
                    wr   cv   wr   s

c. excision of a lung

                                _____/_____
                                 wr   s

16. READ: Pneumonia (nū-MŌ-nē-a) describes a diseased state of the lung and refers to an infection of the lung or, more specifically, the alveoli (air sacs within the lungs). **Bronchopneumonia** (bron-kō-nū-MŌ-nē-a) refers to an infection of the bronchi and the lung. **Pneumonectomy** (nū-mō-NEK-to-mē), excision of the whole lung, is most commonly performed to treat lung cancer.

17. MATCH: *Draw a line to match the combining form or suffix with its definition.*

a. -tomy   chest, chest cavity
b. -centesis   lung, air
c. -thorax, thorac/o   cut into, incision
d. pneum/o   surgical puncture to remove fluid (with a sterile needle)

> **FYI**   While pneumon/o and pneum/o can both be used to mean lung or air, when building and translating terms presented in this text, use **pneum/o** to mean **air** and **pneumon/o** to mean **lung**.

18. BUILD: *Write word parts to build terms using the suffix* **–thorax** *and the combining form* **thorac/o**, *meaning chest, chest cavity.*

a. air in the chest cavity

                               _____/_o_/_____
                                  wr   cv   s

b. incision into the chest cavity

                               _____/_o_/_____
                                  wr   cv   s

c. surgical puncture to remove fluid from the chest cavity

          thora/_____
            wr   s

> **FYI**   The combing vowel "o" and the "c" in **thorac/o** are dropped in the term **thoracentesis**.

19. LABEL: *Write word parts to complete Figure 4.10.*

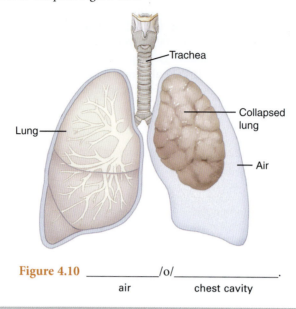

Figure 4.10 _____/o/_____.
air   chest cavity

---

20. READ: Pneumothorax (nū-mō-THOR-aks), directly translated as "air in the chest cavity," specifically refers to air in the pleural space between the membrane covering the lung and the membrane lining the thoracic cavity. Pneumothorax may lead to the collapse of a lung and is often the result of an open chest wound. **Thoracotomy** (tho-ra-KOT-o-mē) is a surgical procedure performed to examine, treat, or excise organs contained in the chest cavity. Procedures involving -**centesis** are performed for therapeutic and diagnostic purposes, facilitating the body's healing processes by removing excess fluid from a body cavity and by obtaining a fluid sample for laboratory analysis, respectively. **Thoracentesis** (thor-a-sen-TĒ-sis) is performed to remove fluid from the chest cavity.

---

21. LABEL: *Write word parts to complete Figure 4.11.*

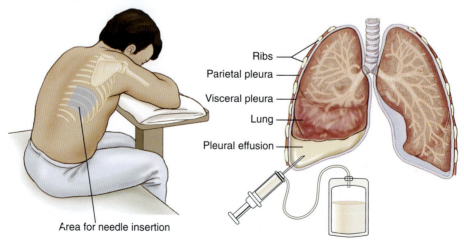

Figure 4.11 A _____/_____ is used for both diagnosis and treatment.
chest cavity   surgical puncture to remove fluid

22. MATCH: *Draw a line to match the combining form, prefix or suffix with its definition.*

a. thorac/o   instrument used for visual examination

b. endo-   visual examination

c. -scope   chest, chest cavity

d. -scopy   within

e. -scopic   pertaining to

f. -ic   pertaining to visual examination

> **FYI** Medical terms ending with the suffix **-scope** and **-scopy** are nouns. Medical terms ending with the suffix **-scopic** are adjectives. For example:
> endoscope = noun, the instrument
> endoscopy = noun, the procedure
> endoscopic = adjective, describes the procedure

23. TRANSLATE: *Complete the definitions of the following terms by using the meaning of word parts to fill in the blanks. Remember, the definition usually starts with the meaning of the suffix. Terms built using the prefix* **endo-**:

a. endo/scope   _____ used for _____ examination _____
                     (a hollow organ or body cavity)

b. endo/scopic   _____ to visual examination _____ (a hollow organ or
                     body cavity)

c. endo/scopy   visual _____ within (a hollow organ or body cavity)

> **FYI** The medical terms endo/scope, endo/scopic, and endo/scopy appear to be made up of a prefix and a suffix. The word root **scop** meaning "to view" is embedded in the suffixes -scope, -scopic, and -scopy.

24. READ: Endoscopy (en-DOS-ko-pē), the visual examination within a hollow organ or body cavity, is performed using an **endoscope** (EN-dō-skōp). **Endoscopic** (en-dō-SKOP-ik) surgery is used for diagnosis and treatment. A small incision is made to accommodate a specialized endoscope fitted with a video camera. Other small incisions are made to hold the surgical instruments. The surgeon uses images displayed on a monitor to perform the surgery. Endoscopic surgery, which causes less pain and reduces recovery time, has replaced many large incision surgeries.

25. BUILD: *Write word parts to build terms using the combining form* **thorac/o**, *meaning chest, chest cavity.*

a. pertaining to the chest

           _____ / _____
                wr   s

b. visual examination of the chest cavity

           _____ / o / _____
                wr   cv   s

c. instrument used for visual examination of the chest cavity

           _____ / o / _____
                wr   cv   s

d. pertaining to visual examination of the chest cavity

           _____ / o / _____
                wr   cv   s

26. READ: Thoracoscopy (thor-a-KOS-ko-pē) is a type of **endoscopy** (en-DOS-ko-pē). **Thoracoscopic** (thor-a-kō-SKOP-ik) surgery, which employs the use of a **thoracoscope** (tho-RAK-ō-skōp), may be performed to obtain a biopsy, remove a portion of the lung, treat cysts, or treat plural effusions. A **thoracic** (thō-RAS-ik) surgeon performs the procedure.

> **FYI**   **Thoracic surgeons** and **pulmonologists** both specialize in treating disorders of the lower respiratory system; however, pulmonologists do not perform surgery.

27. LABEL: *Write word parts to complete Figure 4.12.*

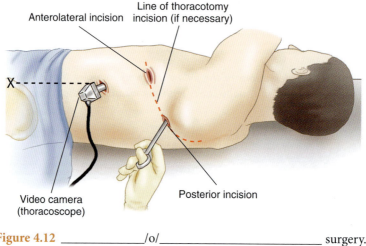

Anterolateral incision   Line of thoracotomy incision (if necessary)

X------

Video camera (thoracoscope)

Posterior incision

Figure 4.12 _____/o/_____ surgery.
              chest cavity   pertaining to visual examination

28. MATCH: *Draw a line to match the word part with its definition.*

a. -graphy   sleep
b. -gram   many
c. poly-   process of recording
d. somn/o   record

29. TRANSLATE: *Complete the definitions of the following terms by using the meaning of word parts to fill in the blanks. Remember, the definition usually starts with the meaning of the suffix.*

a. poly/somn/o/graphy   process of _____ many _____(tests)
b. poly/somn/o/gram   _____ of _____ sleep (tests)

30. **READ: Polysomnography** (pol-ē-som-NOG-rah-fē), abbreviated as **PSG**, is used to diagnose and evaluate sleep disorders, including sleep-related respiratory disorders. A battery of tests are performed during sleep to monitor oxygen levels, heart rate, eye movements, brain waves, and other measures. The resulting **polysomnogram** (pol- ē-SOM-nō-gram) documents information gathered from the various tests.

31. **LABEL:** *Write word parts to complete figure 4.13.*

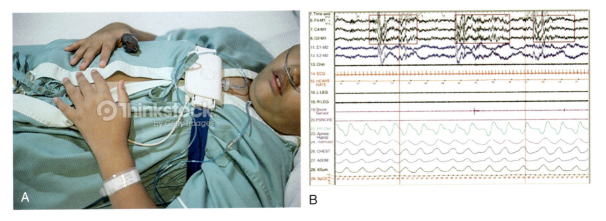

A   B

Figure 4.13   A. _____/_____/o/_____
                         many   sleep (tests)   process of recording

                   B. _____/_____/o/_____
                         many   sleep (tests)   record

32. **REVIEW OF MORE RESPIRATORY SYSTEM TERMS BUILT FROM WORD PARTS:** the following is an alphabetical list of terms built and translated in the previous exercises.

MEDICAL TERMS BUILT FROM WORD PARTS

TERM	DEFINITION	TERM	DEFINITION
1. **bronchitis** (bron-KĪ-tis)	inflammation of the bronchi	6. **endoscopic** (en-dō-SKOP-ik)	pertaining to visual examination within (a hollow organ or cavity)
2. **bronchopneumonia** (bron-kō-nū-MŌ-nē-a)	diseased state of the bronchi and lungs	7. **endoscopy** (en-DOS-ko-pē)	visual examination within (a hollow organ or cavity)
3. **bronchoscope** (BRON-kō-skōp)	instrument used for visual examination of the bronchi	8. **endotracheal (ET)** (en-dō-TRĀ-kē-al)	pertaining to within the trachea
4. **bronchoscopy** (bron-KOS-ko-pē)	visual examination of the bronchi (Figure 4.9)	9. **pneumonectomy** (nū-mō-NEK-to-mē)	excision of a lung
5. **endoscope** (EN-dō-skōp)	instrument used for visual examination within (a hollow organ or cavity)	10. **pneumonia** (nū-MŌ-nē-a)	diseased state of the lungs

MEDICAL TERMS BUILT FROM WORD PARTS—cont'd

TERM	DEFINITION	TERM	DEFINITION
11. pneumothorax (nū-mō-THOR-aks)	air in the chest cavity (Figure 4.10)	18. thoracic (thō-RAS-ik)	pertaining to the chest
12. polysomnography (PSG) (pol-ē-som-NOG-rah-fē)	process of recording many (tests) during sleep; (also called **sleep study**)	19. thoracoscope (tho-RAK-ō-skōp)	instrument used for visual examination of the chest cavity
13. polysomnogram (pol- ē-SOM-nō-gram)	record of many sleep tests	20. thoracoscopic (thor-a-kō-SKOP-ik)	pertaining to visual examination of the chest cavity (Figure 4.12)
14. pulmonary (PUL-mō-nar-ē)	pertaining to the lung	21. thoracoscopy (tho-a-KOS-ko-pē)	visual examination of the chest cavity
15. pulmonologist (pul-mon-OL-o-jist)	physician who studies and treats diseases of the lung	22. thoracotomy (tho-ra-KOT-o-mē)	incision into the chest cavity
16. pulmonology (pul-mon-OL-o-jē)	study of the lung	23. tracheostomy (trā-kē-OS-to-mē)	creation of an artificial opening into the trachea (Figure 4.8)
17. thoracentesis (thor-a-sen-TĒ-sis)	surgical puncture to remove fluid from the chest cavity (Figure 4.11)	24. tracheotomy (trā-kē-OT-o-mē)	incision into the trachea

EXERCISE D   Pronounce and Spell MORE Terms Built from Word Parts

Practice pronunciation and spelling on paper and online.

1. **Practice on Paper**
   a. **Pronounce**: Read the phonetic spelling and say aloud the terms listed in the previous table, Review of MORE Terms Built from Word Parts. Refer to the pronunciation key on p. 9 as necessary.
   b. **Spell**: Have a study partner read the terms aloud. Write the spelling of the terms on a separate sheet of paper.

2. **Practice Online** 🌐
   a. **Access** online learning resources. Go to evolve.elsevier.com > Evolve Resources > Practice Student Resources.
   b. **Pronounce**: Select Audio Glossary > Exercise D. Select a term to hear its pronunciation and repeat aloud.
   c. **Spell**: Select Activities > Spell Terms > Exercise D. Select the audio icon and type the correct spelling of the term.

❏ Check the box when complete.

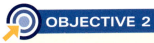

OBJECTIVE 2

Define, pronounce, and spell medical terms NOT built from word parts.

The terms listed below may contain word parts, but are difficult to translate literally.

MEDICAL TERMS NOT BUILT FROM WORD PARTS

TERM	DEFINITION
asthma (AZ-ma)	respiratory disease characterized by coughing, wheezing, and shortness of breath; caused by constriction and inflammation of airways that is reversible between attacks
chronic obstructive pulmonary disease (COPD) (KRON-ik) (ob-STRUK-tive) (PUL-mō-nar-ē) (di ZĒZ)	progressive lung disease blocking air flow, which makes breathing difficult. Chronic bronchitis and emphysema are two main components of COPD. Most COPD is a result of cigarette smoking.
computed tomography (CT) (kom-PU-ted) (tō-MOG-re-fē)	diagnostic imaging test producing scans composed from sectional radiographic images, which can be taken in any of the anatomic planes for a multidimensional view of internal structures. Chest computed tomography is often performed to follow up on abnormalities identified on previous chest radiographs. (Figure 4.14, *B*)
culture and sensitivity (C&S) (KUL-cher) (sen-si-TIV-i-tē)	laboratory test performed on a collected sample to determine the presence of pathogenic bacteria or fungi and to identify the most effective antimicrobial treatment. The test may be performed on sputum, throat cultures, blood, urine, and other fluids. Sputum culture and sensitivity tests are frequently used in the diagnosis of lower respiratory tract infections such as bronchitis and pneumonia.
emphysema (em-fi-SĒ-ma)	loss of elasticity of the alveoli results in distension, causing stretching of the lung. As a result, the body does not receive enough oxygen. (component of COPD)
influenza (flu) (in-flū-EN-za)	highly contagious and often severe viral infection of the respiratory tract
obstructive sleep apnea (OSA) (ob-STRUK-tiv) (slēp) (AP-nē-a)	repetitive pharyngeal collapse during sleep, which leads to short absences of breathing (apnea); can produce daytime drowsiness and elevated blood pressure
radiograph (RĀ-dē-ō-graf)	image created by ionizing radiation; chest radiographs are frequently performed to diagnose respiratory conditions; (also called an **x-ray**) (Figure 4.14, *A*)
sputum (SPŪ-tum)	mucous secretion from the lungs, bronchi, and trachea expelled through the mouth
tuberculosis (TB) (tū-ber-kū-LŌ-sis)	infectious bacterial disease, most commonly spread by inhalation of small particles and usually affecting the lungs (may spread to other organs)
upper respiratory infection (URI) (UP-er) (RES-pi-ra-tor-ē) (in-FEK-shun)	infection of the nasal cavity, pharynx, or larynx, usually caused by a virus; (commonly called a **cold**) (Figure 4.15)

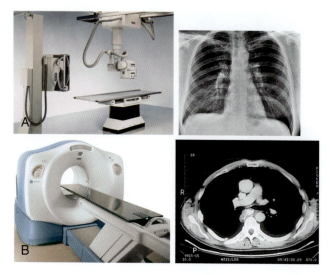

FYI   **Diagnostic imaging**
is a general term referring to procedures that generate images of internal structures, including radiography (also called x-ray), computed tomography (CT), magnetic resonance (MR), nuclear medicine (NM), and sonography (also called ultrasonography abbreviated as US) .

Figure 4.14 Diagnostic imaging. **A,** Radiographic table and chest radiograph (x-ray). **B,** CT scanner and scan of the chest.

EXERCISE E   Label

Write the medical terms pictured and defined using the previous table of Medical Terms NOT Built from Word Parts. Check your work with the Answer Key in Appendix C.

1. _____

diagnostic imaging test producing scans composed from sectional radiographic images, which can be taken in any of the anatomic planes for a multidimensional view of internal structures

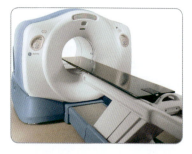

2. _____

image created by ionizing radiation

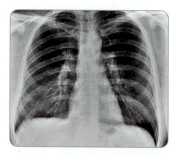

3. _____

repetitive pharyngeal collapse during sleep which leads to short absences of breathing; the lack of activity of the pharyngeal muscle structure allows the airway to close

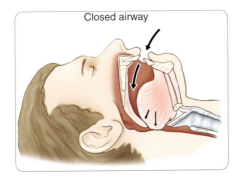

Closed airway

4. _____

loss of elasticity of the alveoli results in distention, causing stretching of the lung

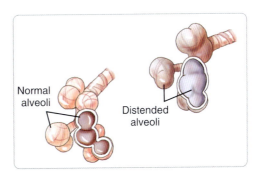

Normal alveoli

Distended alveoli

5. _____

infection of the nasal cavity, pharynx, or larynx, usually caused by a virus and commonly called a cold

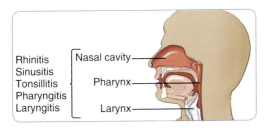

Rhinitis
Sinusitis
Tonsillitis
Pharyngitis
Laryngitis

Nasal cavity
Pharynx
Larynx

6. _____

laboratory test performed on a collected sample to determine the presence of pathogenic bacteria or fungi and to identify the most effective antimicrobial treatment

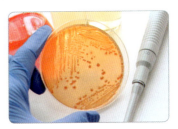

EXERCISE F **Learn Medical Terms NOT Built from Word Parts**

Fill in the blanks with medical terms defined in bold and abbreviations using the Medical Terms NOT Built from Word Parts table. Check your responses with the Answer Key in Appendix C.

1. **COPD** is the abbreviation for the medical term _____.
A person with COPD has dyspnea, especially with physical activity. Emptying the lungs, or exhalation, is particularly difficult; a visible hyperinflation of the chest may be observed. A chest _____, or **image created by ionizing radiation,** abbreviated as CXR, may be used to monitor COPD.

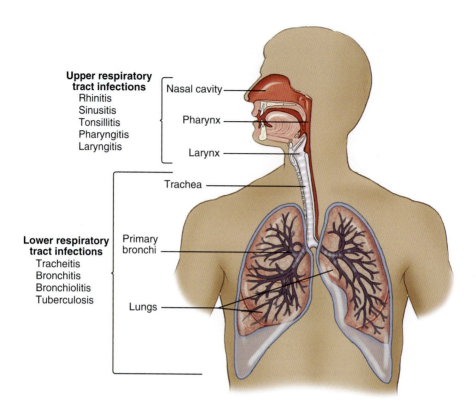

Figure 4.15 Upper and lower respiratory tract infections.

2. In _____, a **respiratory disease characterized by coughing, wheezing, and shortness of breath caused by constriction and inflammation of airways,** there are recurring spasms of the smooth muscles of the bronchial airways. A person with this disease has dyspnea usually triggered by an allergen or exercise. Bringing air into the lungs, or inhalation, is particularly difficult.

> FYI   **SOB** is the abbreviation for "shortness of breath."

3. **An infection of the nasal cavity, pharynx, or larynx is known as a(n)** _____
_____. A patient may have signs and symptoms of a **URI** from a **highly contagious and often severe viral infection** known as _____.

4. A patient with a pulmonary **infectious bacterial disease usually affecting the lungs and which may spread to other organs,** or _____, may be asked to cough to bring up _____, **mucous secretion from the lungs, bronchi, and trachea expelled through the mouth. A laboratory test performed on a collected sample to determine the presence of pathogenic bacteria or fungi,** or _____, may be performed to assess the effectiveness of medication to treat TB.

5. Prolonged cigarette smoking is the most common cause of the **loss of elasticity of the alveoli resulting in distension and causing stretching of the lung** or _____. There is no cure for this disease.

6. Chest _____, a **diagnostic imaging test producing scans composed from sectional radiographic images taken in any of the anatomic planes for a multidimensional view of internal structures**, offers a more detailed image than a chest radiograph. Chest CT scans may be ordered to diagnose unexplained respiratory symptoms such as dyspnea and coughing.

> **FYI**   **Computed tomography** is also used to visualize other anatomic structures, such as the abdomen and brain.

7. **Repetitive pharyngeal collapse during sleep leading to short absences of breathing** or _____ _____, abbreviated as _____, is associated with increased risk for elevated blood pressure, cardiovascular disease, diabetes, and stroke. Nocturnal polysomnography as performed by a sleep technologist is frequently used in the diagnosis of this disorder.

EXERCISE G   Pronounce and Spell Medical Terms NOT Built from Word Parts

Practice pronunciation and spelling on paper and online.

1. **Practice on Paper**
   a. **Pronounce:** Read the phonetic spelling and say aloud the terms listed in the previous table of Medical Terms NOT Built from Word Parts. Refer to the pronunciation key on p. 9 as necessary.
   b. **Spell:** Have a study partner read the terms aloud. Write the spelling of the terms on a separate sheet of paper.

2. **Practice Online** ⊕
   a. **Access** online learning resources. Go to evolve.elsevier.com > Evolve Resources > Practice Student Resources.
   b. **Pronounce:** Select Audio Glossary > Exercise G. Select a term to hear its pronunciation and repeat aloud.
   c. **Spell:** Select Activities > Spell Terms > Exercise G. Select the audio icon and type the correct spelling of the term.

❑ Check the box when complete.

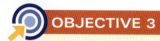

OBJECTIVE 3

Write abbreviations.

ABBREVIATIONS RELATED TO THE RESPIRATORY SYSTEM

Use the online **flashcards** to familiarize yourself with the following abbreviations.

ABBREVIATION	TERM	ABBREVIATION	TERM
ABGs	arterial blood gases	O_2	oxygen
CO_2	carbon dioxide	OSA	obstructive sleep apnea
COPD	chronic obstructive pulmonary disease	PFTs	pulmonary function tests
CPAP	continuous positive airway pressure	PSG	polysomnography
C&S	culture and sensitivity	RT	respiratory therapist
CT	computed tomography	SOB	shortness of breath
CXR	chest radiograph	TB	tuberculosis
ET	endotracheal	URI	upper respiratory infection
flu	influenza	V/Q scan	lung ventilation/perfusion scan

EXERCISE H   Abbreviate Medical Terms

Write the correct abbreviation next to its medical term. Check your responses with the Answer Key in Appendix C.

1. Sign and symptom:

   _____ shortness of breath

2. Diseases and disorders:

   a. _____ tuberculosis

   b. _____ chronic obstructive pulmonary disease

   c. _____ influenza

   d. _____ upper respiratory infection

   e. _____ obstructive sleep apnea

3. Diagnostic tests and equipment:

   a. _____ culture and sensitivity

   b. _____ computed tomography

   c. _____ chest radiograph

   d. _____ lung ventilation/perfusion scan

   e. _____ polysomnography

   f. _____ pulmonary function tests

   g. _____ arterial blood gases

4. Profession:

_____   respiratory therapist

5. Related Terms:

a. _____   continuous positive airway pressure

b. _____   carbon dioxide

c. _____   endotracheal

d. _____   oxygen

 OBJECTIVE 4

Identify medical terms by clinical category.

Now that you have worked through the respiratory system lesson, review and practice medical terms grouped by clinical category. Categories include signs and symptoms, diseases and disorders, diagnostic tests and equipment, surgical procedures, specialties and professions, and other terms related to the respiratory system.

EXERCISE I   **Signs and Symptoms**

Write the medical terms for signs and symptoms next to their definitions.

1. _____   absence of breathing

2. _____   difficult breathing

3. _____   excessive breathing

4. _____   deficient breathing

5. _____   condition of excessive oxygen

6. _____   condition of deficient oxygen

7. _____   condition of deficient carbon dioxide

8. _____   condition of excessive carbon dioxide

9. _____   inflammation of the nose (nasal membranes)

10. _____   rapid flow of blood from the nose

11. _____   discharge from the nose

EXERCISE J Diseases and Disorders

Write the medical terms for diseases and disorders next to their definitions.

1. _____ inflammation of the sinus (membranes)

2. _____ inflammation of the larynx

3. _____ inflammation of the pharynx

4. _____ inflammation of the nose and pharynx

5. _____ infection of the nasal cavity, pharynx, or larynx

6. _____ highly contagious and often severe viral infection of the respiratory tract

7. _____ infectious bacterial disease most commonly spread by inhalation of small particles and usually affecting the lungs (may spread to other organs)

8. _____ air in the chest cavity

9. _____ diseased state of the lungs

10. _____ diseased state of the bronchi and lungs

11. _____ inflammation of the bronchi

12. _____ loss of elasticity of the alveoli results in distension, causing stretching of the lung

13. _____
    _____ progressive lung disease blocking airflow, which makes breathing difficult. Chronic bronchitis and emphysema are two main components.

14. _____ repetitive pharyngeal collapse during sleep, which leads to short absences of breathing; can produce daytime drowsiness and elevated blood pressure

15. _____ respiratory disease characterized by coughing, wheezing, and shortness of breath; caused by constriction and inflammation of airways that is reversible between attacks

EXERCISE K Diagnostic Tests and Equipment

Write the medical terms for diagnostic tests and equipment next to their definitions.

1. _____ instrument used to measure carbon dioxide

2. _____ instrument used to measure oxygen

3. _____ instrument used to measure breathing (lung volume)

4. _____ pertaining to visual examination within (a hollow organ or cavity)

5. _____   visual examination of the chest cavity

6. _____   visual examination of the larynx

7. _____   visual examination of the bronchi

8. _____   instrument used for visual examination within (a hollow organ or cavity)

9. _____   instrument used for visual examination of the larynx

10. _____   instrument used for visual examination of the bronchi

11. _____   instrument used for visual examination of the chest cavity

12. _____   visual examination within (a hollow organ or cavity)

13. _____   pertaining to visual examination of the chest cavity

14. _____   image created by ionizing radiation

15. _____
    _____   diagnostic imaging test producing scans composed from sectional radiographic images, which can be taken in any of the anatomic planes for a multidimensional view of internal structures

16. _____
    _____   laboratory test performed on a collected sample to determine the presence of pathogenic bacteria or fungi and to identify the most effective antimicrobial treatment

17. _____   process of recording many sleep (tests)

18. _____   record of many sleep (tests)

EXERCISE L Surgical Procedures

Write the medical terms for surgical procedures next to their definitions.

1. _____   surgical puncture to remove fluid from the chest cavity

2. _____   incision into the chest cavity

3. _____   incision of a sinus

4. _____   incision into the trachea

5. _____   creation of an artificial opening into the trachea

6. _____   excision of the larynx

7. _____   excision of a lung

EXERCISE M Specialties and Professions

Write the medical terms for specialties and professions next to their definitions.

1. _____   study of the lung

2. _____   physician who studies and treats diseases of the lung

Write the medical terms related to the respiratory system next to their definitions.

1. _____   pertaining to the chest

2. _____   pertaining to the lung

3. _____   pertaining to the nose

4. _____   pertaining to the larynx

5. _____   pertaining to the pharynx

6. _____   pertaining to within the trachea

7. _____   pertaining to mucus

8. _____   mucous secretion from the lungs, bronchi, and trachea expelled through the mouth

OBJECTIVE 5

Use medical language in clinical statements, the case study, and a medical record.

Circle the medical terms and abbreviations defined in the bolded phrases. Medical terms from previous lessons are included. Answers are listed in Appendix C. For pronunciation practice, read the answers aloud.

1. Mrs. Tsunde was experiencing **deficient breathing** (hyperpnea, hypopnea, hypercapnia) and, at times, had periods of **absence of breathing** (apnea, dyspnea, hyperoxia). As a result, she was observed as having **abnormal condition of blue of the extremities** (apnea, asthma, acrocyanosis).

2. The physician performed a **visual examination of the bronchus** (bronchoscopy, bronchoscope) to assist in diagnosing **cancerous tumor** (neoplasm, carcinoma, abscess) in Mrs. Rabin. No **beyond control** (benign, metastasis, malignant) was noted. Treatment included a **surgical puncture to remove fluid from the chest cavity** (thoracoscopy, thoracotomy, thoracentesis) followed by a partial **excision of the lung** (pneumonectomy, pneumothorax, laryngectomy).

3. Sudden sharp chest pain and **difficult breathing** (apnea, dyspnea, asthma) are signs of **air in the chest cavity** (influenza, pneumothorax, tuberculosis). Treatment includes a(n) **incision into the chest cavity** (tracheostomy, thoracentesis, thoracotomy) and insertion of a chest tube to remove the air.

4. **Inflammation of the sinus (membranes)** (Sinusitis, Sinusotomy, Nasopharyngitis) is caused by bacteria, viruses, or fungi. It often occurs after an upper respiratory infection or may follow an acute allergic **inflammation of the nose (nasal membranes)** (rhinorrhagia, rhinorrhea, rhinitis). Symptoms include **discharge from the nose** (rhinorrhagia, rhinorrhea, rhinitis), malaise, pain, and mucopurulent drainage. **Pertaining to visual examination within** (Endoscope, Endoscopic, Endoscopy) surgery, drugs, and heat therapy may be used as treatment.

5. A chest **image created by ionizing radiation** (bronchoscopy, spriometer, radiograph) is used to assist in the diagnosis and monitoring of **an infectious bacterial disease usually affecting the lungs and which may spread to other organs** (tuberculosis, emphysema, influenza), **diseased state of the lung** (pneumothorax, bronchopneumonia, pneumonia), **progressive lung disease that blocks airflow** (COPD, OSA, TB), and other **pertaining to the lung** (pulmonary, laryngeal, pharyngeal) diseases.

6. An **instrument used to measure oxygen** (oximeter, capnometer, spirometer) is used to perform pulse oximetry, which measures the amount of oxygen in the blood. Oximetry, chest **image created by ionizing radiation** (radiograph, polysomnogram, computed tomography), and chest **scans composed from sectional radiographic images** (radiograph, polysomnogram, computed tomography) are often used to diagnose lung disorders such **as loss of elasticity of the alveoli results in distension causing stretching of the lung** (asthma, emphysema, URI). **Condition of excessive carbon dioxide** (Hypercapnia, Hyperoxia, Hyperpnea) can occur with severe emphysema.

7. A patient came to the emergency department of the hospital with **rapid flow of blood from the nose (nosebleed)** (rhinitis, rhinorrhagia, rhinorrhea).

8. The patient had a sore throat, or **inflammation of the throat.** Her physician referred to the condition as (rhinitis, laryngitis, pharyngitis).

9. A **lung ventilation/perfusion scan** (PFTs, V/Q scan, CPAP) is a form of diagnostic imaging often performed to identify a blood clot in the lungs, which is called **pertaining to the lung** (thoracic, endotracheal, pulmonary) embolus.

10. The sleep technologist compiled results of the **process of recording many sleep (tests)** (polysomnography, polysomnogram, PFTs) and forwarded the resulting **record of many sleep (tests)** (polysomnography, polysomnogram, PFTs) to the **physician who studies and treats diseases of the lung** (pulmonology, pulmonologist, respiratory therapist).

EXERCISE P Apply Medical Terms to the Case Study

Think back to Roberta who was introduced in the case study at the beginning of the lesson. After working through Lesson 4 on the respiratory system, consider the medical terms that might be used to describe her experience. List three terms relevant to the case study and their meanings. ▧

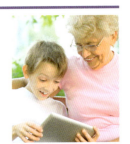

	Medical Term	**Definition**
1.	_____	_____
2.	_____	_____
3.	_____	_____

EXERCISE Q   Use Medical Terms in a Document

Roberta was able to see her primary care physician later that afternoon. Her vital signs were taken, and she was examined by the doctor. Roberta's office visit, test results, and course of care were documented in the following medical record.

Use the definitions in numbers 1-9 to write medical terms within the document on the next page.

1. difficult breathing

2. mucous secretion from the lungs, bronchi, and trachea expelled through the mouth

3. discharge from the nose

4. pertaining to the nose

5. puffy swelling of tissue from the accumulation of fluid

6. abnormal condition of blue

7. image created by ionizing radiation (plural)

8. diseased state of the lungs

9. infection of the nasal cavity, pharynx, or larynx

Refer to the medical record to answer questions 10-13.

10. The term **mucoid**, used in the medical record to describe the sputum observed, is built from word parts. Use your knowledge of word parts to define the term.

    muc/o means _____

    -oid means _____

    Remember, most definitions begin with the suffix.

    muc/oid means _____

11. List two medical terms in the report related to diagnostic tests or equipment:

    _____

    _____

12. PA is the abbreviation for _____, which indicates the x-ray beam for the chest radiograph was projected from the _____ to the _____.

13. Identify two new medical terms in the medical record you would like to investigate. Use your medical dictionary or an online resource to look up the definition.

Medical Term	Definition
1. _____	_____
2. _____	_____

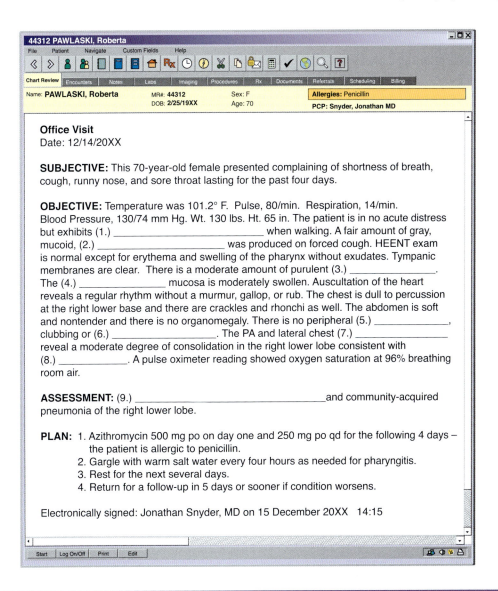

Office Visit
Date: 12/14/20XX

SUBJECTIVE: This 70-year-old female presented complaining of shortness of breath, cough, runny nose, and sore throat lasting for the past four days.

OBJECTIVE: Temperature was 101.2° F. Pulse, 80/min. Respiration, 14/min. Blood Pressure, 130/74 mm Hg. Wt. 130 lbs. Ht. 65 in. The patient is in no acute distress but exhibits (1.) _____ when walking. A fair amount of gray, mucoid, (2.) _____ was produced on forced cough. HEENT exam is normal except for erythema and swelling of the pharynx without exudates. Tympanic membranes are clear. There is a moderate amount of purulent (3.) _____. The (4.) _____ mucosa is moderately swollen. Auscultation of the heart reveals a regular rhythm without a murmur, gallop, or rub. The chest is dull to percussion at the right lower base and there are crackles and rhonchi as well. The abdomen is soft and nontender and there is no organomegaly. There is no peripheral (5.) _____, clubbing or (6.) _____. The PA and lateral chest (7.) _____ reveal a moderate degree of consolidation in the right lower lobe consistent with (8.) _____. A pulse oximeter reading showed oxygen saturation at 96% breathing room air.

ASSESSMENT: (9.) _____and community-acquired pneumonia of the right lower lobe.

PLAN: 1. Azithromycin 500 mg po on day one and 250 mg po qd for the following 4 days – the patient is allergic to penicillin.
2. Gargle with warm salt water every four hours as needed for pharyngitis.
3. Rest for the next several days.
4. Return for a follow-up in 5 days or sooner if condition worsens.

Electronically signed: Jonathan Snyder, MD on 15 December 20XX   14:15

EXERCISE R   Use Medical Language in Online Electronic Health Records

Select the correct medical terms to complete three medical records in one patient's electronic file.

Access online resources at evolve.elsevier.com > Evolve Resources > Practice Student Resources > Activities > Lesson 4 > Electronic Health Records

Topic: COPD
Record 1: Progress Note
Record 2: Radiology Report
Record 3: Pulmonary Function Department Note

❑ Check the box when complete.

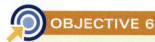

OBJECTIVE 6

Recall and assess knowledge of word parts, medical terms, and abbreviations.

EXERCISE S   **Online Review of Lesson Content**

🌐 *Recall and assess your learning from working through the lesson by completing online learning activities at evolve. elsevier.com > Evolve Resources > Practice Student Resources. Keep track of your progress by placing a check mark next to completed activities.*

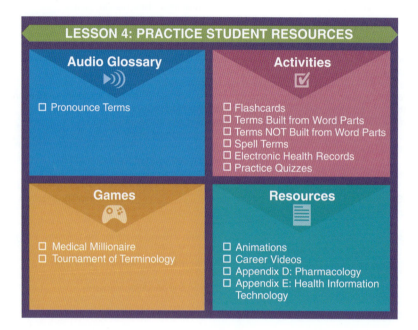

LESSON 4: PRACTICE STUDENT RESOURCES

Audio Glossary ▶))
- ☐ Pronounce Terms

Activities ☑
- ☐ Flashcards
- ☐ Terms Built from Word Parts
- ☐ Terms NOT Built from Word Parts
- ☐ Spell Terms
- ☐ Electronic Health Records
- ☐ Practice Quizzes

Games 🎮
- ☐ Medical Millionaire
- ☐ Tournament of Terminology

Resources 📄
- ☐ Animations
- ☐ Career Videos
- ☐ Appendix D: Pharmacology
- ☐ Appendix E: Health Information Technology

EXERCISE T   **Lesson Content Quiz**

Test your knowledge of the terms and abbreviations introduced in this lesson. Circle the letter for the medical term or abbreviation related to the words in italics.

1. After weeks of experiencing a hoarse voice, the patient underwent a *visual examination of the larynx* performed by an otolaryngologist to determine the cause.
   a. laryngoscope
   b. laryngoscopy
   c. laryngectomy

2. The breathing disorder involving the *absence of spontaneous respiration* is called:
   a. apnea
   b. hypopnea
   c. dyspnea

3. Following a car accident, the occupant experienced chest pain and dyspnea. CXR demonstrated *air in the chest cavity* or:
   a. pneumothorax
   b. thoracentesis
   c. pneumonia

4. A polysomnography test was ordered to rule out *repetitive pharyngeal collapse during sleep* or:
   a. OSA
   b. SOB
   c. C&S

5. During evaluation of the patient presenting with dyspnea, the *condition of excessive carbon dioxide* was discovered.
   a. hyperoxia
   b. hypercapnia
   c. hypoxia

6. After undergoing many diagnostic tests, the patient received the diagnosis of a *progressive lung disease blocking air flow, which makes breathing difficult.*
   a. obstructive sleep apnea
   b. upper respiratory infection
   c. chronic obstructive pulmonary disease

7. To assist with long-term mechanical ventilation of the comatose patient, *a creation of an artificial opening into the trachea* was performed.
   a. thoracotomy
   b. tracheostomy
   c. laryngectomy

8. To rule out tuberculosis in a patient who had been coughing up blood, the pulmonologist ordered a TB *laboratory test performed on a collected sample to determine the presence of pathogenic bacteria or fungi and to identify the most effective antimicrobial treatment.*
   a. culture and sensitivity
   b. computed tomography
   c. bronchoscopy

9. A *physician who treats diseases of the lung* was consulted to treat the patient diagnosed with COPD.
   a. respiratory therapist
   b. pulmonology
   c. pulmonologist

10. A chest *diagnostic imaging test producing scans composed from sectional radiographic images, which can be taken in any of the anatomic planes for a multidimensional view of internal structures* was ordered to monitor growth of a small cell cancer tumor of the lung.
    a. CT
    b. CXR
    c. C&S

LESSON AT A GLANCE RESPIRATORY SYSTEM WORD PARTS

COMBINING FORMS

bronch/o	pneumon/o
capn/o	pulmon/o
laryng/o	rhin/o
muc/o	sinus/o
nas/o	somn/o
ox/i	spir/o
pharyng/o	thorac/o
pneum/o	trache/o

SUFFIXES

-ary	-pnea
-centesis	-rrhagia
-eal	-rrhea
-ectomy	-scope
-gram	-scopic
-graphy	-scopy
-ia	-stomy
-meter	-thorax

PREFIXES

a-, an-
dys-
endo-
hyper-
poly-

LESSON AT A GLANCE | RESPIRATORY SYSTEM MEDICAL TERMS AND ABBREVIATIONS

SIGNS AND SYMPTOMS
apnea
dyspnea
hypercapnia
hyperoxia
hyperpnea
hypocapnia
hypopnea
hypoxia
rhinitis
rhinorrhagia
rhinorrhea

DISEASES AND DISORDERS
asthma
bronchitis
bronchopneumonia
chronic obstructive pulmonary disease
 (COPD)
emphysema
influenza (flu)
laryngitis
nasopharyngitis
obstructive sleep apnea (OSA)
pharyngitis
pneumonia
pneumothorax
sinusitis
tuberculosis (TB)
upper respiratory infection (URI)

DIAGNOSTIC TESTS AND EQUIPMENT
bronchoscope
bronchoscopy
capnometer
computed tomography (CT)
culture and sensitivity (C&S)
endoscope
endoscopic
endoscopy
laryngoscope
laryngoscopy
oximeter
polysomnogram
polysomnography (PSG)
radiograph
spirometer
thoracoscope
thoracoscopic
thoracoscopy

SURGICAL PROCEDURES
laryngectomy
pneumonectomy
sinusotomy
thoracentesis
thoracotomy
tracheostomy
tracheotomy

SPECIALTIES AND PROFESSIONS
pulmonologist
pulmonology

RELATED TERMS
endotracheal (ET)
laryngeal
mucous
nasal
pharyngeal
pulmonary
sputum
thoracic

ABBREVIATIONS

ABGs	CXR	PSG
CO_2	ET	RT
COPD	flu	SOB
C&S	O_2	TB
CPAP	OSA	URI
CT	PFTs	V/Q scan

Urinary System

Tyrone Parker

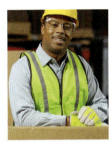

Tyrone Parker was feeling fine until about 3 days ago. He was at his job at a warehouse when he noticed pain in his back, but only on the left side. At first he thought maybe he pulled something when he was moving inventory. He took some over-the-counter pain medicine but this didn't really seem to help. In the past when he had back pain it got better after a night of sleep. When he woke up the next morning the pain was worse and it had spread into the lower part of his belly and his groin, still on the left side. He also noticed blood when he urinated. He was worried that he might have an infection.

■ *Consider Tyrone's situation as you work through the lesson on the urinary system. At the end of the lesson, we will return to this case study and identify medical terms used to document Tyrone's experience and the care he receives.*

OBJECTIVES

1 ■ Build, translate, pronounce, and spell medical terms built from word parts (p. 120).

2 ■ Define, pronounce, and spell medical terms NOT built from word parts (p. 135).

3 ■ Write abbreviations (p. 138).

4 ■ Identify medical terms by clinical category (p. 139).

5 ■ Use medical language in clinical statements, the case study, and a medical record (p. 142).

6 ■ Recall and assess knowledge of word parts, medical terms, and abbreviations (p. 145).

INTRODUCTION TO THE URINARY SYSTEM

Anatomic Structures of the Urinary System

kidneys (KID-nēz)	two bean-shaped organs in the lumbar region that filter the blood to remove waste products and form urine
renal pelvis (RĒ-nal) (PEL-vis)	funnel-shaped reservoir in each kidney that collects urine and passes it to the ureter
ureters (Ū-re-ters)	two slender tubes that carry urine from the kidney to the bladder
urethra (ū-RĒ-thra)	narrow tube that carries urine from the bladder to the outside of the body
urinary bladder (Ū-ri-nar-ē) (BLAD-er)	muscular, hollow organ that temporarily holds urine

Anatomic Structures of the Urinary System—cont'd

urinary meatus (Ū-ri-nar-ē) (mē-Ā-tus)	opening through which urine passes to the outside of the body
urinary tract (Ū-ri-nar-ē) (tract)	organs and ducts responsible for the elimination of urine
urine (Ū-rin)	pale yellow liquid waste product made up of 95% water

Functions of the Urinary System

- Removes waste material from the body
- Regulates fluid volume
- Maintains electrolyte concentration in body fluid
- Assists in blood pressure regulation

How the Urinary System Works

The **kidneys,** fist-sized organs shaped like kidney beans, filter the blood and remove water, salt, amino acids, electrolytes, and other minerals (see Figure 5.1). After filtration, a portion of these materials is reabsorbed into the bloodstream, maintaining optimal levels of each. The remaining amounts are combined with uric acid, ammonia, and other substances to form **urine.** Urine collects in the **renal pelvis,** a funnel-shaped reservoir in each kidney, where it drains into the **ureter,** a tube extending from the kidney. The ureter carries urine to the **urinary bladder,** where it is temporarily stored. Urine is emptied from the bladder and eliminated from the body through the **urethra.** The **urinary meatus** is the opening through which urine passes out of the body.

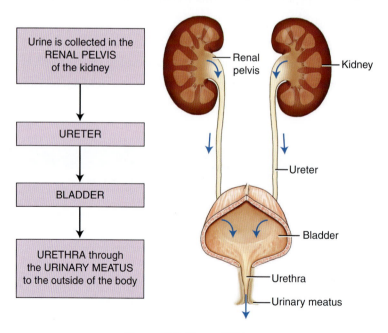

Urine is collected in the RENAL PELVIS of the kidney

↓

URETER

↓

BLADDER

↓

URETHRA through the URINARY MEATUS to the outside of the body

Renal pelvis

Kidney

Ureter

Bladder

Urethra

Urinary meatus

Figure 5.1 Flow of Urine.

CAREER FOCUS Professionals Who Work with the Urinary System

- **Medical/Surgical Nurses** work in hospitals taking care of patients who are ill or who have had surgery. They implement providers' instructions for care and advocate for their patients. They watch for signs of infection, a risk in patients who are catheterized. Pain management is another of their important responsibilities.

- **Nephrology Nurses** play a primary role in health maintenance for those living with kidney disease through patient education and routine assessments. In patients with renal failure, these nurses perform dialysis, a procedure in which the body's liquid wastes are removed with special machinery. Nephrology nurses also perform tasks related to the dialysis process: they manage intravenous lines, change dressings and administer medications.

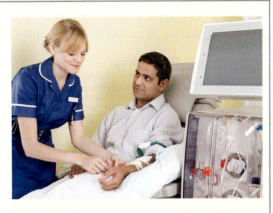

Figure 5.2 Patient Care Technician assisting a patient undergoing dialysis.

- **Dialysis Patient Care Technicians (PCTs)** work under the supervision of nephrology nurses and provide direct care for patients undergoing dialysis treatments (Figure 5.2). They operate the machines and monitor the fluid removal rate of the patients while using sterile techniques to make sure the risk of infection is very low.

- **Urology Technicians** work in laboratories, hospitals and clinics assisting urologists with the diagnosis and treatment of urinary disorders. Their duties include reviewing patient records, explaining procedures, setting up equipment, and assisting with diagnostic testing. Urology technicians might also take ultrasound images of the bladder and perform catheterizations.

🌐 FOR MORE INFORMATION

- To learn more about careers as a dialysis patient care technician, go to the National Kidney Foundation website and search for Renal Career Fact Sheet—*Dialysis Technician*.

- Access online learning resources at evolve.elsevier.com > Practice Student Resources > Other Resources > Career Videos to watch an interview with a **Medical/Surgical Nurse**.

OBJECTIVE 1

Build, translate, pronounce, and spell medical terms built from word parts.

WORD PARTS	Presented with the Urinary System

Use the paper or online **flashcards** to familiarize yourself with the following word parts.

COMBINING FORM (WR + CV)	DEFINITION	COMBINING FORM (WR + CV)	DEFINITION
cyst/o	bladder, sac	noct/i	night
hem/o, hemat/o	blood	olig/o	scanty, few
hydr/o	water	pyel/o	renal pelvis
lith/o	stone(s), calculus (*pl.* calculi)	py/o	pus
		ur/o	urination, urine, urinary tract
meat/o	meatus (opening)	ureter/o	ureter
nephr/o, ren/o	kidney	urethr/o	urethra
SUFFIX (S)	**DEFINITION**	**SUFFIX (S)**	**DEFINITION**
-emia	blood condition	-plasty	surgical repair
-iasis	condition	-tripsy	surgical crushing

WORD PARTS PRESENTED IN PREVIOUS LESSONS		Used to Build Urinary System Terms	
SUFFIX (S)	**DEFINITION**	**SUFFIX (S)**	**DEFINITION**
-al	pertaining to	-logist	one who studies and treats (specialist, physician)
-ectomy	surgical removal, excision		
-gram	record, radiographic image	-logy	study of
-graphy	process of recording, radiographic imaging	-osis	abnormal condition
		-scopic	pertaining to visual examination
-ia	diseased state, condition of	-scopy	visual examination
-itis	inflammation	-stomy	creation of an artificial opening
		-tomy	cut into, incision
PREFIX (P)	**DEFINITION**	**PREFIX (P)**	**DEFINITION**
a-, an-	absence of, without	dys-	difficult, painful, abnormal

Refer to Appendix A, Word Parts Used in *Basic Medical Language*, for alphabetical lists of word parts and their meanings.

EXERCISE A   **Build and Translate Medical Terms Built from Word Parts**

*Use the **Word Parts Tables** to complete the following questions. Check your responses with the Answer Key in Appendix C at the back of the book.*

1. LABEL: *Write the combining forms for anatomical structures of the urinary system on Figure 5.3. These anatomical combining forms will be used to build and translate medical terms in Exercise A.*

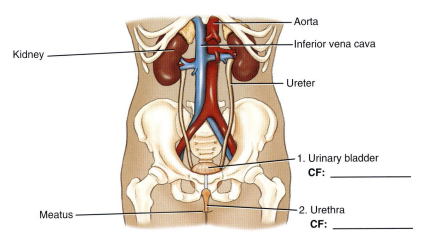

Kidney

Aorta

Inferior vena cava

Ureter

1. Urinary bladder
   CF: _____

2. Urethra
   CF: _____

Meatus

Figure 5.3 The urinary system with combining forms for bladder and urethra.

2. MATCH: *Draw a line to match the word part with its definition.*

a. -gram   inflammation
b. -graphy   stone(s), calculus (*pl.* calculi)
c. -itis   condition
d. -iasis   process of recording, radiographic imaging
e. lith/o   record, radiographic image

3. BUILD: *Using the combining form **cyst/o** and the suffixes reviewed in the previous exercise, build the following terms describing conditions related to the urinary bladder. Remember, the definition usually starts with the meaning of the suffix.*

a. inflammation of the bladder   _____/_____
                                                     wr   s

b. radiographic imaging of the bladder   _____/ o /_____
                                                     wr   cv   s

c. radiographic image of the bladder   _____/ o /_____
                                                     wr   cv   s

d. condition of stone(s) in the bladder   _____/ o /_____/_____
                                                     wr   cv   wr   s

4. **READ:** **Cystitis** (sis-TĪ-tis) is an inflammation of the urinary bladder. **Cystography** (sis-TOG-ra-fē) may identify this inflammation by taking a radiographic image of the bladder. A **cystogram** (SIS-tō-gram) can show whether there are stones present in the bladder. **Cystolithiasis** (sis-tō-lith-Ī-a-sis) is also referred to as bladder stones.

> **FYI**   **Bladder** is a derivative of the Anglo-Saxon **blaeddre**, meaning a **blister** or **windbag**.

5. **LABEL:** *Write word parts to complete Figure 5.4.*

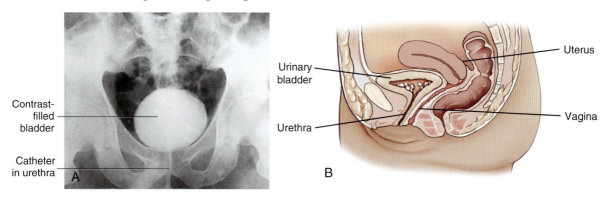

Figure 5.4 A. _____/o/_____.
                       bladder   radiographic image
          B. _____/o/_____/_____.
                       bladder   stone(s)   condition

6. **MATCH:** *Draw a line to match the word part with its definition.*

   a. -stomy   stone(s), calculus (*pl.* calculi)
   b. -scope   cut into, incision
   c. -scopy   instrument used for visual examination
   d. -tomy   surgical repair
   e. -plasty   creation of an artificial opening
   f. lith/o   visual examination

7. **TRANSLATE:** *Complete the definitions of the following terms by filling in the blanks for procedures related to the bladder (**cyst/o**). Remember, the definition usually starts with the meaning of the suffix.*

   a. cyst/o/stomy _____ of an _____ _____ into the _____
   b. cyst/o/scope _____ used for _____ _____ of the _____
   c. cyst/o/scopy _____ _____ of the _____
   d. cyst/o/lith/o/tomy _____ into the _____ to remove stone(s)

8. **READ:** A **cystoscope** (SIS-tō-skōp) is used to examine the inside of the bladder to look for abnormalities such as infection or cancer. **Cystoscopy** (sis-TOS-ko-pē) can also be used to treat abnormalities, such as removal of a small tumor using a tool passed through the scope. **Cystolithotomy** (sis-tō-li-THOT-o-mē) uses an incision low on the belly to access the bladder to remove large stones. A **cystostomy** (sis-TOS-to-mē) creates an artificial opening into the bladder, which allows a tube to be inserted for drainage of urine.

9. **BUILD:** *Write word parts to build terms related to the urethra, using the combining form* **urethr/o**.

   a. instrument used for visual examination of the urethra

   _____ / o / _____
        wr   cv   s

   b. inflammation of the urethra and bladder

   _____ / o / _____ / _____
        wr   cv   wr   s

   c. radiographic imaging of the bladder and urethra

   _____ / o / _____ / o / _____
        wr   cv   wr   cv   s

   d. surgical repair of the urethra

   _____ / o / _____
        wr   cv   s

10. **READ:** **Urethroplasty** (ū-RĒ-thrō-plas-tē) is surgical repair of the urethra and may be necessary to treat severe injury or birth defects. A **urethroscope** (ū-RĒ-thrō-skōp) may be used to diagnose narrowing of the urethra. **Urethrocystitis** (ū-rē-thrō-sis-TĪ-tis) is inflammation of the urethra and bladder and may be diagnosed by **cystourethrography** (sis-tō-ū-rē-THROG-ro-fē).

11. **LABEL:** *Write word parts to complete Figure 5.5.*

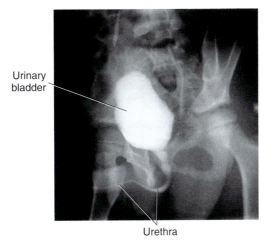

Urinary bladder

Urethra

Figure 5.5 Image generated by _____ / o / _____ / o / _____.
                             bladder   urethra   radiographic imaging

12. MATCH: *Draw a line to match the word part with its definition.*

a. ur/o   pus

b. hem/o, hemat/o   diseased state, condition of

c. py/o   urine, urination, urinary tract

d. dys-   blood

e. -ia   difficult or painful

---

13. TRANSLATE: *Complete the definitions of the following terms built from the combining form **ur/o**.*

a. hemat/ur/ia   _____ of blood in the _____

b. py/ur/ia   condition of _____ in the _____

c. dys/ur/ia   _____ of difficult or _____ urination

---

14. READ: Signs of a bladder infection can include difficult or painful urination, or **dysuria** (dis-Ū-rē-a), as well as blood in the urine, or **hematuria** (hem-a-TU-rē-a). **Pyuria** (pī-Ū-rē-a), a term meaning condition of pus in the urine, can cause urine to appear cloudy and is another sign of infection.

---

15. MATCH: *Draw a line to match the word part with its definition.*

a. a-, an-   urine, urination, urinary tract

b. noct/i   blood condition

c. olig/o   absence of, without

d. -emia   night

e. ur/o   few, scanty

---

16. BUILD: *Write word parts to describe conditions describing urine.*

a. condition of absence of urine   _____ / _____ / _____
                                                     p   wr   s

b. condition of night urination   _____ / _____ / _____
                                                 wr   wr   s

c. condition of scanty urine (amount)   _____ / _____ / _____
                                                 wr   wr   s

d. urine in the blood   _____ / _____
                                                 wr   s

FYI   Sometimes literal translation brings one close to the meaning of the word but does not account for every word in the definition used in the practice of medicine. For example, **anuria** (an-Ū-rē-a) literally means condition of absence of urine. For learning purposes, that will be the meaning used in this text. In practice, the term means failure of the kidneys to produce urine.

17. **READ: Nocturia** (nok-TŪ-rē-a) describes having to get up multiple times during the night to urinate. It may be caused by partial blockage of the urinary tract, as with an enlarged prostate gland. **Oliguria** (ol-i-GŪ-rē-a) refers to the scanty production of urine which can be due to dehydration, blockage, infections, and many other serious causes. **Uremia** (ū-RĒ-mē-a) is a toxic condition resulting from urea in the blood.

> **FYI** For learning purposes, we have allowed the definition of **uremia** to be urine in the blood because urea is present in urine. The term **hematuria** means blood in the urine. Hematuria is a sign, whereas uremia is a serious disorder. Use your medical dictionary or an online source to learn more about these common terms.

18. **LABEL:** *Write the combining forms for anatomical structures of the urinary system on Figure 5.6. These anatomical combining forms will be used to build and translate medical terms in following exercises.*

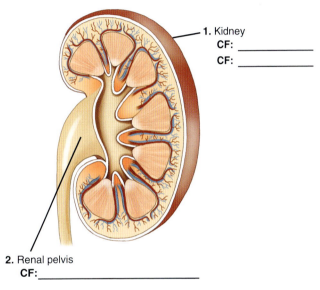

1. Kidney
   CF: _____
   CF: _____

2. Renal pelvis
   CF: _____

Figure 5.6 Kidney and renal pelvis with combining forms

19. **MATCH:** *Draw a line to match the word part with its definition.*

   a. lith/o   condition
   b. nephr/o   surgical crushing
   c. pyel/o   stone(s), calculus (*pl.* calculi)
   d. -tripsy   kidney
   e. -iasis   renal pelvis

20. **TRANSLATE:** *Complete the definitions of the following terms built from the combining form **lith/o,** meaning stone(s) or calculus. Use the meaning of word parts to fill in the blanks.*

   a. lith/o/tripsy   _____ _____ of stone(s)
   b. nephr/o/lith/iasis   condition of _____(s) in the _____
   c. pyel/o/lith/o/tomy   incision into the _____ _____ to remove _____(s)

> **FYI** **Pyelos** is the Greek word for **tub-shaped vessel**, which describes the renal pelvis' shape.

21. READ: **Nephrolithiasis** (nef-rō-lith-Ī-a-sis) is the medical term for kidney stones, a common disorder. **Lithotripsy** (LITH-ō-trip-sē) is a noninvasive procedure that uses shock waves to "crush" or break the stones into smaller pieces that can be passed through the urinary system. If stones are trapped in the renal pelvis, a minor surgery requiring a small incision in the back called **pyelolithotomy** (pī-el-ō-lith-OT-o-mē) can be used to remove the stones.

22. LABEL: *Write word parts to complete Figure 5.7*

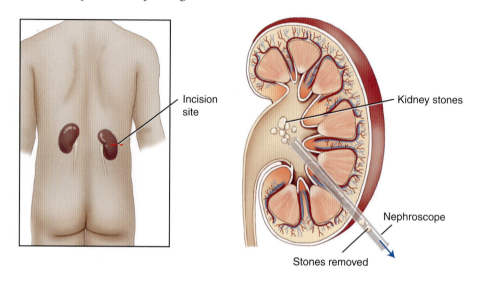

Incision site

Kidney stones

Nephroscope

Stones removed

Figure 5.7 Percutaneous _____/o/_____/o/_____
                              renal pelvis   stone(s)   incision
uses a small incision into the back to remove medium or larger-size kidney stones. A nephroscope is passed into the kidney through the incision; the urologist then removes the stone(s) through the nephroscope.

23. REVIEW OF URINARY SYSTEM TERMS BUILT FROM WORD PARTS: *The following is an alphabetical list of terms built and translated in the previous exercises.*

MEDICAL TERMS BUILT FROM WORD PARTS

TERM	DEFINITION	TERM	DEFINITION
1. **anuria** (an-Ū-rē-a)	condition of absence of urine	4. **cystography** (sis-TOG-ra-fē)	radiographic imaging of the bladder
2. **cystitis** (sis-TĪ-tis)	inflammation of the bladder	5. **cystolithiasis** (sis-tō-lith-Ī-a-sis)	condition of stone(s) in the bladder (Figure 5.4, *B*)
3. **cystogram** (SIS-tō-gram)	radiographic image of the bladder (Figure 5.4, *A*)	6. **cystolithotomy** (sis-tō-li-THOT-o-mē)	incision into the bladder to remove stone(s)

MEDICAL TERMS BUILT FROM WORD PARTS—cont'd

TERM	DEFINITION	TERM	DEFINITION
7. **cystoscope** (SIS-tō-skōp)	instrument used for visual examination of the bladder	15. **nocturia** (nok-TŪ-rē-a)	condition of night urination
8. **cystoscopy** (sis-TOS-ko-pē)	visual examination of the bladder	16. **oliguria** (ol-i-GŪ-rē-a)	condition of scanty urine (amount)
9. **cystostomy** (sis-TOS-to-mē)	creation of an artificial opening into the bladder	17. **pyelolithotomy** (pī-el-ō-lith-OT-o-mē)	incision into the renal pelvis to remove stone(s) (Figure 5.7)
10. **cystourethrography** (sis-tō-ū-rē-THROG-ro-fē)	radiographic imaging of the bladder and urethra (Figure 5.5)	18. **pyuria** (pī-Ū-rē-a)	condition of pus in the urine
11. **dysuria** (dis-Ū-rē-a)	condition of difficult or painful urination	19. **uremia** (ū-RĒ-mē-a)	urine in the blood
12. **hematuria** (hem-a-TU-rē-a)	condition of blood in the urine	20. **urethrocystitis** (ū-rē-thrō-sis-TĪ-tis)	inflammation of the urethra and bladder
13. **lithotripsy** (LITH-ō-trip-sē)	surgical crushing of stone(s)	21. **urethroplasty** (ū-RĒ-thrō-plas-tē)	surgical repair of the urethra
14. **nephrolithiasis** (nef-rō-lith-Ī-a-sis)	condition of stone(s) in the kidney	22. **urethroscope** (ū-RĒ-thrō-skōp)	instrument used for visual examination of the urethra

EXERCISE B   Pronounce and Spell Terms Built from Word Parts

Practice pronunciation and spelling on paper and online.

1. **Practice on Paper**
   a. **Pronounce**: Read the phonetic spelling and say aloud the terms listed in the previous table, Review of Terms Built from Word Parts.
   b. **Spell**: Have a study partner read the terms aloud. Write the spelling of the terms on a separate sheet of paper.

2. **Practice Online** 🌐
   a. **Access** online learning resources. Go to evolve.elsevier.com > Evolve Resources > Practice Student Resources.
   b. **Pronounce**: Select Audio Glossary > Lesson 5 > Exercise B. Select a term to hear its pronunciation and repeat aloud.
   c. **Spell**: Select Activities > Lesson 5 > Spell Terms > Exercise B. Select the audio icon and type the correct spelling of the term.

❏ Check the box when complete.

EXERCISE C   Build and Translate MORE Medical Terms Built from Word Parts

*Use the **Word Parts Tables** to complete the following questions. Check your responses with the Answer Key in Appendix C at the back of the book.*

1. **LABEL:** *Write the combining forms for anatomical structures of the urinary system on Figure 5.8. These anatomical combining forms will be used to build and translate medical terms in Exercise C.*

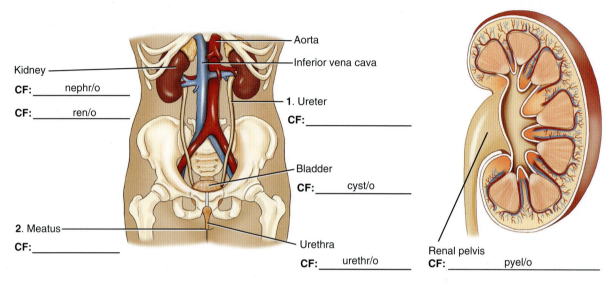

Kidney
CF: _____nephr/o_____
CF: _____ren/o_____

2. Meatus
CF: _____

Aorta
Inferior vena cava
1. Ureter
CF: _____

Bladder
CF: _____cyst/o_____

Urethra
CF: _____urethr/o_____

Renal pelvis
CF: _____pyel/o_____

Figure 5.8 The urinary system with combining forms for ureter and meatus.

2. **MATCH:** *Draw a line to match the word part with its definition.*

   a. -itis   renal pelvis
   b. -osis   water
   c. -al   inflammation
   d. hydr/o   abnormal condition
   e. pyel/o   pertaining to

3. **TRANSLATE:** *Complete the definitions of the following terms by using the meaning of the word parts to fill in the blanks. Remember, the definition usually starts with the meaning of the suffix. Terms built from combining forms **ren/o** and **nephr/o**, meaning kidney:*

   a. nephr/itis   _____ of the _____
   b. ren/al   _____ to the _____
   c. hydr/o/nephr/osis _____ _____ of _____ in the kidney
   d. pyel/o/nephr/itis _____ of the _____ _____ and kidney

4. **READ:** **Nephritis** (ne-FRĪ-tis) refers to inflammation of the kidneys and is frequently caused by infections and medications. Acute **pyelonephritis** (pī-e-lō-ne-FRĪ-tis) is a bacterial infection that causes swelling and enlargement of the kidneys, while chronic **pyelonephritis** can result in scarring and loss of function.

5. **LABEL:** *Write word parts to complete Figure 5.9.*

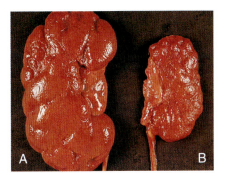

Figure 5.9 **A.** Acute _____/o/_____/_____.
  renal pelvis   kidney   inflammation
B. Normal-sized kidney with some scarring.

6. **READ:** **Hydronephrosis** (hī-drō-ne-FRŌ-sis), literally translated as abnormal condition of water in the kidney, is actually a buildup of urine in the kidney caused by blockage somewhere in the urinary tract, such as a stone in the ureter. This causes distention (swelling) of the renal pelvis.

7. **LABEL:** *Write word parts to complete Figure 5.10.*

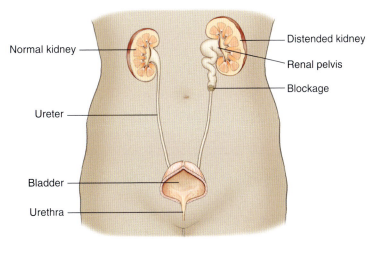

Normal kidney

Distended kidney

Renal pelvis

Blockage

Ureter

Bladder

Urethra

Figure 5.10 _____/o/_____/_____.
  water   kidney   abnormal condition

8. **MATCH:** *Draw a line to match the combining form or suffix with its definition.*

    a. pyel/o   creation of an artificial opening
    b. -ectomy   cut into, incision
    c. -stomy   surgical removal, excision
    d. -tomy   renal pelvis

9. **BUILD:** *Using the combining form **nephr/o** and the suffixes reviewed in the previous exercise, build the following terms describing procedures related to the kidney. Remember, the definition usually starts with the meaning of the suffix*

    a. excision of the kidney   _____ / _____
                                                 wr   **s**

    b. creation of an artificial opening into the kidney   _____ / o / _____
                                                   wr   **cv**   **s**

    c. incision into the kidney   _____ / o / _____
                                                   wr   **cv**   **s**

10. **READ:** A **nephrectomy** (ne-FREK-to-mē) may be performed to treat kidney cancer. A **nephrostomy** (ne-FROS-to-mē) creates an artificial opening into the kidney to relieve hydronephrosis caused by blockage, such as when a stone gets stuck in a ureter. A **nephrotomy** (ne-FROT-o-mē) might be necessary to remove a very large kidney stone.

11. **LABEL:** *Write word parts to complete Figure 5.11.*

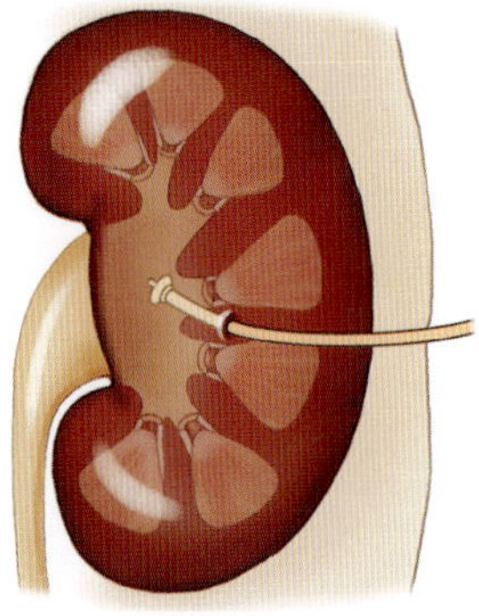

Figure 5.11 _____ / o / _____ .
                         kidney   creation of an artificial opening

12. **MATCH:** *Draw a line to match the word part with its definition.*

    a. -itis   surgical repair
    b. -tomy   stone(s), calculus (*pl.* calculi)
    c. -iasis   inflammation
    d. -plasty   cut into, incision
    e. lith/o   condition

13. **TRANSLATE:** *Complete the definitions of the following terms by using the meaning of the word parts to fill in the blanks. Terms built from the combining form **ureter/o**, meaning ureter:*

   a. ureter/o/lith/iasis _____ of stone(s) in the _____
   b. ureter/o/pyel/o/nephr/itis _____ of the ureter, _____ _____, and kidney
   c. ureter/o/lith/o/tomy _____ into the _____ to remove _____(s)

14. **READ: Ureterolithiasis** (ū-rē-ter-ō-lith-Ī-a-sis) occurs when a stone is stuck in a ureter. The urine flow can become blocked. If bacteria are present, the area above the blockage can become infected. This is known as **ureteropyelonephritis** (ū-rē-ter-ō-pī-e-lō-ne-FRĪ-tis). A **ureterolithotomy** (ū-rē-ter-ō-lith-OT-o-mē) is generally only done if other, less invasive measures fail.

15. **BUILD:** *Using the combining form **ureter/o**, build the following terms describing procedures related to the ureter.*

   a. excision of the ureter

   _____/_____
   wr   s

   b. surgical repair of the ureter

   _____/_o_/_____
   wr   cv   s

16. **READ: Ureterectomy** (ū-rē-ter-EK-to-mē) is generally performed for cancers involving one or both ureters. **Ureteroplasty** (ū-RĒ-ter-ō-plas-tē) may be necessary if the ureter is blocked due to stones, infections, or cancer.

17. **LABEL:** *Write word parts to complete Figure 5.12.*

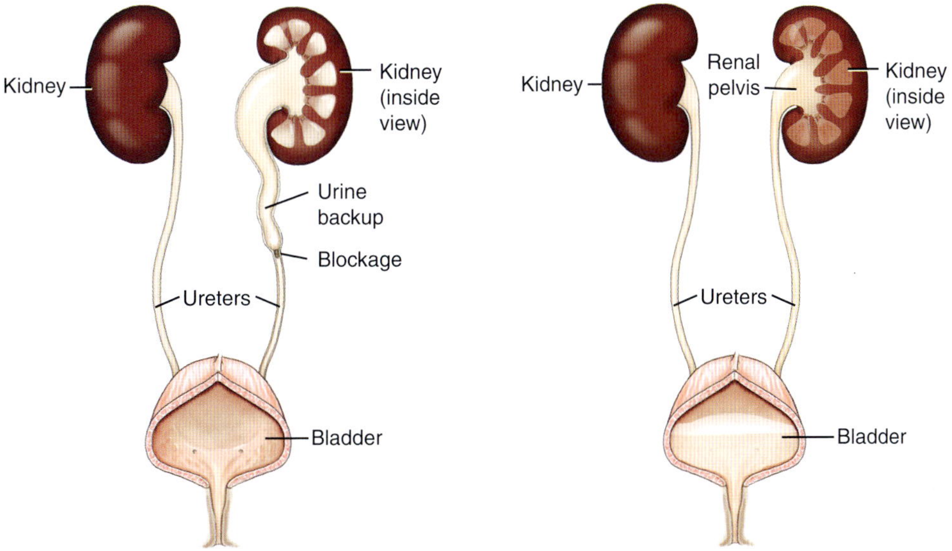

Figure 5.12 A. Left ureter is blocked causing urine to back up in the kidney

   B. After _____/o/_____, the ureter is open and urine flows freely to the bladder.
   ureter   surgical repair

18. MATCH: *Draw a line to match the suffix with its definition.*

    a. -al   cut into, incision

    b. -scopy   pertaining to

    c. -tomy   visual examination

---

19. TRANSLATE: *Complete the definitions of the following terms by using the meaning of the word parts to fill in the blanks. Terms built from the combining form* **meat/o,** *meaning urinary meatus:*

    a. meat/al   _____ to the _____

    b. meat/o/scopy   _____ _____ of the meatus

    c. meat/o/tomy   _____ into the _____ (to enlarge it)

> **FYI**   **Meatus** comes from the Latin **meare** meaning **to pass** or **to go**. Other anatomic passages share the same name, such as the auditory meatus.

---

20. READ: Meatoscopy (mē-a-TOS-ko-pē) uses a special device to see the urethral meatus. **Meatotomy** (mē-a-TOT-o-mē) is performed when the urinary meatus is too narrow, which may be caused by scarring from injury, or from birth defects.

---

21. MATCH: *Draw a line to match the word part with its definition.*

    a. -gram   one who studies and treats (specialist, physician)

    b. -logist   study of

    c. -logy   record, radiographic image

    d. -stomy   creation of an artificial opening

---

22. BUILD: *Write word parts to build the following terms using the combining form* **ur/o,** *meaning urine or urinary tract.*

    a. radiographic image of the urinary tract   _____ / o / _____

                                                         wr   **cv**   **s**

    b. physician who studies and treats diseases of the   _____ / o / _____
urinary tract

                                                         wr   **cv**   **s**

    c. study of the urinary tract   _____ / o / _____

                                                          wr   **cv**   **s**

    d. creation of an artificial opening into the urinary   _____ / o / _____
tract

                                                          wr   **cv**   **s**

---

23. READ: Urology (ū-ROL-o-jē) is the study of the urinary tract. A **urologist** (ū-ROL-o-jist) is a surgeon who specializes in diseases of the urinary tract, including bladder cancer, urinary infections, and ureteral stones. A **urogram** (Ū-rō-gram) obtains an image of the entire urinary tract, from the kidneys to the urinary meatus. The surgical creation of a **urostomy** (ū-ROS-tō-mē) allows for diversion of urine around a blocked or missing portion of the urinary tract.

24. LABEL: *Write word parts to complete Figure 5.13.*

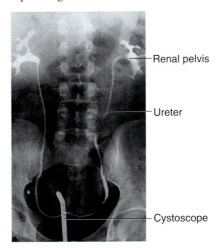

- Renal pelvis
- Ureter
- Cystoscope

Figure 5.13 _____/o/_____.
          urinary tract   radiographic image

---

25. TRANSLATE: *Complete the definitions of the following terms by using the meaning of the word parts to fill in the blanks.*

a. nephr/o/logist   _____ who _____ and _____ _____ of the kidney

b. nephr/o/logy   _____ of the _____

---

26. READ: Nephrology (ne-FROL-o-jē) refers to study of the kidneys and related diseases. A **nephrologist** (ne-FROL-o-jist) is an internal medicine physician who has completed extra years of study to specialize in kidney disease. Nephrologists also treat diseases which affect the kidney, such as hypertension and diabetes.

---

27. REVIEW OF MORE URINARY SYSTEM TERMS BUILT FROM WORD PARTS: *the following is an alphabetical list of terms built and translated in the previous exercises.*

MEDICAL TERMS BUILT FROM WORD PARTS

TERM	DEFINITION	TERM	DEFINITION
1. hydronephrosis (hī-drō-ne-FRŌ-sis)	abnormal condition of water in the kidney (distention of the renal pelvis with urine because of an obstruction) (Figure 5.10)	**4. meatotomy** (mē-a-TOT-o-mē)	incision into the meatus (to enlarge it)
2. meatal (mē-Ā-tal)	pertaining to the meatus	**5. nephrectomy** (ne-FREK-to-mē)	excision of the kidney
3. meatoscopy (mē-a-TOS-ko-pē)	visual examination of the meatus	**6. nephritis** (ne-FRĪ-tis)	inflammation of the kidney

MEDICAL TERMS BUILT FROM WORD PARTS—cont'd

TERM	DEFINITION	TERM	DEFINITION
7. nephrologist (ne-FROL-o-jist)	physician who studies and treats diseases of the kidney	15. ureterolithotomy (ū-rē-ter-ō-lith-OT-o-mē)	incision into the ureter to remove stone(s)
8. nephrology (ne-FROL-o-jē)	study of the kidney	16. ureteroplasty (ū-RĒ-ter-ō-plas-tē)	surgical repair of the ureter (Figure 5.12)
9. nephrostomy (nef-ROS-to-mē)	creation of an artificial opening into the kidney (Figure 5.11)	17. ureteropyelonephritis (ū-rē-ter-ō-pī-e-lō-ne-FRĪ-tis)	inflammation of the ureter, renal pelvis, and kidney
10. nephrotomy (ne-FROT-o-mē)	incision into the kidney	18. urogram (Ū-rō-gram)	radiographic image of the urinary tract (Figure 5.13)
11. pyelonephritis (pī-e-lō-ne-FRĪ-tis)	inflammation of the renal pelvis and kidney (Figure 5.9)	19. urologist (ū-ROL-o-jist)	physician who studies and treats diseases of the urinary tract
12. renal (RĒ-nal)	pertaining to the kidney	20. urology (ū-ROL-o-jē)	study of the urinary tract
13. ureterectomy (ū-rē-ter-EK-to-mē)	excision of the ureter	21. urostomy (ū-ROS-tō-mē)	creation of an artificial opening in the urinary tract
14. ureterolithiasis (ū-rē-ter-ō-lith-Ī-a-sis)	condition of stone(s) in the ureter		

EXERCISE D   Pronounce and Spell MORE Terms Built from Word Parts

Practice pronunciation and spelling on paper and online.

1. **Practice on Paper**
   a. **Pronounce**: Read the phonetic spelling and say aloud the terms listed in the previous table, Review of MORE Terms Built from Word Parts.
   b. **Spell**: Have a study partner read the terms aloud. Write the spelling of the terms on a separate sheet of paper.

2. **Practice Online** 🌐
   a. **Access** online learning resources. Go to evolve.elsevier.com > Evolve Resources > Practice Student Resources.
   b. **Pronounce**: Select Audio Glossary > Lesson 5 > Exercise D. Select a term to hear its pronunciation and repeat aloud.
   c. **Spell**: Select Activities > Lesson 5 > Spell Terms > Exercise D. Select the audio icon and type the correct spelling of the term.

❏   Check the box when complete.

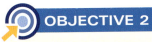

OBJECTIVE 2

Define, pronounce, and spell medical terms NOT built from word parts.

The terms listed below may contain word parts, but are difficult to translate literally.

MEDICAL TERMS NOT BUILT FROM WORD PARTS

TERM	DEFINITION
chronic kidney disease (CKD) (KRON-ik) (KID-nē) (di-ZĒZ)	progressive, irreversible loss of kidney function
dialysis (dī-AL-i-sis)	procedure for removing toxic waste from the blood because of an inability of the kidneys to do so
extracorporeal shock wave lithotripsy (ESWL) (eks-tra-kor-POR-ē-al) (shok) (wāv) (LITH-ō-trip-sē)	noninvasive surgical procedure to crush stone(s) in the kidney or ureter by administration of repeated shock waves. Stone fragments are eliminated from the body in the urine.
incontinence (in-KON-ti-nens)	inability to control the bladder and/or bowels
renal calculi (*sing*. calculus) (RĒ-nal) (KAL-kū-lī), (KAL-kū-lus)	stones in the kidney; (also called **nephrolithiasis**)
renal failure (RĒ-nal) (FĀL-ūr)	loss of kidney function resulting in its inability to remove waste products from the body and maintain fluid balance; can be acute, chronic, or end-stage
renal transplant (RĒ-nal) (TRANS-plant)	surgical implantation of a donor kidney into a patient with inadequate renal function
urinalysis (UA) (ū-rin-AL-i-sis)	laboratory test in which multiple routine tests are performed on a urine specimen
urinary catheterization (Ū-rin-ār-ē) (kath-e-ter-i-ZĀ-shun)	procedure that involves the passage of a catheter into the urinary bladder to withdraw urine
urinary tract infection (UTI) (Ū-rin-ār-ē) (tract) (in-FEK-shun)	infection of one or more organs of the urinary tract
void (voyd)	to pass urine

EXERCISE E   Label

Write the medical terms pictured and defined using the previous table of Medical Terms NOT Built from Word Parts. Check your work with the Answer Key in Appendix C.

1. _____

passage of a catheter into the urinary bladder to withdraw urine

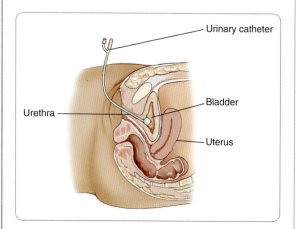

2. _____

noninvasive surgical procedure to crush stone(s) in the kidney or ureter by administration of repeated shock waves

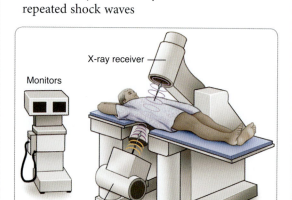

3. _____

procedure for removing toxic waste from the blood because of an inability of the kidneys to do so

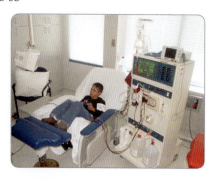

4. _____

stones in the kidney; (also called nephrolithiasis)

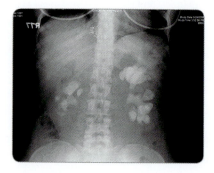

5. _____

laboratory test in which multiple routine tests are performed on a urine specimen

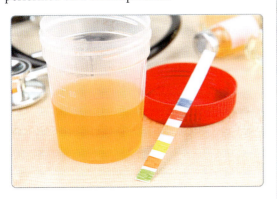

6. _____

surgical implantation of a donor kidney into a patient with inadequate renal function

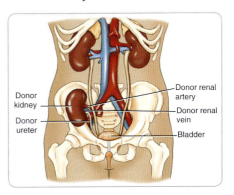

Donor kidney
Donor ureter
Donor renal artery
Donor renal vein
Bladder

EXERCISE F — Learn Medical Terms NOT Built from Word Parts

*Fill in the blanks with medical terms defined in **bold** and abbreviations using the Medical Terms NOT Built from Word Parts table. Check your responses with the Answer Key in Appendix C.*

1. The **inability to control the bladder and/or bowels** is called _____. Urinary incontinence occurs when one loses control over the ability to **pass urine** or _____. This can sometimes be caused by a **UTI** or _____. A **laboratory test which performs multiple routine assessments on a urine specimen**, or _____ (**UA**), can help to diagnose this. In severe cases of incontinence, a _____ may be performed, which is a **procedure that uses a catheter to withdraw urine from the bladder**.

2. Acute renal failure (ARF) is the sudden and severe loss of kidney function that leads to a buildup of waste in the body. Prompt treatment can reverse the condition and recovery can occur. **CKD, or _____ _____**, is a **progressive, irreversible loss of kidney function** that leads to the onset of uremia. Dialysis and kidney transplant are used in treating this disease. Chronic renal failure, or CRF, is an older term that has mostly been replaced by CKD. End-stage renal disease (ESRD) refers to _____, or the **loss of kidney function resulting in its inability to remove waste products from the body and maintain fluid balance**, that has become too severe to sustain life.

3. When kidney failure is advanced, a nephrologist may order _____, a **procedure for removing toxic waste from the blood because of an inability of the kidneys to do so.** This takes over kidney functions by removing waste and extra fluids, helping to keep a safe level of necessary chemicals in the blood, and controlling blood pressure.

> **FYI**   There are two main types of dialysis. **Hemodialysis** uses an external machine (hemodialyzer) which is connected to the patient's blood vessels via a tube. The hemodialyzer then filters the blood and returns it to the body. In **peritoneal dialysis**, the blood is cleaned inside the body using the abdominal lining as a natural filter. Sterile fluid is put into the abdomen through a catheter, then removed the same way.

4. Another term for **nephrolithiasis,** which also means **stones in the kidney**, is _____.
    If stones become large or obstructive, treatment is required. A urologist may order a type of lithotripsy which uses a **noninvasive surgical procedure to crush stone(s) in the kidney or ureter by administration of repeated shock waves** called **ESWL** or _____.

> **FYI**   **Extracorporeal** means occurring outside the body

EXERCISE G   Pronounce and Spell Medical Terms NOT Built from Word Parts

Practice pronunciation and spelling on paper with the textbook and online.

1. **Practice on Paper**
    a. **Pronounce:** Read the phonetic spelling and say aloud the terms listed in the previous Medical Terms NOT Built from Word Parts Table.
    b. **Spell:** Have a study partner read the terms aloud. Write the spelling of the terms on a separate sheet of paper.

2. **Practice Online** 🌐
    a. **Access** online learning resources. Go to evolve.elsevier.com > Evolve Resources > Practice Student Resources.
    b. **Pronounce:** Select Audio Glossary > Exercise G. Select a term to hear its pronunciation and repeat aloud.
    c. **Spell:** Select Activities > Spell Terms > Exercise G. Select the audio icon and type the correct spelling of the term.

❑   Check the box when complete.

OBJECTIVE 3

Write abbreviations.

ABBREVIATIONS RELATED TO THE URINARY SYSTEM

Use the online **flashcards** to familiarize yourself with the following abbreviations.

ABBREVIATION	TERM	ABBREVIATION	TERM
cath	catheterization, catheter	**PCT**	patient care technician
CKD	chronic kidney disease	**PKD**	polycystic kidney disease
ESWL	extracorporeal shock wave lithotripsy	**UA**	urinalysis
HD	hemodialysis	**UTI**	urinary tract infection
OAB	overactive bladder	**VCUG**	voiding cystourethrogram

FYI **Polycystic kidney disease** (PKD) is an inherited disorder that causes cysts (fluid-filled sacs) to form throughout the kidneys. PKD can range from mild to severe, with the worst cases resulting in renal failure.

EXERCISE H Abbreviate Medical Terms

Write the correct abbreviation next to its medical term.

1. Diseases and Disorders:

   a. _____ chronic kidney disease

   b. _____ urinary tract infection

   c. _____ polycystic kidney disease

   d. _____ overactive bladder

2. Diagnostic Tests:

   a. _____ urinalysis

   b. _____ voiding cystourethrogram

3. Surgical Procedures:

   a. _____ extracorporeal shock wave lithotripsy

   b. _____ hemodialysis

4. Specialties and Professions:

   _____ (dialysis) patient care technician

5. Related Term:

   _____ catheterization, catheter

OBJECTIVE 4

Identify medical terms by clinical category.

Now that you have worked through the urinary system lesson, review and practice medical terms grouped by clinical category. Categories include signs and symptoms, diseases and disorders, diagnostic tests and equipment, surgical procedures, specialties and professions, and other terms related to the urinary system.

EXERCISE I Signs and Symptoms

Write the medical terms for signs and symptoms next to their definitions.

1. _____ condition of absence of urine

2. _____ condition of difficult or painful urination

3. _____ condition of blood in the urine

4. _____ condition of night urination

5. _____ condition of scanty urine (amount)

6. _____ condition of pus in the urine

7. _____ inability to control the bladder and/or bowels

EXERCISE J   Diseases and Disorders

Write the medical terms for diseases and disorders next to their definitions.

1. _____ inflammation of the bladder

2. _____ condition of stone(s) in the bladder

3. _____ abnormal condition of water (urine) in the kidney

4. _____ condition of stone(s) in the kidney

5. _____ inflammation of the kidney

6. _____ inflammation of the renal pelvis and kidney

7. _____ inflammation of the urethra and bladder

8. _____ stones in the kidney

9. _____ loss of kidney function resulting in its inability to remove waste products from the body and maintain fluid balance

10. _____ infection of one or more organs of the urinary tract

11. _____ condition of urine in the blood

12. _____ condition of stone(s) in the ureter

13. _____ inflammation of the ureter, renal pelvis, and kidney

14. _____ progressive, irreversible, loss of renal function; leads to the onset of uremia

EXERCISE K   Diagnostic Tests and Equipment

Write the medical terms for diagnostic tests and equipment next to their definitions.

1. _____ radiographic image of the bladder

2. _____ radiographic imaging of the bladder

3. _____ instrument used for visual examination of the bladder

4. _____ visual examination of the bladder

5. _____ radiographic imaging of the bladder and urethra

6. _____ visual examination of the meatus

7. _____ instrument used for visual examination of the urethra

8. _____ laboratory test in which multiple routine tests are performed on a urine specimen

9. _____ radiographic image of the urinary tract

EXERCISE L   Surgical Procedures

Write the medical terms for surgical procedures next to their definitions.

1. _____   incision into the bladder to remove stone(s)

2. _____   creation of an artificial opening into the bladder

3. _____   noninvasive surgical procedure to crush stone(s) in the
   _____   kidney or ureter by administration of repeated shock
                                  waves

4. _____   surgical crushing of stone(s)

5. _____   incision into the meatus (to enlarge it)

6. _____   excision of the kidney

7. _____   surgical repair of the ureter

8. _____   creation of an artificial opening into the kidney

9. _____   incision into the kidney

10. _____   incision into the renal pelvis to remove stone(s)

11. _____   surgical implantation of a donor kidney into a patient
                                   with inadequate renal function

12. _____   excision of the ureter

13. _____   creation of an artificial opening in the urinary tract

14. _____   incision into the ureter to remove stone(s)

15. _____   surgical repair of the urethra

EXERCISE M   Specialties and Professions

Write the medical terms for specialties and professions next to their definitions.

1. _____   study of the kidney

2. _____   physician who studies and treats diseases of the kidney

3. _____   study of the urinary tract

4. _____   physician who studies and treats diseases of the
                                  urinary tract

EXERCISE N   Medical Terms Related to the Urinary System

Write the medical terms related to the urinary system next to their definitions.

1. _____   pertaining to the (urinary) meatus

2. _____   pertaining to the kidney

3. _____   procedure for removing toxic waste from the blood
                                  because of an inability of the kidneys to do so

4. _____   procedure that involves the passage of a catheter into the urinary bladder to withdraw urine

5. _____   to pass urine

 OBJECTIVE 5

Use medical language in clinical statements, the case study, and a medical record.

EXERCISE O   Use Medical Terms in Clinical Statements

Circle the medical terms and abbreviations defined in the bolded phrases. Answers are listed in Appendix C. For pronunciation practice, read the answers aloud.

1. Mr. Yin was admitted to the medical center for a(n) **excision of a kidney** (nephrostomy, nephrectomy, nephrotomy). The kidney will be used as a donor organ for **pertaining to the kidney** (renal, meatal, ureteral) transplant for his brother who is suffering from chronic, bilateral (both) **inflammation of the kidneys** (pyelonephritis, ureteropyelonephritis, nephritis).

2. Mr. Garcia was complaining of **difficult or painful urination** (dysuria, anuria, oliguria) and was noted to have **condition of blood in the urine** (pyuria, hematuria, uremia). The **multiple routine tests done on a urine specimen** (urogram, cystoscopy, urinalysis) revealed **condition of pus in the urine** (nocturia, pyuria, incontinence). He was diagnosed and treated for **inflammation of the bladder** (cystitis, nephritis, pyelonephritis).

3. Tassiana Smith, a 10-year-old girl, has had recurrent (chronic) **inflammation of the bladder** (cystitis, nephritis, cystolithiasis). To determine the cause, the physician ordered a(n) **radiographic image of the bladder** (urogram, cystogram, parallelogram) to be followed by **visual examination of the bladder** (cystourethrography, cystoscopy, urethroscope) if necessary.

4. **Surgical crushing of stone(s)** (Pyelolithotomy, Lithotripsy, Dialysis) was used to treat Mrs. Hand, who was diagnosed as having **condition of stone(s) in the ureter** (ureteropyelonephritis, cystolithiasis, ureterolithiasis).

5. To correct a condition called stress **inability to control the bladder** (incontinence, oliguria, nocturia), a **physician who studies and treats diseases of the urinary tract** (nephrologist, urologist, pulmonologist) may perform a **surgical repair of the urethra** (ureterolithotomy, urethroplasty, ureterectomy).

6. Voiding **radiographic imaging of the bladder and urethra** (urinalysis, cystourethrography, cystography) is performed by instilling radiopaque dye in the bladder. Radiographic images called cystourethrograms are taken of the bladder during voiding of the dye. The test may be performed to find the cause of repeated **infection of one or more organs of the urinary tract** (cystitis, urinary tract infection, uremia).

7. A(n) **physician who studies and treats diseases of the kidney** (dermatologist, oncologist, nephrologist) takes care of patients with **progressive, irreversible loss of kidney function** (UTI, COPD, CKD) and prescribes **procedure for removing toxic waste from the blood because of an inability of the kidneys to do so** (dialysis, incontinence, lithotripsy) therapy. A urologist treats diseases of the male and female urinary system, including urinary **inability to control the bladder and/or bowels** (dialysis, incontinence, lithotripsy) and of the male reproductive system, both medically and surgically.

EXERCISE P   Apply Medical Terms to the Case Study

Think back to Tyrone who was introduced in the case study at the beginning of the lesson. After working through Lesson 5 on the urinary system, consider the medical terms that might be used to describe his experience. List two terms relevant to the case study and their meanings. ■

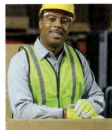

Medical Term   **Definition**

1. _____   _____

2. _____   _____

EXERCISE Q   Use Medical Terms in a Document

Tyrone went to the Urgent Care near his work. A medical assistant saw him, wrote down his problems, and took his vital signs. The physician assistant examined him, ordered tests, then gave him a diagnosis and recommendations for his care. These are documented in the medical record below.

Use the definitions in numbers 1-9 to write medical terms within the following document.

1. condition of blood in the urine

2. stones in the kidney

3. infection of one or more organs of the urinary tract

4. pertaining to the kidney

5. procedure for removing toxic waste from the blood because of an inability of the kidneys to do so

6. laboratory test in which multiple routine tests are performed on a urine specimen

7. condition of pus in the urine

8. condition of stone(s) in the ureter

9. abnormal condition of water (urine) in the kidney

Refer to the medical record to answer questions 10-14.

10. The term **hematuria**, used in the medical record to describe findings on the urinalysis, is also often described as a sign or symptom. Use your knowledge of word parts to review this term.

    ur/o means _____

    -ia means _____

    hem/o, hemat/o means _____

    Thus, **hematuria** means _____ of _____ in the _____

```
0045689 PARKER, Tyrone                                                    _ □ X
File    Patient    Navigate    Custom Fields    Help
```

| Chart Review | Encounters | Notes | Labs | Imaging | Procedures | Rx | Documents | Referrals | Scheduling | Billing |

Name: **PARKER, Tyrone**   MR#: **0045689**   Sex: M   **Allergies: Demerol**
                            DOB: 10/17/19XX   Age: 38   PCP: Pearson, Michael, PA-C

Urgent Care Visit
Date of visit: 12/15/20XX
Patient Care Provider: Michael Pearson, PA-C

SUBJECTIVE: The patient is a 38-year-old man who was in his usual state of good health when he began to experience left-sided flank pain accompanied by gross (1.) _____ three days ago. He denies chills or fever. He has no prior history of (2.) _____ but was treated for (3.) _____ one year ago. He had an appendectomy as a child. His father had chronic (4.) _____ failure requiring (5.) _____.

OBSERVATION: T 98.6 F, BP 140/80 mm Hg, P 72, R 16. He is oriented and in no acute distress. Abdomen is soft with mild tenderness over the left flank. No organomegaly. (6.) _____ showed hematuria without (7.) _____. CT scan of the abdomen revealed (8.) _____ of the distal left ureter. There is no (9.) _____ of the left kidney.

ASSESSMENT: Left distal ureterolithiasis.

PLAN: 1. Strain urine.
2. Increase fluid intake.
3. Oxycodone 5 mg/acetaminophen 500 mg, one tablet orally every four hours as needed for pain.
4. Return for office visit in one week. Call if pain worsens or fever or chills develop.

Electronically signed: Michael Pearson, PA-C 12/16/20XX 16:15

```
Start    Log On/Off    Print    Edit
```

11. List two other terms that use **ur/o** and **–ia** to describe signs or symptoms related to urine:

_____

_____

12. CKD is the abbreviation for _____, which has also been called chronic renal failure.

13. Left distal ureterolithiasis means that a stone is located in the _____ section of the left _____.

14. Identify two new medical terms in the medical record you would like to investigate. Use your medical dictionary or an online resource to look up the definition.

Medical Term	**Definition**
1. _____	_____
2. _____	_____

EXERCISE R   **Use Medical Language in Electronic Health Records Online**

Select the correct medical terms to complete three medical records in one patient's electronic file.

 Access online resources at evolve.elsevier.com > Evolve Resources > Practice Student Resources > Activities > Lesson 5 > Electronic Health Records

Topic: Renal Calculus
Record 1: Encounter Visit
Record 2: Operative Report
Record 3: Post-operative Office Visit

OBJECTIVE 6

Recall and assess knowledge of word parts, medical terms, and abbreviations.

EXERCISE S   **Online Review of Lesson Content**

Recall and assess your learning from working through the lesson by completing online learning activities at evolve. elsevier.com > Evolve Resources > Practice Student Resources. Keep track of your progress by placing a check mark next to completed activities.

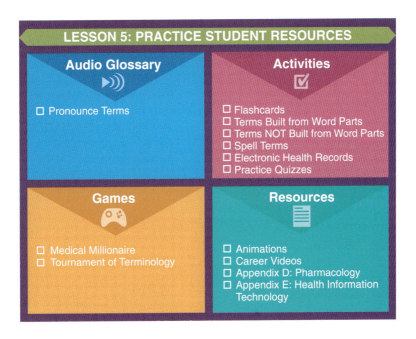

LESSON 5: PRACTICE STUDENT RESOURCES

Audio Glossary
- ☐ Pronounce Terms

Activities
- ☐ Flashcards
- ☐ Terms Built from Word Parts
- ☐ Terms NOT Built from Word Parts
- ☐ Spell Terms
- ☐ Electronic Health Records
- ☐ Practice Quizzes

Games
- ☐ Medical Millionaire
- ☐ Tournament of Terminology

Resources
- ☐ Animations
- ☐ Career Videos
- ☐ Appendix D: Pharmacology
- ☐ Appendix E: Health Information Technology

EXERCISE T   Lesson Content Quiz

Test your knowledge of the terms and abbreviations introduced in this lesson. Circle the letter for the medical term or abbreviation related to the words in italics.

1. *Condition of night urination* is more common in men over the age of 50, and may be associated with an enlarged prostate.
   a. oliguria
   b. nocturia
   c. dysuria

2. *Incision into the renal pelvis to remove stone(s)* may be necessary if ESWL is not possible.
   a. pyelolithotomy
   b. cystolithotomy
   c. urereterectomy

3. *Loss of kidney function resulting in its inability to remove waste products from the body and maintain fluid balance* can be due to diabetes, high blood pressure, or a number of other acute and chronic conditions.
   a. renal transplant
   b. renal calculi
   c. renal failure

4. Autosomal dominant *polycystic kidney disease* is the most common type of cystic disease of the kidneys; it usually appears during the third decade of life.
   a. PKD
   b. CKD
   c. PCT

5. Percutaneous *creation of an artificial opening into the kidney* may be necessary if there is blockage that is preventing urine flow from the kidney; *abnormal condition of water (urine) in the kidney* is often present in these cases.
   a. nephrotomy, nephritis
   b. nephroplasty, ureterolithiasis
   c. nephrostomy, hydronephrosis

6. A urologist uses a(n) *instrument used for visual examination of the bladder* to aid in the diagnosis of conditions such as cystolithiasis, cystitis, and bladder cancers.
   a. cystogram
   b. cystoscope
   c. cystoscopy

7. If a patient has a *UTI* in addition to renal calculi, it must be eliminated with antibiotics prior *to noninvasive surgical procedure to crush stone(s) in the kidney or ureter by administration of repeated shock waves.*
   a. urinary tract infection, extracorporeal shock wave lithotripsy
   b. urinalysis, lithotripsy
   c. urogram, ureterolithotomy

8. During voiding *radiographic imaging of the bladder and urethra*, a catheter is passed through the meatal opening, dye is placed into the bladder through this tube, and images are obtained.
   a. cystography
   b. cystourethrography
   c. meatoscopy

9. *Urine in the blood* can be a serious complication of chronic kidney disease, and may require dialysis.
   a. anuria
   b. hematuria
   c. uremia

10. Suprapubic *creation of an artificial opening into the bladder* is used when a patient is unable to empty his or her bladder, and the use of urinary catheterization is either not desirable or not possible.
    a. meatotomy
    b. cystostomy
    c. ureterocutaneostomy

LESSON AT A GLANCE URINARY SYSTEM WORD PARTS

COMBINING FORMS

cyst/o
hem/o, hemat/o
hydr/o
lith/o
meat/o
nephr/o, ren/o
noct/i

olig/o
pyel/o
py/o
ur/o
ureter/o
urethr/o

SUFFIXES

-emia
-iasis
-plasty
-tripsy

LESSON AT A GLANCE URINARY SYSTEM MEDICAL TERMS AND ABBREVIATIONS

SIGNS AND SYMPTOMS

anuria
dysuria
hematuria
incontinence
nocturia
oliguria
pyuria

DISEASES AND DISORDERS

chronic kidney disease (CKD)
cystitis
cystolithiasis
hydronephrosis
nephritis
nephrolithiasis
pyelonephritis
renal calculi
renal failure
uremia
ureterolithiasis
ureteropyelonephritis
urethrocystitis
urinary tract infection (UTI)

DIAGNOSTIC TESTS AND EQUIPMENT

cystogram
cystography
cystoscope
cystoscopy
cystourethrography
meatoscopy
urethroscope
urinalysis (UA)
urogram

SURGICAL PROCEDURES

cystolithotomy
cystostomy
extracorporeal shock wave lithotripsy
  (ESWL)
lithotripsy
meatotomy
nephrectomy
nephrostomy
nephrotomy
pyelolithotomy
renal transplant
ureterectomy
ureterolithotomy
ureteroplasty
urethroplasty
urostomy

SPECIALTIES AND PROFESSIONS

nephrologist
nephrology
urologist
urology

RELATED TERMS

dialysis
meatal
renal
urinary catheterization
void

ABBREVIATIONS

cath	OAB	UTI
CKD	PCT	VCUG
ESWL	PKD	
HD	UA	

Reproductive Systems

Cindy Collier and Rajive Modi

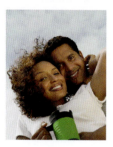

Cindy and Rajive want to have a baby. They have been trying for over a year, but Cindy hasn't gotten pregnant. Cindy worries something is wrong. Even though she has her period every month, it is very painful, and she bleeds a lot. She often has pain low in her belly. She had sexual partners before Rajive, and she is worried that one may have given her a disease. Rajive is also concerned, and wonders if something might be wrong with him that is keeping Cindy from getting pregnant. When he was born only one of his testicles was down, and they had to do surgery to fix the other one. He hasn't had any problems with it since then. He had partners before Cindy. Now he is worried that he may have passed something on to Cindy.

■ *Consider Cindy and Rajive's situation as you work through the lesson on reproductive systems. We will return to this case study and identify medical terms used to describe and document their experiences.*

OBJECTIVES

1 ■ Build, translate, pronounce, and spell medical terms built from word parts (p. 151).

2 ■ Define, pronounce, and spell medical terms NOT built from word parts (p. 166).

3 ■ Write abbreviations (p. 171).

4 ■ Identify medical terms by clinical category (p. 172).

5 ■ Use medical language in clinical statements, the case study, and a medical record (p. 176).

6 ■ Recall and assess knowledge of word parts, medical terms, and abbreviations (p. 179).

INTRODUCTION TO THE REPRODUCTIVE SYSTEMS

Anatomic Structures of the Female Reproductive System

breasts (brests)	milk-producing glands (also called **mammary glands**)
cervix (SER-vicks)	narrow lower portion of the uterus
endometrium (en-dō-MĒ-trē-um)	inner lining of the uterus
ovaries (Ō-var-ēs)	almond-shaped organs located in the pelvic cavity; form and store ova; produce the hormones estrogen and progesterone
ovum (*pl.* ova) (Ō-vam), (Ō-va)	female reproductive (egg) cell produced by the ovaries

Anatomic Structures of the Female Reproductive System—cont'd

uterine tubes (Ū-ter-in) (toobz)	tubes attached to the uterus that provide a passageway for the ovum to move from the ovary to the uterus (also called **fallopian tubes**)
uterus (Ū-ter-us)	pear-sized and shaped muscular organ that lies in the pelvic cavity, except during pregnancy when it enlarges and extends up into the abdominal cavity; its functions are menstruation, pregnancy, and labor
vagina (va-JĪ-nah)	passageway between the uterus and the outside of the body

Anatomic Structures of the Male Reproductive System

epididymis (ep-i-DID-a-mis)	coiled tube attached to each of the testes that provides for storage, transit, and maturation of sperm
penis (PĒ-nis)	male organ of urination and coitus (sexual intercourse)
prostate gland (PROS-tāt) (gland)	encircles the upper end of the urethra; secretes fluid that aids in the movement of sperm and ejaculation
scrotum (SKRŌ-tem)	sac containing the testes and epididymis, suspended on both sides of and just behind the penis
semen (SĒ-men)	composed of sperm, seminal fluids, and other secretions
seminal vesicles (SEM-e-nel) (VES-i-kelz)	main glands located at the base of the urinary bladder that open into the vas deferens; secrete a thick fluid that forms part of the semen
sperm (spurm)	male reproductive cell produced by the testes
testis, testicle (*pl.* testes, testicles) (TES-tis), (TES-ti-kel); (TES-tēs), (TES-ti-kelz)	primary male sex organ; oval-shaped and enclosed within the scrotum; produce sperm and the hormone testosterone
urethra (ū-RĒ-thra)	narrow tube that carries semen from the vas deferens to the outside of the body; also connects to the urinary bladder in the male (a circular muscle constricts during intercourse to prevent urination)
vas deferens (vas) (DEF-ar-enz)	duct carrying the sperm from the epididymis to the urethra

Functions of the Reproductive Systems

- Produce egg and sperm cells
- Secrete hormones
- Provide for conception and pregnancy

How the Reproductive Systems Work

Male and female reproductive organs do not fully develop and begin performing reproductive functions until the individual is approximately 11 years of age. Puberty is the time during which the reproductive organs mature. Hormones initiate puberty and play a key role in all the reproductive cycles. Hormones secreted by the reproductive systems produce feminine and masculine physical traits.

At birth, the **female reproductive system** (Figure 6.2) contains all the ova that will be produced. Upon puberty, a mature **ovum** is released from an **ovary** in a cyclical manner, usually every 28 days. Once released, the ovum travels through the **uterine tube** to the **uterus.** Because this is approximately a seven-day journey, conception or fertilization of the ovum with sperm usually occurs in the uterine tube. If the egg is not fertilized, layers of the endometrium detach and pass through the **vagina** along with blood as menstrual flow. The menstrual cycle occurs from puberty until women reach menopause, the cessation of the female reproductive cycles occurring sometime in middle age.

In contrast, the **male reproductive system** (Figure 6.9) generally remains functional from puberty to the end of life. **Sperm** is produced in the **testes** and passes through the **epididymis, vas deferens,** and **urethra.** The sperm matures as it travels through this series of ducts. Additional fluid, produced by the **prostate gland** and **seminal vesicles,** is contributed along the way to produce **semen.** Semen is ejaculated from the **penis** into the vagina for potential creation of offspring.

CAREER FOCUS **Professionals Who Work with the Reproductive Systems**

- **Obstetric Technicians (OB/GYN tech)** assist during vaginal births, sterilize equipment, and maintain medical records. Training requirements may include certification in nursing assisting and surgical technology.

- **Certified Nurse Midwives (CNM)** are registered nurses who hold a master's degree in nursing and certification in midwifery. CNMs work closely with gynecologists and specialize in the care of pregnant women, childbirth, and care of infants.

- **Direct-Entry Midwives** are trained in midwifery but are not nurses. Types include Certified Professional Midwives (CPMs) and Certified Midwives (CMs). They usually practice in non-hospital settings, including birthing centers and the patient's home.

- **Mammographers,** also called mammography technologists, obtain diagnostic images of breast tissue using special x-ray equipment. They are responsible for positioning patients correctly for imaging. They also take a medical history and answer patient questions.

- **Sonographers** use high frequency sound waves directed at a specific part of the body. These are captured as moving images, which are recorded and provided to the physician for diagnosis. They also explain the procedure to patients and may need to help calm them due to anxieties about the exam or the diagnosis.

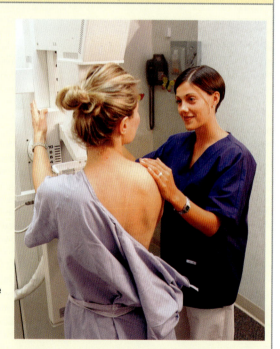

Figure 6.1 A mammographer assisting a patient with her screening exam.

🌐 **FOR MORE INFORMATION**

- To view a video on the careers of **Gynecologists** and **Obstetricians** go the Career One Stop's webpage and search under Health Science Videos.

- Access online learning resources at evolve.elsevier.com > Practice Student Resources > Other Resources > Career Videos to watch interviews with a **Mammography Technologist** and a **Sonographer**.

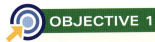

OBJECTIVE 1

Build, translate, pronounce, and spell medical terms built from word parts.

WORD PARTS   Presented with the Reproductive Systems

Use the paper or online **flashcards** to familiarize yourself with the following word parts.

Combining Form (WR + CV)	DEFINITION	COMBINING FORM (WR + CV)	DEFINITION
FEMALE REPRODUCTIVE SYSTEM		**MALE REPRODUCTIVE SYSTEM**	
cervic/o	cervix (or neck)	**orchi/o**	testis (testicle)
colp/o, vagin/o	vagina	**prostat/o**	prostate gland
endometri/o	endometrium	**scrot/o**	scrotum
gynec/o	woman	**vas/o**	vessel, duct (in the male reproductive system, vas/o refers to the vas deferens)
hyster/o	uterus		
mamm/o, mast/o	breast		
men/o	menstruation, menstrual		
oophor/o	ovary		
salping/o	uterine tube (fallopian tube)		
son/o	sound		

SUFFIX (S)	DEFINITION	SUFFIX (S)	DEFINITION
-cele	hernia, protrusion	**-rrhaphy**	suturing, repairing
-pexy	surgical fixation, suspension	**-rrhexis**	rupture

WORD PARTS PRESENTED IN PREVIOUS LESSONS   Used to Build Terms for the Reproductive Systems

COMBINING FORM (WR+CV)	DEFINITION	COMBINING FORM (WR + CV)	DEFINITION
cyst/o	bladder, sac	**lith/o**	stone(s), calculus (*pl.* calculi)

SUFFIX (S)	DEFINITION	SUFFIX (S)	DEFINITION
-al, -ic	pertaining to	**-itis**	inflammation
-ectomy	surgical removal, excision	**-logist**	one who studies and treats (specialist, physician)
-gram	record, radiographic image	**-logy**	study of
-graphy	process of recording, radiographic imaging	**-osis**	abnormal condition

WORD PARTS PRESENTED IN PREVIOUS LESSONS		Used to Build Terms for the Reproductive Systems—cont'd	
SUFFIX (S)	**DEFINITION**	**SUFFIX (S)**	**DEFINITION**
-plasty	surgical repair	-scope	instrument used for visual examination
-rrhagia	rapid flow of blood; excessive bleeding	-scopy	visual examination
-rrhea	flow, discharge	-tomy	cut into, incision
PREFIX (P)	**DEFINITION**	**PREFIX (P)**	**DEFINITION**
a-	absence of, without	dys-	difficult, painful, abnormal

Refer to Appendix A, Word Parts Used in *Basic Medical Language* for alphabetical lists of word parts and their meanings.

EXERCISE A   Build and Translate Terms Built from Word Parts

*Use the **Word Parts Tables** to complete the following questions. Check your responses with the Answer Key in Appendix C.*

1. **LABEL:** *Write the combining forms for anatomical structures of the female reproductive system on Figure 6.2. These anatomical combining forms will be used to build and translate medical terms in Exercise A.*

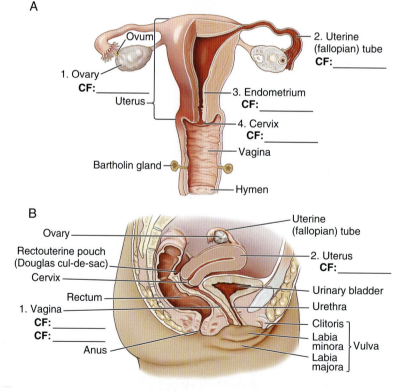

A

Ovum
2. Uterine (fallopian) tube
CF: _____
1. Ovary
CF: _____
Uterus
3. Endometrium
CF: _____
4. Cervix
CF: _____
Vagina
Bartholin gland
Hymen

B

Ovary
Uterine (fallopian) tube
Rectouterine pouch (Douglas cul-de-sac)
2. Uterus
CF: _____
Cervix
Urinary bladder
Rectum
Urethra
1. Vagina
CF: _____
CF: _____
Clitoris
Labia minora
Vulva
Anus
Labia majora

Figure 6.2 Female reproductive system with combining forms. **A,** Frontal view; **B,** Sagittal view.

FYI **Uterine tubes** are often presented as **fallopian tubes.** Gabriele Fallopius, 1523-1563, was a famous anatomist. An accurate dissector, Fallopius is remembered for his precise descriptions of the ovaries, round ligaments, and uterine tubes.

2. MATCH: *Draw a line to match the suffix with its definition.*

   a. -al   inflammation
   b. -itis   abnormal condition
   c. -osis   pertaining to

---

3. BUILD: *Using the suffix **-itis**, build terms describing inflammation of female reproductive organs. Remember, the definition usually starts with the meaning of the suffix.*

   a. inflammation of the vagina (*HINT:*   _____/_____
          *use the combining form starting with a **v.**)*   wr   s

   b. inflammation of the uterine tube   _____/_____
                                                                      wr   s

   c. inflammation of an ovary   _____/_____
                                                                      wr   s

   d. inflammation of the cervix   _____/_____
                                                                      wr   s

> **FYI**   **Cervic/o** is also used to denote the neck or any part of a body organ resembling a neck. By examining the other word parts in the medical term, you can determine whether the term applies to the cervix of the uterus or another body organ. For example, **cervic/o/thorac/ic** means pertaining to the neck and thorax. Locate **cervic/o** in your medical dictionary or an online source and read the definitions of the many medical terms containing the combining form **cervic/o.**

---

4. TRANSLATE: *Complete the definitions of the following terms by using the meaning of word parts to fill in the blanks. Remember, the definition usually starts with the meaning of the suffix.*

   a. vagin/al   _____ to the _____
   b. cervic/al   pertaining _____ the _____
   c. endometri/al   _____ to the _____
   d. endometr/itis   _____ of the endometrium
   e. endometri/osis   abnormal _____ of the _____
                            (growth of endometrial tissue outside of the uterus)

> **FYI**   Embedded within the combining form **endometri/o** are the prefix **endo-,** meaning within, and the word root **metr,** meaning uterus.

---

5. READ: Noninfectious **vaginitis** (vaj-i-NĪ-tis) may occur after menopause as a result of dryness caused by reduced estrogen, or may be the result of irritation caused by use of **vaginal** (VAJ-i-nal) sprays, perfumed soap and detergent, and some methods of birth control, such as spermicides. Infectious vaginitis may be caused by bacteria, yeast, or parasites. A **cervical** (SER-vi-kal) infection may cause **cervicitis** (ser-vi-SĪ-tis) and may spread to the uterus and uterine tubes causing **endometritis** (en-dō-mē-TRĪ-tis) and **salpingitis** (sal-pin-JĪ-tis). In severe infections, **oophoritis** (ō-of-o-RĪ-tis) may also occur. Infections of one or more of the female reproductive organs, including the cervix, uterus, uterine tubes, and ovaries are called pelvic inflammatory disease (PID).

6. LABEL: *Write word parts to complete Figure 6.3.*

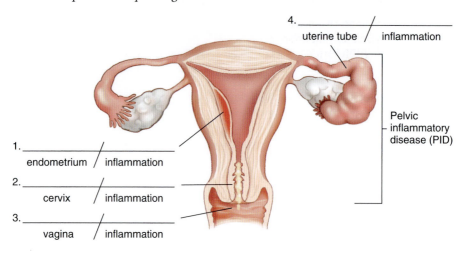

4. _____
   uterine tube / inflammation

1. _____
   endometrium / inflammation

2. _____
   cervix / inflammation

3. _____
   vagina / inflammation

Pelvic inflammatory disease (PID)

Figure 6.3 Ascending infection of the female reproductive system as seen in pelvic inflammatory disease.

7. READ: Endometriosis (en-dō-mē-trē-Ō-sis) is an abnormal condition in which **endometrial** (en-dō-MĒ-trē-l) tissue grows outside of the uterus in various areas of the pelvic cavity, including the surfaces of the ovaries, uterine tubes, uterus, and intestines.

8. LABEL: *Write word parts to complete Figure 6.4.*

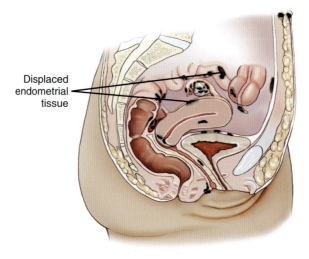

Displaced endometrial tissue

Figure 6.4 _____ / _____ .
           endometrium   abnormal condition

9. MATCH: *Draw a line to match the combining form or suffix with its definition.*

a. -logy   woman (women)
b. -logist   visual examination
c. -scope   one who studies and treats (specialist, physician)
d. -scopy   study of
e. gynec/o   instrument used for visual examination

10. BUILD: *Build the following terms, using the word parts from the previous exercise and the combining form* **colp/o** *for vagina:*

a. instrument used for visual examination of the vagina

_____/ o /_____
                wr   cv   s

b. visual examination of the vagina

_____/ o /_____
                wr   cv   s

c. study of women (female reproductive system)

_____/ o /_____
                wr   cv   s

d. physician who studies and treats disease of women
   (female reproductive system)

_____/ o /_____
                wr   cv   s

11. READ: Colposcopy (kol-POS-ko-pē) is performed by a **gynecologist** (gīn-ek-OL-o-jist) to provide a closer look at vaginal tissue, the vulva, and the cervix. It is performed with a **colposcope** (KOL-pō-skōp) equipped with a light and microscope. A biopsy may be performed during colposcopy if abnormal tissue is present. Colposcopy can be used to diagnose cancers of the vulva, vagina, and cervix, as well as genital warts and cervicitis.

12. MATCH: *Draw a line to match the suffix with its definition.*

a. -cele   surgical fixation
b. -pexy   hernia, protrusion

13. TRANSLATE: *Complete the definitions of the following terms by using the meaning of word parts to fill in the blanks. (HINT: use a the definition that starts with a* **p** *for the first term)*

a. cyst/o/cele   _____ of the (urinary) _____
                    (through anterior vaginal wall)

b. hyster/o/pexy   surgical _____ of the _____

14. READ: Weakening of pelvic muscles and ligaments resulting from traumatic vaginal childbirth, straining during bowel movements, and normal aging can lead to displacement of pelvic organs as seen in **cystocele** (SIS-tō-sēl), and rectocele. Cystocele refers to the protrusion of the urinary bladder into the vagina through the anterior vaginal wall, while rectocele describes protrusion of the rectum against the posterior wall of the vagina. **Hysteropexy** (HIS-ter-ō-pek-sē) may be performed when the uterus is dropping into the superior portion of the vagina (uterovaginal prolapse).

15. LABEL: *Write word parts to complete Figure 6.5.*

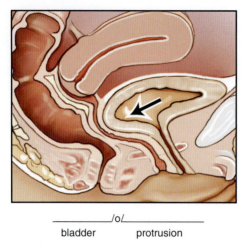

_____/o/_____
    bladder   protrusion

Figure 6.5 Protrusion of the bladder through the anterior wall of the vagina.

16. MATCH: *Draw a line to match the suffix with its definition.*

a. -gram   surgical removal, excision
b. -pexy   record, radiographic image
c. -ectomy   suturing, repairing
d. -rrhexis   surgical fixation
e. -rrhaphy   rupture

> **FYI**   All four **–rrh** suffixes have now been introduced: **-rrhea**, **-rrhagia**, **-rrhaphy**, and **-rrhexis**. Can you recall their definitions?

17. BUILD: *Write word parts to build terms describing procedures used to diagnose and treat abnormalities of the uterus, the uterine tubes, and the ovaries.*

a. excision of the uterus

                                          _____/_____
                                                    wr   **s**

b. surgical fixation of the ovary

                                          _____/_o_/_____
                                                    wr   **cv**   **s**

c. rupture of the uterus

                                          _____/_o_/_____
                                                    wr   **cv**   **s**

d. suturing of the uterus

                                          _____/_o_/_____
                                                    wr   **cv**   **s**

18. **READ: Hysterorrhexis** (his-ter-ō-REK-sis), while rare, is a risk factor in a vaginal birth after a previous birth by Cesarean section. Any suturing of the uterus may be referred to as **hysterorrhaphy** (his-ter-OR-a-fē). Hysteroptosis, or uterine prolapse, may be treated surgically by **hysteropexy** (HIS-ter-ō-pek-sē) and, in more severe cases, by **hysterectomy** (his-te-REK-to-mē). **Oophoropexy** (ō-OF-ō-rō-pek-sē), where the ovaries are positioned outside the radiation field, may be performed to preserve fertility in cancer patients receiving radiation to the pelvic area.

19. **TRANSLATE:** *Complete the definitions of the following terms by using the meaning of word parts to fill in the blanks.*

   a. cervic/ectomy   _____ of the _____

   b. oophor/ectomy   _____ of the _____

   c. hyster/o/salping/o/–oophor/ectomy   excision of the _____, uterine _____(s), and _____ (plural)

   d. hyster/o/salping/o/gram   _____ image of the _____ and _____ tubes

> **FYI** A hyphen is often used between two word parts when one ends and the other begins with the same vowel, as in the term **salpingo-oophoritis**.

20. **READ:** A **hysterosalpingogram** (his-ter-ō-sal-PING-gō-gram), which is often performed in fertility studies, provides a radiographic image of the inside of the uterus and the uterine tubes. The image is analyzed by a radiologist and may be used to assess the patency (openness) of uterine tubes and to diagnose uterine abnormalities.

21. **LABEL:** *Write word parts to complete Figure 6.6.*

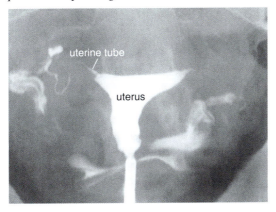

uterine tube

uterus

> **FYI** Use your medical dictionary or a reliable online source to learn more about **hysterosalpingogram** and the use of **fluoroscopy** in obtaining the image.

Figure 6.6 _____/o/_____/o/_____.
                uterus   uterine tube   radiographic image

22. **READ: Cervicectomy** (ser-vi-SEK-to-mē), hysterectomy, **oophorectomy** (ō-of-o-REK-to-mē), and **hysterosalpingo-oophorectomy** (his-ter-ō-sal-ping-gō-ō-of-ō-REK-to-mē) are surgical procedures used to treat cancer and other pelvic abnormalities.

23. **LABEL:** *Write word parts to complete Figure 6.7.*

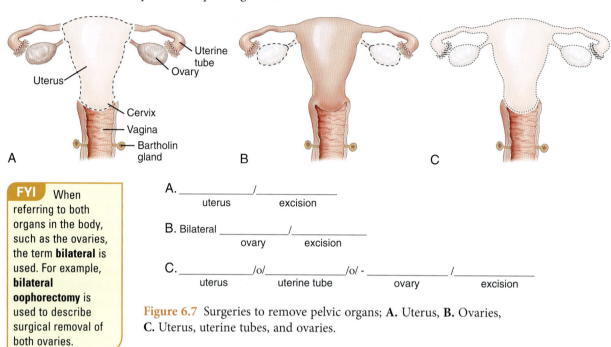

FYI   When referring to both organs in the body, such as the ovaries, the term **bilateral** is used. For example, **bilateral oophorectomy** is used to describe surgical removal of both ovaries.

A. _____/_____
         uterus   excision

B. Bilateral _____/_____
                        ovary   excision

C. _____/o/_____/o/ - _____/_____
         uterus   uterine tube   ovary   excision

Figure 6.7 Surgeries to remove pelvic organs; **A.** Uterus, **B.** Ovaries, **C.** Uterus, uterine tubes, and ovaries.

---

24. **MATCH:** *Draw a line to match the word part with its definition.*

    a. a-   rapid flow of blood; excessive bleeding
    b. dys-   flow, discharge
    c. men/o   without, absence of
    d. -rrhea   difficult, painful, abnormal
    e. -rrhagia   menstruation, menstrual

FYI   The combining form **men/o** is used in medicine to describe the monthly or menstrual cycle in women. It is derived from the Greek word **mene**, or moon, which refers to the lunar month.

---

25. **TRANSLATE:** *Complete the definitions of the following terms built from the combining form **men/o**, meaning menstruation, menstrual. Hints: use **flow** for the definition of -rrhea, and begin the definition with the prefix if present.*

    a. a/men/o/rrhea   _____ menstrual _____

    b. dys/men/o/rrhea   _____ flow

    c. men/o/rrhea   flow at _____

    d. men/o/rrhagia   _____ flow of blood at _____

26. **READ: Menorrhea** (men-ō-RĒ-a) refers to normal discharge during menstruation. Primary **dysmenorrhea** (dis-men-ō-RĒ-a) refers to pelvic cramping occurring with normal menstruation. Secondary dysmenorrhea refers to pelvic cramping resulting from a disease process, such as endometriosis. **Menorrhagia** (men-ō-RĀ-jea) indicates heavy menstrual bleeding and may be caused by fibroid tumors, hormonal imbalance, ectopic pregnancy, and abnormal conditions of pregnancy. **Amenorrhea** (a-men-ō-RĒ-a) is the absence of menstruation as seen with pregnancy, menopause, some medications, excessive weight loss or exercise, and stress.

27. **MATCH:** *Draw a line to match the suffix or combining form with its definition.*

    a. -gram
    b. -graphy
    c. -plasty
    d. -ectomy
    e. mamm/o, mast/o
    f. son/o
    g. -pexy

    surgical repair
    breast
    record, radiographic image
    process of recording, radiographic imaging
    surgical removal, excision
    surgical fixation
    sound

> **FYI**   **Mamm** is of Latin origin, and **mast** is of Greek origin. With practice, you will become familiar with their use in medical terms.

28. **BUILD:** *Write word parts to build terms describing diagnosis and treatment of the breast. Hint: use **mast/o** to build the first two terms, and **mamm/o** for any remaining terms that relate to the breast.*

    a. excision of the breast

    _____ / _____
                    wr   s

    b. surgical fixation of the breast

    _____ / o / _____
                wr   cv   s

    c. radiographic image of the breast

    _____ / o / _____
                wr   cv   s

    d. radiographic imaging of the breast

    _____ / o / _____
                wr   cv   s

    e. surgical repair of the breast

    _____ / o / _____
                wr   cv   s

    f. process of recording sound

    _____ / o / _____
                wr   cv   s

29. **READ: Mammography** (ma-MOG-ra-fē) is a radiography procedure that uses specialized equipment to obtain an image of the breast for examination. The resulting image is a **mammogram** (MAM-ō-gram). Mammography is used for screening when no symptoms are present and for diagnosis when a lump has been detected, nipple discharge is present, or as warranted based on findings of a screening mammogram. **Sonography** (so-NOG-rah-fē), also called ultrasound, is a diagnostic imaging procedure that can be used to determine whether a lump is cystic (fluid-filled) or solid. **Mastectomy** (mas-TEK-tō-mē) is a surgical procedure used to prevent and treat breast cancer. **Mammoplasty** (MAM-ō-plas-tē) is a surgical procedure to alter the

size and shape of the breast through augmentation, reduction, or for reconstruction after mastectomy. **Mastopexy** (MAS-tō-pek-sē), a surgical procedure to lift sagging breast tissue, may be performed after weight loss, pregnancy, or removal of an implant.

> **FYI**   Refer back to the table in Lesson 2 for a review of diagnostic imaging procedures, including radiography and sonography.

30.   LABEL: *Write word parts to complete Figure 6.8.*

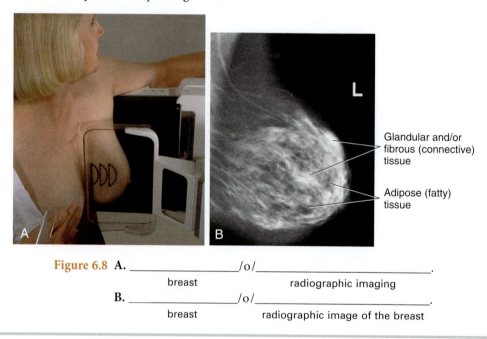

Figure 6.8 **A.** _____ /o/ _____.
                        breast   radiographic imaging
             B. _____ /o/ _____.
                        breast   radiographic image of the breast

31.   REVIEW OF FEMALE REPRODUCTIVE SYSTEM TERMS BUILT FROM WORD PARTS: the following is an alphabetical list of terms built and translated in the previous exercises.

MEDICAL TERMS BUILT FROM WORD PARTS

TERM	DEFINITION	TERM	DEFINITION
1. amenorrhea (a-men-ō-RĒ-a)	without menstrual flow	**5. colposcope** (KOL-pō-skōp)	instrument used for visual examination of the vagina
2. cervical (SER-vi-kal)	pertaining to the cervix	**6. colposcopy** (kol-POS-ko-pē)	visual examination of the vagina
3. cervicectomy (ser-vi-SEK-to-mē)	excision of the cervix (also called **trachelectomy**)	**7. cystocele** (SIS-tō-sēl)	protrusion of the bladder (through anterior vaginal wall) (Figure 6.5)
4. cervicitis (ser-vi-SĪ-tis)	inflammation of the cervix (Figure 6.3, 2)	**8. dysmenorrhea** (dis-men-ō-RĒ-a)	painful menstrual flow

MEDICAL TERMS BUILT FROM WORD PARTS—cont'd

TERM	DEFINITION	TERM	DEFINITION
9. **endometrial** (en-dō-MĒ-trē-l)	pertaining to the endometrium	22. **mammoplasty** (MAM-ō-plas-tē)	surgical repair of the breast
10 **endometriosis** (en-dō-mē-trē-Ō-sis)	abnormal condition of the endometrium (growth of endometrial tissue outside of the uterus) (Figure 6.4)	23. **mastectomy** (mas-TEK-tō-mē)	excision of the breast
11. **endometritis** (en-dō-mē-TRĪ-tis)	inflammation of the endometrium (Figure 6.3, *1*)	24. **mastopexy** (MAS-tō-pek-sē)	surgical fixation of the breast (performed to lift sagging breast tissue or to create symmetry)
12. **gynecologist** (gīn-ek-OL-o-jist)	physician who studies and treats diseases of women	25. **mastitis** (mas-TĪ-tis)	inflammation of the breast
13. **gynecology** (gīn-ek-OL-o-jē)	study of women (the branch of medicine focused on the health and diseases of the female reproductive system)	26. **menorrhagia** (men-ō-RĀ-jea)	rapid flow of blood at menstruation
14. **hysterectomy** (his-te-REK-to-mē)	excision of the uterus (Figure 6.7, *A*)	27. **menorrhea** (men-ō-RĒ-a)	flow at menstruation
15. **hysteropexy** (HIS-ter-ō-pek-sē)	surgical fixation of the uterus	28. **oophorectomy** (ō-of-o-REK-tō-mē)	excision of the ovary (Figure 6.7, *B*)
16. **hysterorrhaphy** (his-ter-OR-a-fē)	suturing of the uterus	29. **oophoritis** (ō-of-o-RĪ-tis)	inflammation of the ovary
17. **hysterorrhexis** (his-ter-ō-REK-sis)	rupture of the uterus	30. **oophoropexy** (ō-OF-ō-rō-pek-sē)	surgical fixation of the ovary
18. **hysterosalpingogram** (his-ter-ō-sal-PING-gō-gram)	radiographic image of the uterus and uterine tubes (Figure 6.6)	31. **salpingitis** (sal-pin-JĪ-tis)	inflammation of the uterine tube (Figure 6.3, *4*)
19. **hysterosalpingo-oophorectomy** (his-ter-ō-sal-ping-gō-ō-of-ō-REK-to-mē)	excision of the uterus, uterine tubes, and ovaries (Figure 6.7, *C*)	32. **sonography** (so-NOG-rah-fē)	process of recording sound (also called **ultrasonography**)
20. **mammogram** (MAM-ō-gram)	radiographic image of the breast (Figure 6.8, *B*)	33. **vaginal** (VAJ-i-nal)	pertaining to the vagina
21. **mammography** (ma-MOG-ra-fē)	radiographic imaging of the breast (Figure 6.8, *A*)	34. **vaginitis** (vaj-i-NĪ-tis)	inflammation of the vagina (Figure 6.3, *3*)

EXERCISE B   **Pronounce and Spell Terms Built from Word Parts**

Practice pronunciation and spelling on paper and online.

1. **Practice on Paper**
   a. **Pronounce:** Read the phonetic spelling and say aloud the terms listed in the previous table, Review of Female Reproductive System Terms Built from Word Parts.
   b. **Spell:** Have a study partner read the terms aloud. Write the spelling of the terms on a separate sheet of paper.

2. **Practice Online** 🌐
   a. **Access** online learning resources. Go to evolve.elsevier.com > Evolve Resources > Practice Student Resources.
   b. **Pronounce:** Select Audio Glossary > Lesson 6 > Exercise B. Select a term to hear its pronunciation and repeat aloud.
   c. **Spell:** Select Activities > Lesson 6 > Spell Terms > Exercise B. Select the audio icon and type the correct spelling of the term.

❏   Check the box when complete.

EXERCISE C   **Build and Translate MORE Medical Terms Built from Word Parts**

1. **LABEL:** *Write the combining forms for anatomical structures of the male reproductive system on Figure 6.9. These anatomical combining forms will be used to build and translate medical terms in Exercise C.*

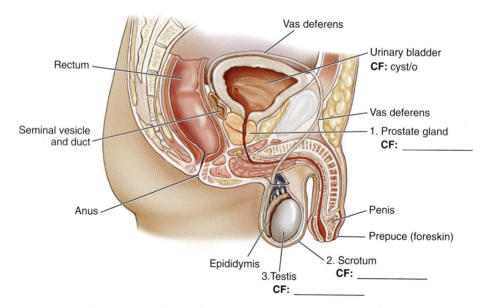

Figure 6.9 Male reproductive system with combining forms.

2. MATCH: *Draw a line to match the combining form or suffix with its definition.*

    a. cyst/o   inflammation
    b. lith/o   bladder, sac
    c. -itis   pertaining to
    d. -ectomy   stone(s), calculus (*pl.* calculi)
    e. -ic   surgical removal, excision

3. TRANSLATE: *Complete the definitions of the following terms built from the combining form **prostat/o**, meaning prostate gland.*

    a. prostat/itis   _____ of the _____ gland
    b. prostat/o/cyst/itis   inflammation of the prostate _____ and the (urinary) _____
    c. prostat/ic   _____ to the _____ gland
    d. prostat/o/lith   _____(s) in the prostate _____
    e. prostat/ectomy   _____ of the prostate gland

4. READ: Bacterial **prostatitis** (pros-ta-TĪ-tis) may be acute, characterized by a sudden onset of symptoms, or chronic, as seen with recurring urinary tract infections. In **prostatocystitis** (pros-ta-tō-sis-TĪ-tis) the prostate gland and the bladder are affected. The formation of one or more **prostatoliths** (pros-TAT-ō-liths) may contribute to **prostatic** (pros-TAT-ik) inflammation. **Prostatectomy** (pros-ta-TEK-to-mē) is a surgical procedure used to treat prostate cancer.

5. LABEL: *Write word parts to complete Figure 6.10.*

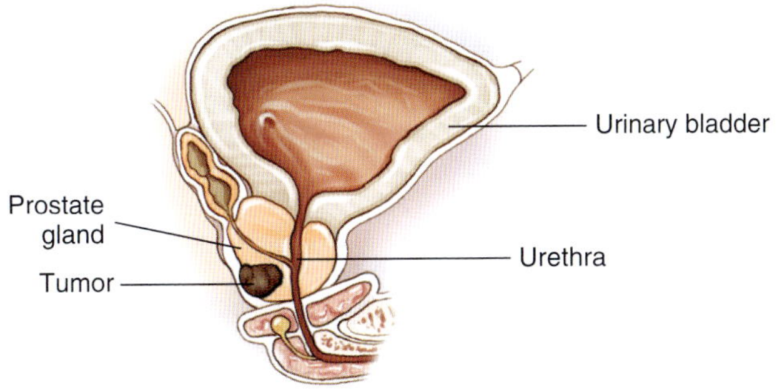

          Urinary bladder
     Prostate gland
     Urethra
     Tumor

Figure 6.10 _____/_____ cancer.
               prostate   pertaining to

6. MATCH: *Draw a line to match the prefix or suffix with its definition.*

    a. -itis   surgical fixation
    b. -ectomy   inflammation
    c. -pexy   surgical removal, excision
    d. -al   surgical repair
    e. -plasty   pertaining to

7. **BUILD:** *Write word parts to build the following terms using the combining forms* **orchi/o**, *meaning testis (testicle), and* **scrot/o**, *meaning scrotum.*

a. inflammation of the testis

_____/_____
wr   s

b. surgical fixation of the testis

_____/_o_/_____
wr   cv   s

c. excision of the testis

_____/_____
wr   s

d. pertaining to the scrotum

_____/_____
wr   s

e. surgical repair of the scrotum

_____/_o_/_____
wr   cv   s

8. **READ: Orchitis** (or-KĪ-tis) results from a viral infection, as seen in mumps, or a bacterial infection, as seen in sexually transmitted infections such as gonorrhea and chlamydia. The infection may be unilateral, involving one testicle or bilateral, involving both testicles. **Orchiopexy** (OR-kē-ō-pek-sē) is a surgical procedure that may be performed to bring an undescended testicle into the scrotum. **Orchiectomy** (or-kē-EK-to-mē) is a surgical procedure performed to treat testicular cancer and may be unilateral or bilateral. **Scrotoplasty** (SKRŌ-tō-plas-tē) describes surgical procedures to repair the **scrotal** (SKRŌT-al) sac, including placement of testicular implants after an orchiectomy.

9. **MATCH:** *Draw a line to match the combining form or the suffix with its definition.*

a. vas/o   creation of an artificial opening
b. -ectomy   surgical removal, excision
c. -stomy   vessel, duct (refers to vas deferens in the context of the male reproductive system)

10. **TRANSLATE:** *Complete the definitions of surgical terms by using the meaning of word parts to fill in the blanks:*

a. vas/ectomy   _____ of the _____ (vas deferens)
b. vas/o/vas/o/stomy   _____ of an artificial _____ between _____(s)

11. **READ: Vasectomy** (va-SEK-to-mē) is a surgical procedure to remove a portion of the vas deferens for the purpose of birth control by preventing the flow of sperm to the outside of the body. A **vasovasostomy** (vas-ō-vā-ZOS-to-mē) may be performed at a later time to reverse the vasectomy and to reconnect the vas deferens, potentially returning male fertility.

12. **LABEL:** *Write word parts to complete Figure 6.11.*

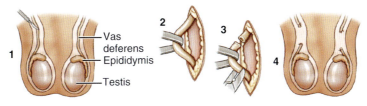

1. incision is made into the covering of the vas deferens
2. vas deferens is exposed
3. segment of vas deferens is excised
4. vas deferens is repositioned and skin is sutured

Figure 6.11 _____ / _____ .
          duct   excision

13. **REVIEW OF MALE REPRODUCTIVE SYSTEM TERMS BUILT FROM WORD PARTS:** the following is an alphabetical list of terms built and translated in the previous exercises.

MEDICAL TERMS BUILT FROM WORD PARTS

TERM	DEFINITION	TERM	DEFINITION
1. **orchiectomy** (or-kē-EK-to-mē)	excision of the testis	7. **prostatocystitis** (pros-ta-tō-sis-TĪ-tis)	inflammation of the prostate gland and the bladder
2. **orchitis** (or-KĪ-tis)	inflammation of the testis	8. **prostatolith** (pros-TAT-ō-lith)	stone(s) in the prostate gland
3. **orchiopexy** (OR-kē-ō-pek-sē)	surgical fixation of the testis	9. **scrotal** (SKRŌT-al)	pertaining to the scrotum
4. **prostatectomy** (pros-ta-TEK-to-mē)	excision of the prostate gland	10. **scrotoplasty** (SKRŌ-tō-plas-tē)	surgical repair of the scrotum
5. **prostatic** (pros-TAT-ik)	pertaining to the prostate gland (Figure 6.10)	11. **vasectomy** (va-SEK-to-mē)	excision of the duct (vas deferens) (Figure 6.11)
6. **prostatitis** (pros-ta-TĪ-tis)	inflammation of the prostate gland	12. **vasovasostomy** (vas-ō-vā-ZOS-to-mē)	creation of an artificial opening between ducts

EXERCISE D   Pronounce and Spell MORE Terms Built from Word Parts

Practice pronunciation and spelling on paper and online.

1. **Practice on Paper**
   a. **Pronounce:** Read the phonetic spelling and say aloud the terms listed in the previous table, Review of Male Reproductive System Terms Built from Word Parts.
   b. **Spell:** Have a study partner read the terms aloud. Write the spelling of the terms on a separate sheet of paper.

2. **Practice Online** 🌐

   a. **Access** online learning resources. Go to evolve.elsevier.com > Evolve Resources > Practice Student Resources.
   b. **Pronounce:** Select Audio Glossary > Lesson 6 > Exercise D. Select a term to hear its pronunciation and repeat aloud.
   c. **Spell:** Select Activities > Lesson 6 > Spell Terms > Exercise D. Select the audio icon and type the correct spelling of the term.

❏ Check the box when complete.

OBJECTIVE 2

Define, pronounce, and spell medical terms NOT built from word parts.

The terms listed below may contain word parts, but are difficult to translate literally.

FYI **Pap test** is named after Dr. George N. Papanicolaou (1883–1962), who in 1943 developed the original method of "smearing" cervical cells directly on a microscopic slide to evaluate for the possibility of cancer. This may be used for tissue specimens from any organ, but is most commonly used in cervical and vaginal secretions. More recently, a Pap test has been developed which involves releasing the cells into a vial of liquid preservative, and then transferring them to a microscopic slide in the lab. Both tests are excellent at detecting pre-cancerous abnormalities, and have contributed to a 70% decrease in cervical cancer deaths in the United States over the last 50 years.

FEMALE REPRODUCTIVE SYSTEM TERMS NOT BUILT FROM WORD PARTS

TERM	DEFINITION
dilation and curettage (D&C) (dī-LĀ-shun) (and) (kū-re-TAHZH)	surgical procedure to widen the cervix and scrape the endometrium with an instrument called a curette
obstetrics (ob-STET-riks)	branch of medicine that deals with the management of pregnancy, labor, and the post-partum period (approximately 6 weeks after giving birth)
Pap test (pap) (test)	laboratory test involving cytological study of cervical and vaginal secretions used to determine the presence of abnormal or cancerous cells (also called **Pap smear**)
pelvic inflammatory disease (PID) (PEL-vik) (in-FLAM-a-tor-ē) (di-ZĒZ)	inflammation of some or all of the female reproductive organs; can be caused by many different pathogens
uterine fibroid (Ū-ter-in) (FĪ-broyd)	benign tumor of the uterine muscle (also called **myoma and leiomyoma**)
uterovaginal prolapse (ū-ter-ō-VAG-i-nal) (PRO-laps)	downward displacement of the uterus into the vagina

FYI **Cancers of the Reproductive Systems** affect the organs of the female and male reproductive systems. Consult the Merck Manual Home Edition at merckmanual.com/home/ for more information about specific cancers.

Female Reproductive System	*Male Reproductive System*
breast cancer	penile cancer
vulvar cancer	testicular cancer
vaginal cancer	prostate cancer
cervical cancer	
uterine cancer	
uterine tube cancer	
ovarian cancer	

MALE REPRODUCTIVE SYSTEM TERMS NOT BUILT FROM WORD PARTS

TERM	DEFINITION
benign prostatic hyperplasia (**BPH**) (be-NĪN) (pros-TAT-ik) (hī-per-PLĀ-zha)	nonmalignant enlargement of the prostate gland
circumcision (ser-kum-SI-shun)	surgical removal of all or part of the foreskin of the penis
digital rectal examination (**DRE**) (DIJ-i-tal) (REK-tal) (eg-zam-i-NĀ-shun)	physical examination in which the healthcare provider inserts a gloved finger into the rectum and palpates the size and shape of the prostate gland through the rectal wall; used to screen for BPH and prostate cancer. BPH usually presents as a uniform, nontender enlargement, whereas cancer usually presents as a stony hard nodule.
erectile dysfunction (**ED**) (e-REK-tīl) (dis-FUNK-shun)	inability of the male to attain or maintain an erection sufficient to perform sexual intercourse (formerly called impotence)
prostate-specific antigen (**PSA**) **assay** (PROS-tāt) (spe-SIF-ik) (AN-ti-gen) (AS-ā)	blood test that measures the level of prostate-specific antigen, a protein produced by the prostate gland
semen analysis (SĒ-men) (a-NAL-i-sis)	laboratory test involving microscopic observation of ejaculated semen, revealing the size, structure, and movement of sperm; used to evaluate male infertility and to determine the effectiveness of a vasectomy (also called **sperm count** and **sperm test**)
sexually transmitted infection (**STI**) (SEKS-ū-al-ē) (TRANS-mi-ted) (in-FEK-shun)	infection spread through sexual contact (also called **sexually transmitted disease (STD)**)
transurethral resection of the prostate gland (**TURP**) (trans-ū-RĒ-thral) (rē-SEK-shun) (of) (the) (PROS-tāt)	surgical removal of pieces of the prostate gland tissue by using an instrument inserted through the urethra

FYI   **Sexually Transmitted Infection (STI) vs. Sexually Transmitted Disease(STD): what's the difference?** Usually, a "disease" refers to a clear medical problem, often with signs or symptoms. But patients with an infection may have no signs or symptoms and still have the problem. While **STI** is medically more accurate, you will also frequently hear the term **STD**. These infections affect both females and males, causing damage to reproductive organs and potentially serious health consequences if left untreated. Any sexual behavior involving contact with the body fluids of another person puts an individual at risk for infection.

Consult the Centers for Disease Control and Prevention website at cdc.gov/std/ or your medical dictionary for more information about the following common sexually transmitted diseases:

Parasitic
- pubic lice
- trichomoniasis

Bacterial
- chlamydia
- gonorrhea
- syphilis
- vaginosis

Viral
- cytomegalovirus
- genital herpes
- hepatitis B
- human immunodeficiency virus (HIV)/AIDS
- human papillomavirus (HPV)

EXERCISE E   Label

Write the medical terms pictured and defined using the previous table of Medical Terms NOT Built from Word Parts. Check your work with the Answer Key in Appendix C.

1. _____

surgical procedure to widen the cervix and scrape the endometrium with an instrument called a curette

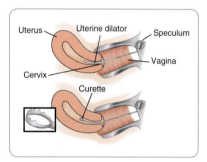

2. _____

benign tumor of the uterine muscle

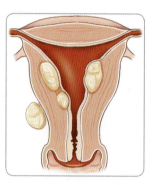

3. _____

nonmalignant enlargement of the prostate gland

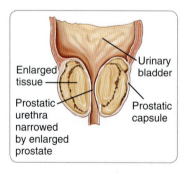

4. _____

inflammation of some or all of the female reproductive organs; can be caused by many different pathogens

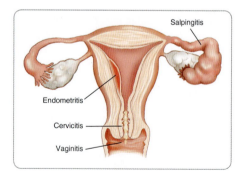

5. _____

surgical removal of pieces of the prostate gland tissue by using an instrument inserted through the urethra

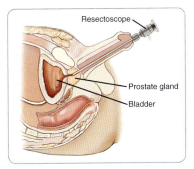

Resectoscope

Prostate gland

Bladder

6. _____

surgical removal of all or part of the foreskin of the penis

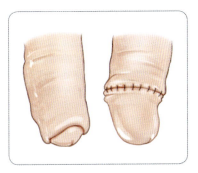

7. _____

laboratory test involving cytological study of cervical and vaginal secretions used to determine the presence of abnormal or cancerous cells

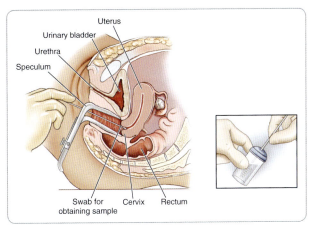

Uterus

Urinary bladder

Urethra

Speculum

Swab for obtaining sample   Cervix   Rectum

EXERCISE F **Learn Medical Terms NOT Built from Word Parts**

Fill in the blanks with medical terms defined and abbreviated in bold using the Female and Male Reproductive Systems Terms Not Built from Word Parts tables. Check your responses with the Answer Key in Appendix C.

1. A **cytologic study of cervical and vaginal secretions,** or _____, is used to detect cancers of the cervix and is generally recommended for women between the ages of 21 and 65.

2. Human papillomavirus (HPV) is a common **infection spread through sexual contact** _____ _____, which is associated with the development of cervical cancer. Penile, anal, vulvar, vaginal, and throat cancers are also linked to HPV infection.

> **FYI**   The Food and Drug Administration (FDA) approved the first vaccine against **human papillomavirus (HPV)** in 2006, directly impacting the prevention of cervical cancer. The vaccine is highly effective in protecting against a majority of forms of HPV as long as it is administered before a male or female becomes sexually active. Because vaccination is not 100% effective, periodic cervical cancer screening is recommended.

3. Although sometimes asymptomatic, **benign tumors of the uterine muscle** _____ made up of mainly fibrous tissue may cause pelvic pain, heavy bleeding, miscarriage, or pregnancy loss.

4. **PID,** or _____, characterized by inflammation of some or all of the female reproductive organs, is caused by an infection. The patient may have fever, foul-smelling vaginal discharge, and pain in the lower abdomen. PID may result in infertility if left untreated.

5. A **D&C,** or _____, is performed to diagnose disease, correct bleeding, or empty uterine contents, such as tissue remaining after a miscarriage.

6. A **blood test that measures the level of PSA,** or _____, is used for early detection of prostate cancer along with a **DRE,** or _____. An elevated PSA level or a palpated, stony hard nodule may indicate cancer. The assay is also used to monitor the disease after treatment.

7. A patient with a **nonmalignant enlargement of the prostate gland,** or _____ _____, may have difficulty with urination. As a result, the bladder may retain urine, causing the patient to be more susceptible to bladder infections. Treatment may include **surgical removal of pieces of the prostate gland tissue using an instrument inserted through the urethra,** or _____ _____.

8. **ED,** or _____, is common in men who have undergone prostate surgery. Other causes of ED include diabetes and cardiovascular disease. Medications that work by relaxing smooth muscle cells and increasing the flow of blood to the genital area are the current first-line treatment.

9. **Surgical removal of all or part of the foreskin of the penis,** or _____, is practiced by many cultures throughout the world for religious or health reasons. The Latin term translates as "a cutting around."

10. A **laboratory test involving microscopic observation of ejaculated semen, revealing the size, structure, and movement of sperm,** or _____, is one of the first steps in evaluating a couple for infertility, which is usually described as a failure to achieve pregnancy after twelve months or more of regular, unprotected sexual intercourse.

11. **Branch of medicine that deals with the management of pregnancy, labor, and the post-partum period,** or _____ is a field that centers around pregnancy, while gynecology addresses the health and diseases of females outside of pregnancy. An obstetrician/gynecologist specializes in both forms of care.

12. Downward displacement of the uterus into the vagina, or _____, is caused by weakening of the pelvic muscles and ligaments, often due to previous childbirth, straining, or loss of estrogen during normal aging. Nonsurgical treatment may include pelvic strengthening exercises or a pessary (a device inserted into the vagina to keep the uterus in place). Hysteropexy and hysterectomy are surgical treatments for this disorder.

EXERCISE G **Pronounce and Spell Terms NOT Built from Word Parts**

Practice pronunciation and spelling on paper and online.

1. **Practice on Paper**
   a. **Pronounce:** Read the phonetic spelling and say aloud the terms listed in the previous Medical Terms NOT Built from Word Parts tables.
   b. **Spell:** Have a study partner read the terms aloud. Write the spelling of the terms on a separate sheet of paper.

2. **Practice Online** 🌐
   a. **Access** online learning resources. Go to evolve.elsevier.com > Evolve Resources > Practice Student Resources.
   b. **Pronounce:** Select Audio Glossary > Lesson 6 > Exercise G. Select a term to hear its pronunciation and repeat aloud.
   c. **Spell:** Select Activities > Lesson 6 > Spell Terms > Exercise G. Select the audio icon and type the correct spelling of the term.

❏ Check the box when complete.

OBJECTIVE 3

Write abbreviations.

ABBREVIATIONS FOR THE REPRODUCTIVE SYSTEMS

Use the online **flashcards** to familiarize yourself with the following abbreviations.

ABBREVIATION	TERM	ABBREVIATION	TERM
BPH	benign prostatic hyperplasia	PID	pelvic inflammatory disease
Cx	cervix	PSA	prostate-specific antigen
D&C	dilation and curettage	RP	radical prostatectomy
DRE	digital rectal examination	STD	sexually transmitted disease
ED	erectile dysfunction	STI	sexually transmitted infection
HPV	human papillomavirus	TAH/BSO	total abdominal hysterectomy/ bilateral salpingo-oophorectomy
HSG	hysterosalpingogram	TRUS	transrectal ultrasound
OB/GYN	obstetrician-gynecologist	TURP	transurethral resection of the prostate gland

EXERCISE H   Abbreviate Medical Terms

Write the correct abbreviation next to its medical term.

1. Diseases and Disorders:

   a. _____   sexually transmitted infection

   b. _____   sexually transmitted disease

   c. _____   pelvic inflammatory disease

   d. _____   benign prostatic hyperplasia

   e. _____   human papillomavirus

   f. _____   erectile dysfunction

2. Diagnostic Tests:

   a. _____   digital rectal examination

   b. _____   prostate-specific antigen

   c. _____   hysterosalpingogram

   d. _____   transrectal ultrasound

3. Surgical Procedures:

   a. _____   dilation and curettage

   b. _____   transurethral resection of the prostate gland

   c. _____   total abdominal hysterectomy/bilateral salpingo-oophorectomy

   d. _____   radical prostatectomy

4. Specialties and Professions:

   _____   obstetrician-gynecologist

5. Related Terms:

   _____   cervix

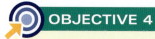 **OBJECTIVE 4**

Identify medical terms by clinical category.

Now that you have worked through the reproductive systems lesson, review and practice medical terms grouped by clinical category. Categories include signs and symptoms, diseases and disorders, diagnostic tests and equipment, surgical procedures, specialties and professions, and related terms related to the female and male reproductive systems. Check your responses with the Answer Key in Appendix C.

EXERCISE I   **Signs and Symptoms**

Write the medical terms for signs and symptoms next to their definitions.

1. _____   rapid flow of blood at menstruation

2. _____   without menstrual flow

3. _____   painful menstrual flow

EXERCISE J   **Diseases and Disorders**

Write the medical terms for diseases and disorders next to their definitions.

1. _____   nonmalignant enlargement of the prostate gland

2. _____   inability of the male to attain or maintain an erection sufficient to perform sexual intercourse

3. _____   infection spread through sexual contact (also called **sexually transmitted disease**)

4. _____   inflammation of the cervix

5. _____   protrusion of the bladder (through anterior vaginal wall)

6. _____   inflammation of the endometrium

7. _____   abnormal condition of the endometrium (growth of endometrial tissue outside of the uterus)

8. _____   downward displacement of the uterus into the vagina.

9. _____   inflammation of the breast

10. _____   inflammation of the ovary

11. _____   inflammation of the uterine tube

12. _____   inflammation of the vagina

13. _____   inflammation of the testis

14. _____   inflammation of the prostate gland

15. _____   inflammation of the prostate gland and the bladder

16. _____   stone(s) in the prostate gland

17. _____   inflammation of some or all of the female reproductive organs; can be caused by many different pathogens

18. _____   benign tumor of the uterine muscle (also called **myoma** and **leiomyoma**)

EXERCISE K   Surgical Procedures

Write the medical terms for surgical procedures next to their definitions.

1. _____   excision of the testis

2. _____   surgical fixation of the testis

3. _____   excision of the prostate gland

4. _____   surgical repair of the scrotum

5. _____   excision of the duct (vas deferens)

6. _____   creation of an artificial opening between ducts

7. _____   excision of the cervix (also called **trachelectomy**)

8. _____   excision of the uterus

9. _____   surgical fixation of the uterus

10. _____   suturing of the uterus

11. _____   rupture of the uterus

12. _____   excision of the uterus, uterine tubes, and ovaries

13. _____   surgical repair of the breast

14. _____   excision of the breast

15. _____   excision of the ovary

16. _____   surgical fixation of the ovary

17. _____   surgical removal of pieces of the prostate gland tissue by using
    _____   an instrument inserted through the urethra

18. _____   surgical procedure to widen the cervix and scrape the
    endometrium with an instrument called a curette

19. _____   surgical fixation of the breast (performed to lift sagging breast
    tissue or to create symmetry)

EXERCISE L   Diagnostic Tests and Equipment

Write the medical terms for diagnostic tests and equipment next to their definitions.

1. _____   instrument used for visual examination of the vagina

2. _____   visual examination of the vagina

3. _____   radiographic image of the uterus and uterine tubes

4. _____   radiographic image of the breast

5. _____   radiographic imaging of the breast

6. _____ laboratory test involving cytological study of cervical and vaginal secretions used to determine the presence of abnormal or cancerous cells (also called **Pap smear**)

7. _____ physical examination in which the healthcare provider inserts a gloved finger into the rectum and palpates the size and shape of the prostate gland through the rectal wall

8. _____ blood test that measures the level of a protein produced by the _____ prostate gland

9. _____ laboratory test involving microscopic observation of ejaculated semen, revealing the size, structure, and movement of sperm

10. _____ process of recording sound

EXERCISE M   **Specialties and Professions**

Write the medical terms for specialties and professions next to their definitions.

1. _____ study of women (the branch of medicine focused on the health and diseases of the female reproductive system)

2. _____ physician who studies and treats diseases of women

3. _____ branch of medicine that deals with the management of pregnancy, labor, and the and the post-partum period (approximately 6 weeks after giving birth)

EXERCISE N   **Medical Terms Related to the Reproductive Systems**

Write the medical terms related to the reproductive systems next to their definitions.

1. _____ flow at menstruation

2. _____ pertaining to the vagina

3. _____ pertaining to the cervix

4. _____ pertaining to the endometrium

5. _____ pertaining to the scrotum

6. _____ pertaining to the prostate gland

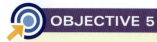

OBJECTIVE 5

Use medical language in clinical statements, the case study, and a medical record.

EXERCISE O | **Use Medical Terms in Clinical Statements**

Circle the medical terms and abbreviations defined in the bolded phrases. Medical terms from previous lessons are included. Answers are listed in Appendix C. For pronunciation practice, read the answers aloud.

1. A **visual examination of the vagina** (hysterosalpingogram, colposcopy, colposcope) is used to further evaluate abnormal **cytologic study of the cervical and vaginal secretions** (Pap test, PSA assay, DRE) results to identify suspicious lesions. A biopsy of the tissue is used to diagnose the condition.

2. Mariana Esteban was experiencing **pertaining to the vagina** (endometrial, cervical, vaginal) itching, burning, and excessive discharge. She was diagnosed with **inflammation of the vagina** (cervicitis, vaginitis, endometritis) caused by *Candida albicans,* a yeastlike fungus.

3. After Lin Xiang's routine **process of radiographic imaging of the breast** (mammogram, mammography) exam, the radiologist discovered a breast lesion on the **radiographic image of the breast** (mammogram, mammography). A biopsy revealed a malignant tumor. A(n) **excision of the breast** (mastectomy, mammoplasty, mastopexy) was performed. The patient is scheduled, at a later date, for reconstructive **surgical repair of the breast** (mastectomy, mammoplasty, mastopexy) with an implant.

4. When **nonmalignant enlargement of the prostate gland** (BPH, PID, ED), chronic **inflammation of the prostate gland** (scrotal, prostatic, prostatitis) or **pertaining to the prostate gland** (prostatolith, prostatitis, prostatic) cancer fails to respond to medical treatment, **excision of the prostate gland** (prostatectomy, scrotoplasty, orchiopexy) may be necessary.

5. A 14-year-old male was admitted to the emergency department with abdominal pain and unilateral **pertaining to the scrotum** (prostatic, scrotoplasty, scrotal) swelling. Testicular torsion was diagnosed; treatment included a unilateral **excision of the testis** (orchitis, orchiopexy, orchiectomy) to remove the damaged testicle and **surgical fixation of the testis** (orchitis, orchiopexy, orchiectomy) of the remaining testicle to prevent future occurrence of testicular torsion.

EXERCISE P | **Apply Medical Terms to the Case Study**

Think back to Cindy and Rajive introduced in the case study at the beginning of the lesson. After working through Lesson 6 on the reproductive systems, consider the medical terms that might be used to describe their experiences. List three terms relevant to the case study and their meanings. ▪

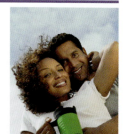

Medical Term **Definition**

1. _____ _____

2. _____ _____

3. _____ _____

EXERCISE Q **Use Medical Terms in a Document**

Cindy and Rajive finally had a heart-to-heart talk about their feelings and decided it was time to reach out for help. Cindy checked in with her gynecologist who referred the couple to the fertility clinic at the local hospital.

Use the definitions in numbers 1-11 to write medical terms within the following consultation report.

1. surgical fixation of the testis

2. flow at menstruation

3. painful menstrual flow

4. rapid flow of blood at menstruation

5. cytological examination of the cervical and vaginal secretions

6. inflammation of the prostate gland

7. infection spread through sexual contact (plural)

8. inflammation of the cervix

9. inflammation of some or all of the female reproductive organs

10. microscopic observation of ejaculated semen, revealing the size, structure, and movement of sperm

11. radiographic image of the uterus and uterine tubes

Refer to the medical record to answer questions 12-14.

12. The term **scrotocele** appears in the medical record. Use your knowledge of word parts to define the term.

    scrot/o means _____

    -cele means _____

    Remember, most definitions begin with the suffix.

    scrot/o/cele means _____

13. Identify the abbreviations used in the Physical Exam section of the report.

    Abbreviation   **Medical Term**

    _____   _____

    _____   _____

14. Identify two new medical terms in the medical record you would like to investigate. Use your medical dictionary or an online resource to look up the definition.

    Medical Term   **Definition**

    1. _____   _____

    2. _____   _____

    3. _____   _____

0120890 COLLIER, Cindy

File   Patient   Navigate   Custom Fields   Help

Chart Review | Encounters | Notes | Labs | Imaging | Procedures | Rx | Documents | Referrals | Scheduling | Billing

| Name: **COLLIER, Cindy** | MR#: 0120890 | Gender: F | **Allergies:** None |
| | DOB: 05/13/19XX | Age: 31 | **PCP:** Alvaro, Belinha MD |

Fertility Clinic Consultation
Encounter Date: 11/03/20XX

History:
Cindy, 31-year-old female and her husband Rajive, a 32-year-old male, present for workup and treatment for infertility. They have been trying to conceive for 14 months. Cindy has never been pregnant and Rajive has never fathered a child. Prior to 14 months ago they used oral contraceptive pills and condoms as their birth control method. Rajive's past medical history is significant for an undescended testicle at birth; this was repaired by (1.) _____ at age 2. He denies any other significant medical history. Cindy had the onset of (2.) _____ at age 14, she has symptoms of (3.) _____ and (4.) _____, both of which have worsened since discontinuing birth control pills. Her menstrual cycles are approximately 26 days long. She had a normal (5.) _____ approximately 1 year ago. Cindy is taking folic acid but no other medications. Rajive is not taking any medications or supplements. They do not smoke cigarettes, drink alcohol or use any other drugs.

Physical Examination:
Rajive has previously had a physical examination with his family doctor. According to the records his genitourinary exam revealed an uncircumcised male with normal external genitalia, no evidence of testicular masses, scrotocele, or hernias. DRE revealed no evidence of BPH or (6.) _____.
Cindy's gynecologic exam today reveals normal external genitalia. Examination of the vagina reveals a small amount of discharge and a slightly inflamed cervix. Vaginal and cervical cultures were obtained to test for (7.)_____
Bimanual exam of the uterus and ovaries reveals diffuse tenderness to palpation with slight fullness in the left adnexa.

Diagnostic Studies:
A complete blood count (CBC) was ordered as well as serum tests for thyroid stimulating hormone, follicle stimulating hormone, and prolactin level. A urine pregnancy test was negative.

Impression:
Primary infertility; cause undetermined. Possible chlamydial (8.) _____ and possible (9.) _____.

Recommendation:
We will await culture results and treat both partners with antibiotics if necessary. If labs are normal, we will proceed with a (10.) _____ for Rajive. We should consider a (11.) _____ for Cindy based on her history and physical exam findings.

Electronically signed: Elyse Conner, MD; Department of Obstetrics and Gynecology

Start | Log On/Off | Print | Edit

EXERCISE R **Use Medical Language in Electronic Health Records Online**

Select the correct medical terms to complete three medical records in one patient's electronic file.

 Access online resources at evolve.elsevier.com > Evolve Resources > Practice Student Resources > Activities > Lesson 6 > Electronic Health Records

Topic: Prostate Cancer
Record 1: Office Visit
Record 2: Pathology Report
Record 3: Progress Note

OBJECTIVE 6

Recall and assess knowledge of word parts, medical terms, and abbreviations.

EXERCISE S **Online Review of Lesson Content**

Recall and assess your learning from working through the lesson by completing online learning activities at evolve. elsevier.com > Evolve Resources > Practice Student Resources. Keep track of your progress by placing a check mark next to completed activities.

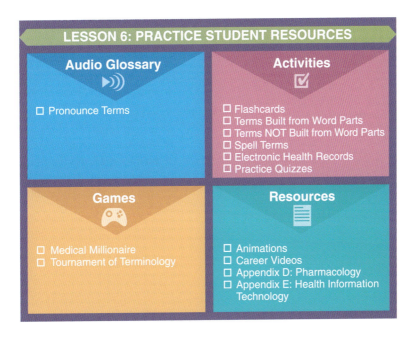

LESSON 6: PRACTICE STUDENT RESOURCES

Audio Glossary
☐ Pronounce Terms

Activities
☐ Flashcards
☐ Terms Built from Word Parts
☐ Terms NOT Built from Word Parts
☐ Spell Terms
☐ Electronic Health Records
☐ Practice Quizzes

Games
☐ Medical Millionaire
☐ Tournament of Terminology

Resources
☐ Animations
☐ Career Videos
☐ Appendix D: Pharmacology
☐ Appendix E: Health Information Technology

EXERCISE T Lesson Content Quiz

Test your knowledge of the terms and abbreviations introduced in this lesson. Circle the letter for the medical term or abbreviation related to the words in italics.

1. *Surgical removal of all or part of the foreskin of the penis* may be performed for cultural or health purposes.
   a. scrotoplasty
   b. circumcision
   c. cervicectomy

2. A *surgical repair of the breast* to reduce size is called reduction:
   a. mammoplasty
   b. mastopexy
   c. mastectomy

3. A *laboratory test involving microscopic observation of ejaculated semen* was ordered after the patient's *excision of a duct (vas deferens)* to evaluate the success of the procedure.
   a. prostate-specific antigen, vasovasostomy
   b. digital rectal examination, orchiopexy
   c. semen analysis, vasectomy

4. Radical *excision of the prostate gland* is used to treat prostate cancer.
   a. prostatectomy
   b. orchiectomy
   c. vasectomy

5. The *surgical procedure to widen the cervix and remove contents from the uterus* can be used for treatment and for diagnostics.
   a. D&C
   b. DRE
   c. HSG

6. *Inflammation of some or all of the female reproductive organs* is often the result of an STI.
   a. endometritis
   b. prostatitis
   c. pelvic inflammatory disease

7. *Surgical fixation of the testis* may be necessary in cases of testicular torsion, in which the spermatic cord becomes twisted, depriving the testicle of its blood supply.
   a. oophoropexy
   b. orchiopexy
   c. hysteropexy

8. For a *cytological study of cervical and vaginal secretions to detect abnormal and cancerous cells,* a scraping of cells from the *pertaining to the cervix* area is obtained for evaluation
   a. Pap test, cervical
   b. mammogram, vaginal
   c. colposcopy, endometrial

9. *Surgical removal of pieces of the prostate gland tissue by using an instrument inserted through the urethra* is associated with a small risk of *inability of the male to attain or maintain an erection sufficient to perform sexual intercourse.*
   a. digital rectal examination; benign prostatic hyperplasia
   b. transurethral resection of the prostate gland (TURP); erectile dysfunction
   c. hysterectomy; hysterorrhexis

10. *Painful menstrual flow* is a common symptom of *abnormal condition of the endometrium (growth of endometrial tissue outside of the uterus).*
    a. amenorrhea; uterine fibroid
    b. menorrhagia; hysterorrhexis
    c. dysmenorrhea; endometriosis

LESSON AT A GLANCE | REPRODUCTIVE SYSTEMS WORD PARTS

COMBINING FORMS
cervic/o	oophor/o
colp/o	orchi/o
endometri/o	prostat/o
gynec/o	salping/o
hyster/o	scrot/o
mamm/o	son/o
mast/o	vagin/o
men/o	vas/o

SUFFIXES
-cele
-pexy
-rrhaphy
-rrhexis

LESSON AT A GLANCE | REPRODUCTIVE SYSTEMS MEDICAL TERMS AND ABBREVIATIONS

SIGNS AND SYMPTOMS
amenorrhea
dysmenorrhea
menorrhagia

DISEASE AND DISORDERS
benign prostatic hyperplasia (BPH)
cervicitis
cystocele
endometriosis
endometritis
erectile dysfunction (ED)
hysterorrhexis
mastitis
oophoritis
orchitis
pelvic inflammatory disease (PID)
prostatitis
prostatocystitis
prostatolith
salpingitis
sexually transmitted infection (STI)
uterine fibroid
uterovaginal prolapse
vaginitis

SURGICAL PROCEDURES
cervicectomy
circumcision
dilation and curettage (D&C)
hysterectomy
hysteropexy
hysterorrhaphy
hysterosalpingo-oophorectomy
mammoplasty
mastectomy
mastopexy
oophorectomy
oophoropexy
orchiectomy
orchiopexy
prostatectomy
scrotoplasty
transurethral resection of the
  prostate gland (TURP)
vasectomy
vasovasostomy

DIAGNOSTIC TESTS AND EQUIPMENT
colposcope
colposcopy
digital rectal examination (DRE)
hysterosalpingogram
mammogram
mammography
Pap test
prostate-specific antigen (PSA) assay
semen analysis
sonography

SPECIALITIES AND PROFESSIONS
gynecologist
gynecology
obstetrics

RELATED TERMS
cervical
endometrial
menorrhea
prostatic
scrotal
vaginal

ABBREVIATIONS
BPH	ED	PID	STI
Cx	HPV	PSA	TAH/BSO
DRE	HSG	RP	TRUS
D&C	OB/GYN	STD	TURP

Cardiovascular and Lymphatic Systems

Natalia Krouse

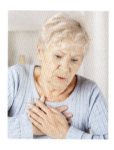

Natalia has not been feeling well lately. She seems to feel "wiped out" most of the time. She wonders if maybe her blood pressure medicine isn't working as well as it used to. Tonight she went for her usual walk with her dogs after dinner. She had barely made it down the driveway when she started feeling pressure in her chest. It felt like something pushing down on her and squeezing her. She noticed pain in her left arm and even in her jaw. She noticed her heart was racing, and she was breathing faster than usual. She was also feeling dizzy at the same time and was afraid she might pass out. She stopped to sit down and after about 5 minutes she started feeling a little better. Her neighbor saw her and called 911. An ambulance came and took her to the Emergency Department of her local hospital.

■ *Consider Natalia's situation as you work through the lesson on the cardiovascular and lymphatic systems. At the end of the lesson, we will return to this case study and identify medical terms used to document Natalia's experience and the care she receives.*

OBJECTIVES

1 ■ Build, translate, pronounce, and spell medical terms built from word parts (p. 186).

2 ■ Define, pronounce, and spell medical terms NOT built from word parts (p. 201).

3 ■ Write abbreviations (p. 207).

4 ■ Identify medical terms by clinical category (p. 208).

5 ■ Use medical language in clinical statements, the case study, and a medical record (p. 211).

6 ■ Recall and assess knowledge of word parts, medical terms, and abbreviations (p. 215).

INTRODUCTION TO THE CARDIOVASCULAR AND LYMPHATIC SYSTEMS

Anatomic Structures of the Cardiovascular System

arteries (AR-te-rēs)	blood vessels that carry blood away from the heart
blood (blud)	fluid circulated through the heart, arteries, capillaries, and veins; composed of plasma and formed elements such as erythrocytes, leukocytes, and thrombocytes (platelets) (Figure 7.1)
blood vessels (blud) (VES-els)	tubelike structures that carry blood throughout the body, including arteries, veins, and capillaries
capillaries (KAP-i-lar-ēs)	microscopic blood vessels; materials are passed between blood and tissues through capillary walls
heart (hart)	muscular, cone-shaped organ the size of a fist, located behind the sternum (breast bone) and between the lungs; pumping action circulates blood throughout the body

Anatomic Structures of the Cardiovascular System—cont'd

plasma
(PLAZ-ma)

clear, straw-colored, liquid portion of blood in which cells are suspended; composed of approximately 90% water and is about 55% of total blood volume

veins
(vānz)

blood vessels that carry blood back to the heart

Functions of the Cardiovascular System

- Pumps blood
- Transports oxygen, nutrients, immune substances, hormones, and other chemicals to and from organs
- Carries waste products away from tissues

Anatomic Structures of the Lymphatic System

lymph
(limf)

transparent, colorless tissue fluid; contains white blood cells and flows in a one-way direction to the heart

lymph nodes
(limf) (nōdz)

small, spherical bodies composed of lymphoid tissue; may be singular or grouped together along the path of lymphatic vessels; filter lymph to keep bacteria and other foreign agents from entering blood

lymphatic vessels
(lim-FAT-ik) (VES-els)

transport lymph from body tissues to a large vein in the chest

spleen
(splēn)

lymphatic organ located in the upper left abdominal cavity between the stomach and the diaphragm; filters blood and acts as a blood reservoir

thymus
(THĪ-mus)

lymphatic organ with two lobes located behind the sternum between the lungs; plays an important role in development of the body's immune system, particularly from infancy to puberty

Functions of the Lymphatic System

- Returns excess fluid from tissues to blood
- Helps maintain blood volume and pressure
- Absorbs fats and fat-soluble vitamins from the small intestine and transports them to the blood
- Filters lymph, trapping and destroying harmful cells
- Generates disease-fighting cells

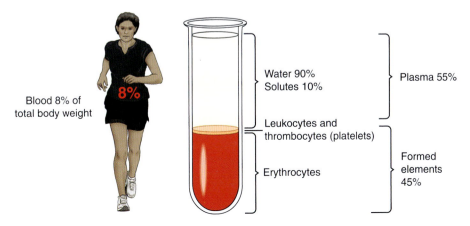

Figure 7.1 Composition of blood.

How the Cardiovascular and Lymphatic Systems Work

The cardiovascular and lymphatic systems are closely related. They work together to maintain an internal balance in the body—transporting nutrients and waste, protecting against infection, and regulating fluid and electrolyte levels. Each system circulates fluid: blood in the cardiovascular system, and lymph in the lymphatic system.

Blood is composed of plasma and formed elements (Figure 7.1). Plasma is the liquid portion of the blood in which the cells are suspended. The formed elements contain erythrocytes (red blood cells), leukocytes (white blood cells), and thrombocytes (platelets).

The cardiovascular system (Figure 7.2) pumps blood from the heart through a closed system of vessels composed of arteries, capillaries, and veins. The heart functions as two pumps operating simultaneously. The left side of the heart pumps blood to the arteries, which carry blood rich in oxygen and other nutrients to replenish organs, tissues, and cells. The exchange of gases, nutrients, and waste between the blood and body tissues takes place in the capillaries. Along the way, blood passes through the organs of other body systems transporting chemical substances, such as hormones, that are essential for body functioning. Veins carry blood back to the right side of the heart, which pumps blood containing carbon dioxide to the lungs to be replenished with oxygen. This oxygen-rich blood then returns to the left side of the heart, to begin the process again.

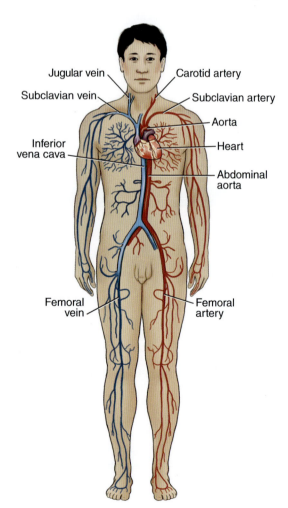

Figure 7.2 Cardiovascular System.

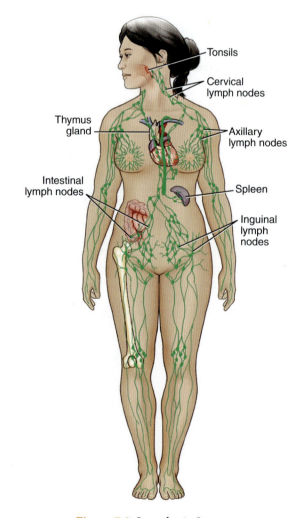

Figure 7.3 Lymphatic System.

The lymphatic system (Figure 7.3) does not have a pump; it passively absorbs fluid called lymph (composed of fluid that passes from capillaries into tissue) and passes it through lymphatic vessels, whose duty it is to return lymph to the blood. Lymph nodes, which filter lymphatic fluid, are located along the paths of these collecting vessels. Infectious agents, cancerous cells, and other debris may be trapped and destroyed. The thymus, a lymphatic organ, generates disease-fighting white blood cells and releases them into the blood for delivery to the specific body site in need. The spleen filters blood, much like lymph nodes filter lymph, and acts as a reservoir.

CAREER FOCUS   **Professionals Who Work with the Cardiovascular and Lymphatic Systems**

- **Phlebotomists** draw blood from patients using a process called venipuncture to collect the blood into special tubes, which is then processed and tested using specialized machines (Figure 7.4). Phlebotomists can also sample blood through a skin puncture, such as pricking a finger to test a patient's blood sugar.

- **Cardiovascular Perfusionists,** also called **Certified Clinical Perfusionists (CCPs),** operate the heart-lung machine for cardiopulmonary bypass during open-heart surgery.

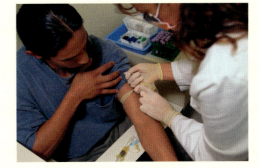

Figure 7.4 Phlebotomist performing venipuncture to withdraw blood from a patient.

- **Cardiovascular Technologists and Technicians** Cardiovascular technologists are trained to prepare patients and assist physicians during procedures such as cardiac catheterization, balloon angioplasty, and open heart surgery. They also monitor patients' blood pressure and heart rate. Cardiovascular technicians conduct electrocardiograms (ECG) and assist with cardiac stress tests and other monitoring.

- **Echocardiography Technicians** are specialized cardiovascular technicians that perform ultrasounds of the heart. The ultrasound collects reflected echoes and Doppler signals from images and spectral tracings of the heart.

🌐 **FOR MORE INFORMATION**

- Access online resources at evolve.elsevier.com > Practice Student Resources > Other Resources > Career Videos to watch interviews with a **Perfusionist** and a **Phlebotomist**.

OBJECTIVE 1

Build, translate, pronounce, and spell medical terms built from word parts.

WORD PARTS | Presented with the Cardiovascular and Lymphatic Systems

Use the paper or online **flashcards** to familiarize yourself with the following word parts.

COMBINING FORM (WR + CV)	DEFINITION	COMBINING FORM (WR + CV)	DEFINITION
aden/o	gland(s); (nodes when combined with lymph/o)	lymph/o	lymph, lymphatic tissue
angi/o	blood vessel(s)	phleb/o	vein(s)
arteri/o	artery (s.), arteries (pl.)	splen/o	spleen
cardi/o	heart	thromb/o	blood clot
ech/o	sound	ven/o	vein(s)
electr/o	electrical activity		

SUFFIX (S)	DEFINITION	SUFFIX (S)	DEFINITION
-ac	pertaining to	-penia	abnormal reduction (in number)
-graph	instrument used to record		
-megaly	enlargement	-sclerosis	hardening

PREFIX (P)	DEFINITION	PREFIX (P)	DEFINITION
brady-	slow	tachy-	rapid, fast

WORD PARTS PRESENTED IN PREVIOUS LESSONS | Used to Build Cardiovascular and Lymphatic System Terms

COMBINING FORM (WR + CV)	DEFINITION	COMBINING FORM (WR + CV)	DEFINITION
cyt/o	cell(s)	my/o	muscle
hem/o, hemat/o	blood	path/o	disease

SUFFIX (S)	DEFINITION	SUFFIX (S)	DEFINITION
-a, -e, -y	no meaning	-logy	study of
-al, -ous	pertaining to	-lysis	dissolution, separating
-ectomy	surgical removal, excision	-oma	tumor
-gram	record, radiographic image	-osis	abnormal condition
-graphy	process of recording, radiographic imaging	-plasty	surgical repair
-ia	diseased state, condition of	-pnea	breathing
-itis	inflammation	-stasis	control, stop
-logist	one who studies and treats (specialist, physician)	-tomy	cut into, incision

PREFIX (P)	DEFINITION	PREFIX (P)	DEFINITION
a-, an-	absence of, without	endo-	within

Refer to Appendix A, Word Parts Used in *Basic Medical Language*, for alphabetical lists of word parts and their meanings.

EXERCISE A   **Build and Translate Medical Terms Built from Word Parts**

*Use the **Word Parts Tables** to complete the following questions. Check your responses with the Answer Key in Appendix C at the back of the book.*

1. **LABEL:** *Write the combining forms for anatomical structures of the cardiovascular system on Figure 7.5. These anatomical combining forms will be used to build and translate medical terms in Exercise A.*

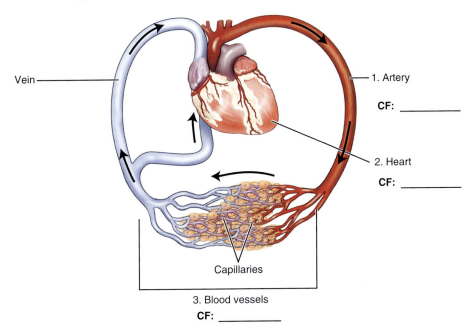

Vein

1. Artery
   CF: _____

2. Heart
   CF: _____

Capillaries

3. Blood vessels
   CF: _____

Figure 7.5 Heart and blood vessels with combining forms.

2. **MATCH:** *Draw a line to match the word part with its definition.*

   a. -logist   enlargement
   b. -logy   study of
   c. -ac   one who studies and treats (specialist, physician)
   d. -megaly   pertaining to

3. **BUILD:** *Using the combining form **cardi/o** and the word parts reviewed in the previous exercise, build the following terms related to the heart. Remember, the definition usually starts with the meaning of the suffix.*

   a. pertaining to the heart
   _____ / _____
   wr   s

   b. study of the heart
   _____ / o / _____
   wr   cv   s

   c. physician who studies and treats diseases of the heart
   _____ / o / _____
   wr   cv   s

   d. enlargement of the heart
   _____ / o / _____
   wr   cv   s

4. **READ: Cardiology** (kar-dē-OL-o-jē) is the field of medicine related to the study of the heart. A **cardiologist** (kar-dē-OL-o-jist) is a physician with special training to diagnose and treat heart disease. **Cardiomegaly** (kar-dē-ō-MEG-a-lē) may be caused by high blood pressure or other **cardiac** (KAR-dē-ak) disorders.

5. **MATCH:** *Draw a line to match the word part with its definition.*

   a. -gram   process of recording, radiographic imaging
   b. -graph   record, radiographic image
   c. -graphy   instrument used to record

6. **TRANSLATE:** *Complete the definitions of the following terms built from the combining form **electr/o** meaning electrical activity. Use the meaning of word parts to fill in the blanks. Remember, the definition usually starts with the meaning of the suffix.*

   a. electr/o/cardi/o/gram   _____ of the electrical activity of the _____

   b. electr/o/cardi/o/graph   instrument used to record the _____ of the heart

   c. electr/o/cardi/o/graphy   _____ of _____ the electrical activity of the heart

7. **READ:** An **electrocardiogram** (ē-lek-trō-KAR-dē-ō-gram) may be ordered by the physician when a patient has chest pain, a symptom of cardiac disease. **Electrocardiography** (ē-lek-trō-kar-dē-OG-ra-fē) records electrical currents generated by the heart and is frequently used for cardiac assessment. Cardiac technicians are trained to use the **electrocardiograph** (ē-lek-trō-KAR-dē-ō-graf); they place sensors on the patient to record these electrical impulses.

> **FYI**   Compare the three suffixes **-gram**, **-graph**, and **-graphy**. The suffix **-gram** is the record. It may be a paper record or radiographic image. The suffix **-graph** is the machine or instrument used to make the record. The suffix **-graphy** is the process of recording.

8. **LABEL:** *Write word parts to complete Figure 7.6.*

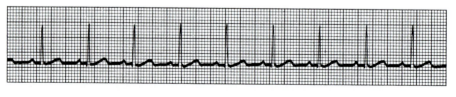

Figure 7.6 _____/o/_____/o/_____.
          electrical activity   heart   record

9. MATCH: *Draw a line to match the word part with its definition.*

a. my/o   no meaning
b. ech/o   breathing
c. tachy-   muscle
d. brady-   sound
e. -pnea   rapid, fast
f. path/o   slow
g. -a, -y   disease

---

10. BUILD: *Using the combining form **cardi/o** and the word parts reviewed in the previous exercise, build the following terms related to the heart:*

a. record of the heart using sound   _____ / o / _____ / o / _____
                                        wr   cv   wr   cv   s

b. slow heart rate   _____ / _____ /a
                                          p   wr   s

c. disease of the heart muscle   _____ / o / _____ / o / _____ /y
                                        wr   cv   wr   cv   wr   s

---

11. READ: Bradycardia (brad-ē-KAR-dē-a) may be caused by medications that slow the heart rate, or by diseases that affect the electrical impulses in the heart. In dilated **cardiomyopathy** (kar-dē-ō-mī-OP-a-thē) the heart muscle stretches and becomes thinner, and the heart doesn't pump as well. An **echocardiogram** (ek-ō-KAR-dē-ō-gram) uses sound waves to show the structure and motion of the heart, and is often used to diagnose cardiomyopathies.

---

12. LABEL: *Write word parts to complete Figure 7.7.*

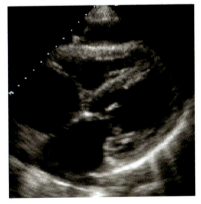

Figure 7.7 _____ /o/ _____ /o/ _____ in a patient with cardiomyopathy.
              sound   heart   record

13. **TRANSLATE:** *Complete the definitions of the following terms:*

    a. my/o/cardi/al   pertaining to the_____ of the heart

    b. tachy/cardi/a   rapid _____ rate

    c. tachy/pnea   _____ breathing

---

14. **READ:** **Tachycardia** (tak-i-KAR-dē-a) can be detected either by a physical exam or by electrocardiography. **Tachypnea** (tak-IP-nē-a) occurs when an adult takes more than twenty breaths in one minute. **Myocardial** (mī-ō-KAR-dē-al) events can cause both tachycardia and tachypnea.

---

15. **MATCH:** *Draw a line to match the word part with its definition.*

    a. -ectomy   record, radiographic image

    b. -al   hardening

    c. -gram   within

    d. -sclerosis   surgical removal, excision

    e. endo-   pertaining to

---

16. **BUILD:** *Using the combining form **arteri/o** and the word parts reviewed in the previous exercise, build the following terms related to arteries:*

    a. excision within the artery   _____ / _____ / _____

                                         p   wr   s

    b. pertaining to the arteries   _____ / _____

                                          wr   s

    c. hardening of the arteries   _____ / o / _____

                                          wr   cv   s

    d. radiographic image of the arteries   _____ / o / _____

                                          wr   cv   s

---

17. **READ:** In **arteriosclerosis** (ar-tēr-ē-ō-skle-RŌ-sis), the **arterial** (ar-TĒ-rē-al) walls become thickened and lose their elasticity. This is usually due to plaque formation. An **arteriogram** (ar-TĒR-ē-ō-gram), which uses injected contrast media to outline arteries, may be performed to determine the extent of disease. An **endarterectomy** (end-ar-ter-EK-to-mē) is a procedure performed to remove plaque from the interior wall of a diseased artery.

18. LABEL: *Write word parts to complete Figures 7.8 and 7.9.*

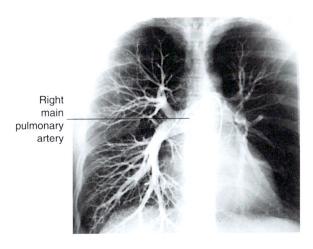

Right
main
pulmonary
artery

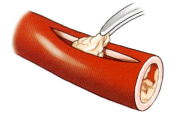

Figure 7.8 _____/o/_____   Figure 7.9 _____/_____/_____.
　　　　　 artery　　　　 radiographic image　　　　　　　 within　　　 artery　　 excision
　　　 showing the right main pulmonary artery.

19. MATCH: *Draw a line to match the word part with its definition.*

a. -graphy　　　　　　 surgical repair
b. -plasty　　　　　　　 process of recording, radiographic imaging

20. TRANSLATE: *Complete the definitions of the following terms using the word root **angi/o** meaning blood vessel.*

a. angi/o/graphy　　　　　 _____ imaging of the blood _____

b. angi/o/plasty　　　　　 surgical _____ of the blood _____

21. READ: Coronary **angiography** (an-jē-OG-ra-fē) is an invasive procedure in which a catheter is inserted into a vessel in the arm or groin and passed all the way into the coronary arteries. Contrast media is injected and images are recorded. **Angioplasty** (AN-jē-ō-plas-tē) is a procedure to restore blood flow through blocked vessels. Coronary angioplasty can be done at the same time as coronary angiography.

> **FYI**   In **percutaneous transluminal coronary angioplasty** (PTCA), also called balloon angioplasty, a balloon is passed through a blood vessel into the coronary artery. Inflation of the balloon compresses the obstructing plaque against the vessel wall, expands the inner diameter of the blood vessel, and allows the blood to circulate more freely.

22. LABEL: *Write word parts to complete Figure 7.10.*

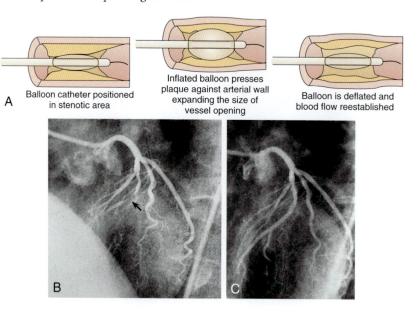

A, Balloon catheter positioned in stenotic area

Inflated balloon presses plaque against arterial wall expanding the size of vessel opening

Balloon is deflated and blood flow reestablished

Figure 7.10 Percutaneous transluminal coronary _____/o/_____ (PTCA).
                                                                                   blood vessel   surgical repair
A, Balloon dilation. **B,** Coronary arteriogram before PTCA. The arrow indicates the area with approximately 95% blockage. **C,** Coronary arteriogram after PTCA in the same patient, now showing increased blood flow through the previously blocked area.

23. REVIEW OF CARDIOVASCULAR AND LYMPHATIC SYSTEM TERMS BUILT FROM WORD PARTS: *the following is an alphabetical list of terms built and translated in the previous exercises.*

MEDICAL TERMS BUILT FROM WORD PARTS

TERM	DEFINITION	TERM	DEFINITION
1. angiography (an-jē-OG-ra-fē)	radiographic imaging of the blood vessels	**5. arteriosclerosis** (ar-tēr-ē-ō-skle-RŌ-sis)	hardening of the arteries
2. angioplasty (AN-jē-ō-plas-tē)	surgical repair of the blood vessels (Figure 7.10)	**6. bradycardia** (brad-ē-KAR-dē-a)	slow heart rate
3. arterial (ar-TĒ-rē-al)	pertaining to the arteries	**7. cardiac** (KAR-dē-ak)	pertaining to the heart
4. arteriogram (ar-TĒR-ē-ō-gram)	radiographic image of the arteries (after an injection of contrast media) (Figure 7.8)	**8. cardiologist** (kar-dē-OL-o-jist)	physician who studies and treats diseases of the heart

MEDICAL TERMS BUILT FROM WORD PARTS—cont'd

TERM	DEFINITION	TERM	DEFINITION
9. **cardiology** (kar-dē-OL-o-jē)	study of the heart	15. **electrocardiography** (ē-lek-trō-kar-dē-OG-ra-fē)	process of recording electrical activity of the heart
10. **cardiomegaly** (kar-dē-ō-MEG-a-lē)	enlargement of the heart	16. **endarterectomy** (end-ar-ter-EK-to-mē)	excision within the artery (excision of plaque from the arterial wall) (Figure 7.9)
11. **cardiomyopathy** (kar-dē-ō-mī-OP-a-thē)	disease of the heart muscle	17. **myocardial** (mī-ō-KAR-dē-al)	pertaining to the muscle of the heart
12. **echocardiogram (ECHO)** (ek-ō-KAR-dē-ō-gram)	record of the heart using sound (Figure 7.7)	18. **tachycardia** (tak-i-KAR-dē-a)	rapid heart rate
13. **electrocardiogram (ECG/EKG)** (ē-lek-trō-KAR-dē-ō-gram)	record of electrical activity of the heart (Figure 7.6)	19. **tachypnea** (tak-IP-nē-a)	rapid breathing
14. **electrocardiograph** (ē-lek-trō-KAR-dē-ō-graf)	instrument used to record electrical activity of the heart		

EXERCISE B   Pronounce and Spell Terms Built from Word Parts

Practice pronunciation and spelling on paper and online.

1. **Practice on Paper**
   a. Pronounce: Read the phonetic spelling and say aloud the terms listed in the previous table, Review of Terms Built from Word Parts.
   b. Spell: Have a study partner read the terms aloud. Write the spelling of the terms on a separate sheet of paper.

2. **Practice Online** 🌐
   a. **Access** online learning resources. Go to evolve.elsevier.com > Evolve Resources > Practice Student Resources.
   b. **Pronounce:** Select Audio Glossary > Lesson 7 > Exercise B. Select a term to hear its pronunciation and repeat aloud.
   c. **Spell:** Select Activities > Lesson 7 > Spell Terms > Exercise B. Select the audio icon and type the correct spelling of the term.

❏ Check the box when complete.

EXERCISE C   Build and Translate MORE Medical Terms Built from Word Parts

*Use the **Word Parts Tables** near the beginning of the lesson to complete the following questions. Check your responses with the Answer Key in Appendix C at the back of the book.*

1. **LABEL:** *Write the combining forms for anatomical structures of the cardiovascular system on Figure 7.11. These anatomical combining forms will be used to build and translate medical terms in Exercise C.*

FYI Though the combining form **angi/o** usually refers to blood vessels, it can also refer to lymphatic vessels. In these instances **lymph/o** appears before **angi/o** to specify the lymphatic vessels. Examples include lymphangitis and lymphangioma.

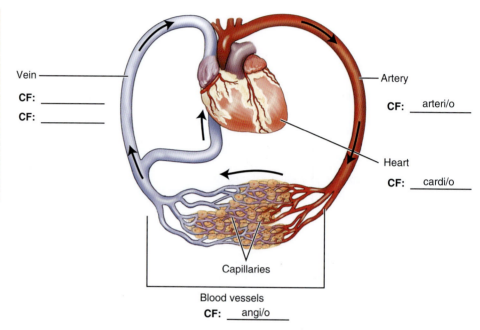

Vein
CF: _____
CF: _____

Artery
CF: ___arteri/o___

Heart
CF: ___cardi/o___

Capillaries

Blood vessels
CF: ___angi/o___

Figure 7.11 Heart and blood vessels with combining forms.

2. **MATCH:** *Draw a line to match the word part with its definition.*

   a. -ous   within
   b. -gram   pertaining to
   c. intra-   record, radiographic image

3. **BUILD:** *Using the combining form **ven/o** and the word parts reviewed in the previous exercise, build the following terms related to veins.*

   a. pertaining to within the veins   _____/_____/_____
                                            p   wr   s

   b. radiographic image of the veins   _____/_o_/_____
                                            wr   cv   s

4. **READ:** An **intravenous** (in-tra-VĒ-nus) catheter is used to inject substances directly into a vein. This may be done for therapy (such as the injection of medications), or for diagnosis (such as the injection of radiographic dyes). During a leg **venogram** (VĒ-nō-gram), contrast media is injected intravenously into a vein in the foot. The radiograph (x-ray) captures images of the contrast media traveling through the leg veins. This allows the physician to see if there is any blockage or other damage to the veins.

5. **LABEL:** *Write word parts to complete Figure 7.12, A and B.*

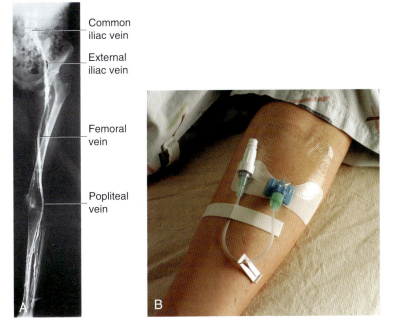

Common iliac vein

External iliac vein

Femoral vein

Popliteal vein

Figure 7.12 A. _____/o/_____ of the left leg.
                        vein   radiographic image

B. Patient's arm with an _____/_____/_____ (IV) catheter.
                                within   vein   pertaining to

6. **MATCH:** *Draw a line to match the word part with its definition.*

   a. -itis   cut into, incision
   b. -tomy   blood clot
   c. thromb/o   inflammation
   d. -osis   abnormal condition

7. TRANSLATE: *Complete the definitions of the following terms by using the meaning of the word parts to fill in the blanks. Terms built from the combining form **phleb/o**, meaning vein:*

a. phleb/itis   _____ of the veins

b. phleb/o/tomy   incision into the _____ (with a needle to remove or instill fluid)

c. thromb/osis   _____ of a blood clot

d. thromb/o/phleb/itis   inflammation of the veins associated with _____

8. READ: Phlebotomy (fle-BOT-o-mē), also called **venipuncture**, is a method of obtaining blood for laboratory testing. **Phlebitis** (fle-BĪ-tis) occurs when a vein becomes inflamed and can cause pain and swelling. Superficial phlebitis occurring in veins close to the skin is usually not dangerous. **Thrombophlebitis** (throm-bō-fle-BĪ-tis) that occurs in the deeper veins can be dangerous, especially if a blood clot breaks off the venous wall and travels through the bloodstream into the lungs. **Thrombosis** (throm-BŌ-sis) refers to the formation of blood clots in the blood vessels.

9. LABEL: *Write word parts to complete Figure 7.13.*

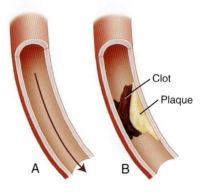

Clot

Plaque

A   B

Figure 7.13 A. Healthy artery with smooth blood flow.

B. Blocked artery due to: _____/_____ and atherosclerosis.
                            blood clot   abnormal condition

10. MATCH: *Draw a line to match the word part with its definition.*

    a. cyt/o   abnormal reduction (in number)
    b. -e   blood clot
    c. -penia   cell
    d. leuk/o   no meaning
    e. thromb/o   white

11. TRANSLATE: *Complete the definitions of the following terms by using the meaning of the word parts to fill in the blanks.*

    a. thromb/o/cyt/e   blood clotting _____

    b. thromb/o/cyt/o/penia   _____ of blood clotting cells

    c. leuk/o/cyt/o/penia   abnormal reduction of _____ blood cells

12. READ: A **thrombocyte** (THROM-bō-sīt) is also called a **platelet**. These blood cells aid in the clotting process. If **thrombocytopenia** (throm-bō-sī-tō-PĒ-nē-a) becomes severe, spontaneous bleeding can occur. **Leukocytopenia** (lū-kō-sī-tō-PĒ-nē-a) can be caused by diseases of the bone marrow, where leukocytes are produced. It can also be caused by infections, drugs, or autoimmune diseases, all of which destroy the white cells once they are circulating.

13. LABEL: *Write the combining forms for anatomical structures of the lymphatic system on Figure 7.14.*

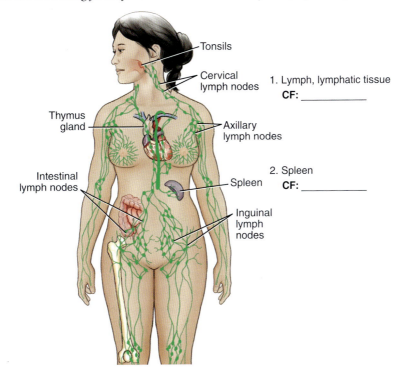

Tonsils

Cervical lymph nodes

1. Lymph, lymphatic tissue
   CF: _____

Thymus gland

Axillary lymph nodes

Intestinal lymph nodes

2. Spleen
   CF: _____

Spleen

Inguinal lymph nodes

Figure 7.14 Lymphatic system and combining forms for lymph nodes and spleen.

14. MATCH: *Draw a line to match the word part with its definition.*

    a. -ectomy   enlargement

    b. -megaly   surgical removal, excision

---

15. BUILD: *Use the combining form **splen/o** along with the word parts reviewed in the previous exercise, to build terms related to the spleen. Note that the medical term spleen has two e's; the combining form **splen/o** has one.*

    a. enlargement of the spleen   _____/ o /_____

                                                   wr   **cv**   **s**

    b. excision of the spleen   _____/_____

                                                     wr   **s**

---

16. READ: The spleen is the largest lymphatic organ. It filters and stores blood. **Splenomegaly** (splē-nō-MEG-a-lē) may be caused by infections such as mononucleosis, cancers such as lymphoma, or other diseases which cause the spleen to retain blood. This can occasionally lead to splenic rupture, which usually requires a **splenectomy** (splē-NEK-to-mē). While people can live without their spleens, their risk of infection is increased.

---

17. MATCH: *Draw a line to match the word part with its definition.*

    a. -itis   no meaning

    b. path/o   gland(s); node(s)

    c. -oma   disease

    d. aden/o   inflammation

    e. -y   tumor

> **FYI**   When the combining forms **lymph/o** and **aden/o** are used together (**lymph/aden/o**), it refers to a collection of tissue called a lymph node, rather than a lymph gland.

---

18. TRANSLATE: *Complete the definitions of the following terms by using the meaning of the word parts to fill in the blanks.*

    a. lymph/aden/o/path/y   _____ of the lymph nodes

    b. lymph/aden/itis   inflammation of the _____

    c. lymph/oma   _____ of lymphatic tissue

---

19. READ: Lymph nodes trap and filter bacteria, viruses, cancer cells, and other unwanted substances. **Lymphadenopathy** (lim-fad-e-NOP-a-thē), or swollen lymph nodes, can be caused by infection, autoimmune diseases, or (infrequently) cancer. When swollen lymph nodes are caused by an infection, this is known as **lymphadenitis** (lim-fad-e-NĪ-tis). **Lymphoma** (lim-FŌ-ma) is a cancer that begins in the lymphatic system. Hodgkin lymphoma is a type of lymphatic cancer.

20. MATCH: *Draw a line to match the word part with its definition.*

a. -logist   tumor
b. -logy   control, stop
c. -oma   dissolution, separating
d. -stasis   one who studies and treats (specialist, physician)
e. -lysis   study of

21. BUILD: *Use the combining forms **hem/o**, **hemat/o** (Hint: **hem/o** for d and e) along with the word parts reviewed in the previous exercise, to build terms related to blood.*

a. study of blood

_____ / o / _____
wr   cv   s

b. physician who studies and treats diseases of the blood

_____ / o / _____
wr   cv   s

c. tumor of blood (usually a collection of blood)

_____ / _____
wr   s

d. stopping (the flow of) blood

_____ / o / _____
wr   cv   s

e. dissolution of (red) blood (cells)

_____ / o / _____
wr   cv   s

22. READ: The specialty of **hematology** (hē-ma-TOL-o-jē) concerns the study of the blood, bone marrow, and lymphatic system. A **hematologist** (hē-ma-TOL-o-jist) treats disorders of abnormal blood cells, as well as bleeding and clotting disorders. The ability to stop bleeding is known as **hemostasis** (hē-mō-STĀ-sis). A **hematoma** (hē-ma-TŌ-ma) is a condition in which blood has leaked out of a broken vessel into the surrounding tissue. **Hemolysis** (hē-MOL-i-sis) refers to the abnormal destruction of erythrocytes, which can lead to anemia.

23. LABEL: *Write word parts to complete Figure 7.15*

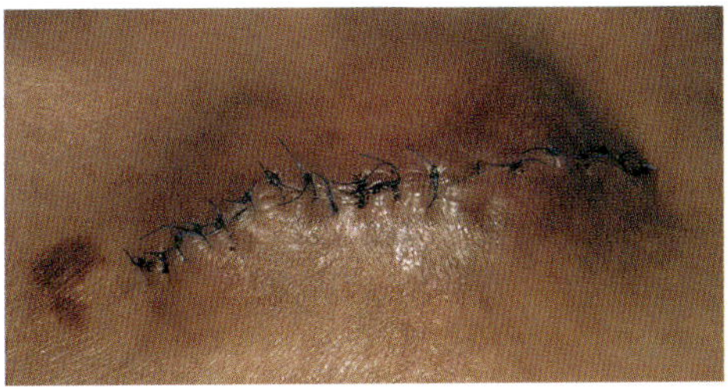

Figure 7.15 Post-surgical site displaying swelling and formation of a _____ / _____ .
                                                                         blood   tumor

24. REVIEW OF MORE CARDIOVASCULAR AND LYMPHATIC SYSTEM TERMS BUILT FROM WORD PARTS: *the following is an alphabetical list of terms built and translated in the previous exercises.*

MEDICAL TERMS BUILT FROM WORD PARTS

TERM	DEFINITION	TERM	DEFINITION
1. hematologist (hē-ma-TOL-o-jist)	physician who studies and treats diseases of the blood	11. phlebitis (fle-BĪ-tis)	inflammation of the veins
2. hematology (hē-ma-TOL-o-jē)	study of blood	12. phlebotomy (fle-BOT-o-mē)	incision into the vein (with a needle to remove blood or instill fluid); (also called **venipuncture**)
3. hemolysis (hē-MOL-i-sis)	dissolution of (red) blood (cells)		
4. hematoma (hē-ma-TŌ-ma)	tumor of blood (collection of blood that has leaked out of a broken vessel into the surrounding tissue) (Figure 7.15)	13. splenectomy (splē-NEK-to-mē)	excision of the spleen
		14. splenomegaly (splē-nō-MEG-a-lē)	enlargement of the spleen
		15. thrombocyte (THROM-bō-sīt)	blood clotting cell (also called **platelet**)
5. hemostasis (hē-mō-STĀ-sis)	stopping (the flow of) blood	16. thrombocytopenia (throm-bō-sī-tō-PĒ-nē-a)	abnormal reduction in number of blood clotting cells
6. intravenous (IV) (in-tra-VĒ-nus)	pertaining to within the veins (Figure 7.12, *B*)		
7. leukocytopenia (lū-kō-sī-tō-PĒ-nē-a)	abnormal reduction of white (blood) cells	17. thrombophlebitis (throm-bō-fle-BĪ-tis)	inflammation of the veins associated with blood clots
8. lymphadenitis (lim-fad-e-NĪ-tis)	inflammation of the lymph nodes	18. thrombosis (throm-BŌ-sis)	abnormal condition of a blood clot (Figure 7.13, *B*)
9. lymphadenopathy (lim-fad-e-NOP-a-thē)	disease of the lymph nodes	19. venogram (VĒ-nō-gram)	radiographic image of the veins (after an injection of contrast media) (Figure 7.12, *A*)
10. lymphoma (lim-FŌ-ma)	tumor of the lymphatic tissue		

EXERCISE D   Pronounce and Spell MORE Terms Built from Word Parts

Practice pronunciation and spelling on paper and online.

1. **Practice on Paper**
   a. **Pronounce**: Read the phonetic spelling and say aloud the terms listed in the previous table, Review of MORE Cardiovascular and Lymphatic System Terms Built from Word Parts.
   b. **Spell**: Have a study partner read the terms aloud. Write the spelling of the terms on a separate sheet of paper.

2. **Practice Online** 🌐

   a. **Access** online learning resources. Go to evolve.elsevier.com > Evolve Resources > Practice Student Resources.

   b. **Pronounce:** Select Audio Glossary > Lesson 7 > Exercise D. Select a term to hear its pronunciation and repeat aloud.

   c. **Spell:** Select Activities > Lesson 7 > Spell Terms > Exercise D. Select the audio icon and type the correct spelling of the term.

❑ Check the box when complete.

OBJECTIVE 2

Define, pronounce, and spell medical terms NOT built from word parts.

The terms listed below may contain word parts, but are difficult to translate literally.

MEDICAL TERMS NOT BUILT FROM WORD PARTS

TERM	DEFINITION
anemia (a-NĒ-mē-a)	condition in which there is a reduction in the number of erythrocytes (RBCs). Anemia may be caused by blood loss, by decreased production of RBCs, or by increased destruction of RBCs.
aneurysm (AN-ū-rizm)	condition in which there is a ballooning of a weakened portion of the arterial wall (Figure 7.17)
blood pressure (BP) (blud) (PRES-ūr)	pressure exerted by the blood against the blood vessel walls; a blood pressure measurement written as systolic pressure (120) and diastolic pressure (80) is commonly recorded as 120/80 mm Hg
cardiac catheterization (KAR-dē-ak) (kath-e-ter-i-ZĀ-shun)	diagnostic procedure performed by passing a catheter into the heart from a blood vessel in the groin or arm to examine the condition of the heart and surrounding blood vessels (Figure 7.16)
cardiopulmonary resuscitation (CPR) (kar-dē-ō-PUL-mo-nar-ē) (rē-sus-i-TĀ-shun)	emergency procedure consisting of artificial ventilation and external cardiac compressions
complete blood count (CBC) (com-PLĒT) (blud) (kownt)	laboratory test for basic blood screening that measures various aspects of erythrocytes, leukocytes, and thrombocytes (platelets); this automated test quickly provides a tremendous amount of information about the blood
coronary artery bypass graft (CABG) (KOR-o-nar-ē) (AR-ter-ē) (BĪ-pas) (graft)	surgical technique to bring a new blood supply to the heart muscle (myocardium) by detouring around blocked arteries
coronary artery disease (CAD) (KOR-o-nar-ē) (AR-ter-ē) (di-ZĒZ)	condition that reduces the flow of blood through the coronary arteries to the heart muscle (myocardium) that may progress to depriving the heart tissue of sufficient oxygen and nutrients to function normally
embolus (*pl.* emboli) (EM-bō-lus), (EM-bō-lī)	blood clot or foreign material, such as air or fat, that enters the bloodstream and moves until it lodges at another point in the circulation
heart failure (HF) (hart) (FĀL-ūr)	condition in which there is an inability of the heart to pump enough blood through the body to supply the tissues and organs with nutrients and oxygen (also called **congestive heart failure [CHF]**)

MEDICAL TERMS NOT BUILT FROM WORD PARTS—cont'd

TERM	DEFINITION
hemorrhage (HEM-ō-rij)	rapid loss of blood, as in bleeding
hypertension (HTN) (hī-per-TEN-shun)	blood pressure that is above normal (generally greater than 130/80 mm Hg in adults)
hypotension (hī-pō-TEN-shun)	blood pressure that is below normal (generally less than 90/60 mm Hg in adults)
leukemia (lū-KĒ-mē-a)	malignant disease characterized by excessive increase in abnormal leukocytes formed in the bone marrow
myocardial infarction (MI) (mī-ō-KAR-dē-al) (in-FARK-shun)	death (necrosis) of a portion of the heart muscle caused by lack of oxygen resulting from an interrupted blood supply (also called **heart attack**)
pulse (P) (puls)	contraction of the heart, which can be felt with a fingertip. The pulse is most commonly felt over the radial artery (in the wrist); however, the pulsations can be felt over a number of sites, including the femoral (groin) and carotid (neck) arteries.
sphygmomanometer (sfig-mō-ma-NOM-e-ter)	device used for measuring blood pressure
stethoscope (STETH-ō-skōp)	instrument used to hear internal body sounds; used for performing auscultation and blood pressure measurement
varicose veins (VAR-i-kōs) (vānz)	condition demonstrated by distended or tortuous veins usually found in the lower extremities

EXERCISE E   Label

Write the medical terms pictured and defined using the previous table of Medical Terms NOT Built from Word Parts. Check your work with the Answer Key in Appendix C.

1. _____

diagnostic procedure performed by passing a catheter into the heart from a blood vessel in the groin or arm to examine the condition of the heart and surrounding blood vessels

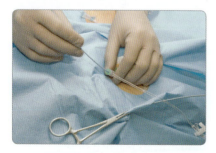

2. _____

surgical technique to bring a new blood supply to the heart muscle by detouring around blocked arteries

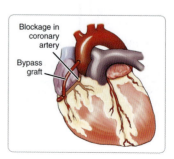

3. _____

distended or tortuous veins

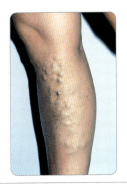

4. _____

laboratory test for basic blood screening that measures various aspects of erythrocytes, leukocytes, and thrombocytes (platelets)

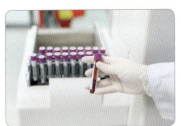

5. _____

ballooning of a weakened portion of the arterial wall

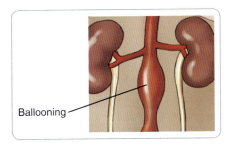

Ballooning

6. _____

emergency procedure consisting of artificial ventilation and external cardiac compressions

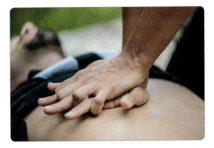

7. _____

instrument used to hear internal body sounds

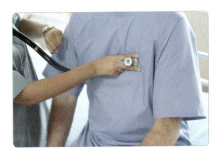

8. _____

pressure exerted by the blood against the blood vessel walls; measurement is written as systolic pressure (120) and diastolic pressure (80), commonly recorded as 120/80 mm Hg

Sphygmomanometer

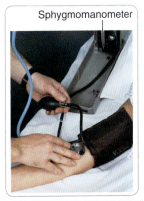

EXERCISE F   Learn Medical Terms NOT Built from Word Parts

Fill in the blanks with medical terms defined in bold using the Medical Terms NOT Built from Word Parts table. Answers are listed in Appendix C.

1. To evaluate the extent of a hemorrhage, a physician may order a **basic blood screening that measures aspects of erythrocytes, leukocytes, and thrombocytes (platelets)**, or _____ _____ _____ abbreviated as _____. This basic blood test will help determine whether a blood transfusion is necessary.

> **FYI**   **Hemorrhage** is a commonly misspelled word. Think of the word part **hem** for blood and the -rrh suffix **-rrhagia**. Together they spell hemorrhagia. Change the suffix -ia to -e and you have the term **hem/o/rrhag/e**.

2. In a physical exam, **pressure exerted by the blood against the blood vessel walls**, or _____ _____ abbreviated as _____, is usually measured when vital signs are assessed. Vital signs include the measurement of temperature, respiration rate, and **contraction of the heart that can be felt with a fingertip**, or _____ abbreviated as _____. The pulse can be felt through the skin at many points including the wrist, neck, or groin.

3. Tools needed to evaluate blood pressure include an **instrument used to hear internal body sounds, which is used for performing auscultation and blood pressure measurement**, or_____, and a **device used for measuring blood pressure**, or _____. To record a blood pressure measurement, the systolic (when the ventricles are contracting) pressure is listed over the diastolic (when the ventricles are relaxing) pressure, such as in a normal blood pressure of 120/80 mm Hg. A reading greater than 130/80 mm Hg generally signifies **blood pressure that is above normal**, or_____, abbreviated _____. A reading less than 90/60 mm Hg generally signifies **blood pressure that is below normal**, or _____.

4. A patient with a **condition that reduces the flow of blood through the coronary arteries to the heart muscle (myocardium)**, or _____ _____ _____ abbreviated as _____, may have angina pectoris, pain in the thoracic region sometimes radiating to the left arm and neck. This can be a warning sign for an upcoming **death of a portion of the heart muscle caused by an interrupted blood supply (also called heart attack)** _____ _____, abbreviated as _____. A physician may order a **diagnostic procedure performed by passing a catheter into the heart from a blood vessel in the groin or arm to examine the condition of the heart and surrounding blood vessels**, or _____ _____ (Figure 7.16).

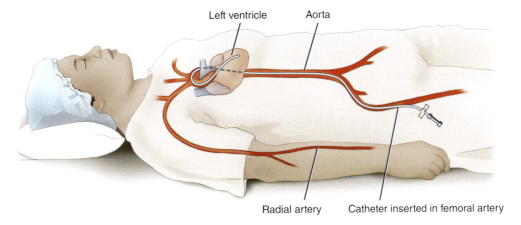

Left ventricle   Aorta

Radial artery   Catheter inserted in femoral artery

Figure 7.16 Cardiac catheterization.

5. The most common site for **ballooning of a weakened portion of the arterial wall**, or _____ is the abdominal aorta, the main blood vessel that transports blood away from the heart (Figure 7.17). While surgery may be needed for larger abdominal aortic aneurysms (AAA), many patients with smaller ones may never need surgery, and are periodically monitored to make sure the aneurysms don't get larger.

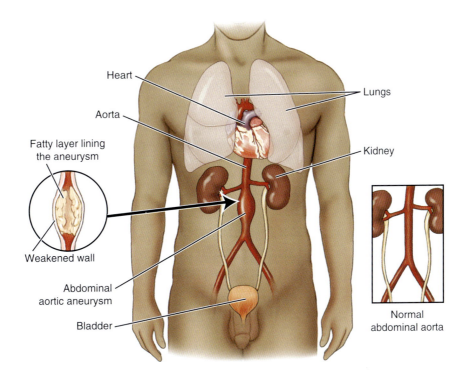

Heart

Lungs

Aorta

Fatty layer lining
the aneurysm

Kidney

Weakened wall

Abdominal
aortic aneurysm

Bladder

Normal
abdominal aorta

Figure 7.17 Abdominal aortic aneurysm.

6. A **reduction in the number of erythrocytes**, or _____, can be caused by low production in the bone marrow, destruction of circulating red blood cells, or **rapid loss of blood, or** _____. **Malignant disease characterized by excessive increase in abnormal leukocytes formed in the bone marrow**, or _____, can also cause anemia by replacing normal red cells with abnormal white cells.

7. In extreme cases, **condition in which there is an inability of the heart to pump enough blood through the body to supply the tissues and organs with nutrients and oxygen**, or _____ _____ abbreviated as _____, can lead to cardiac arrest, in which the heart stops beating. If recognized quickly, **emergency procedure consisting of artificial ventilation and external cardiac compressions**, or _____ _____ abbreviated as _____, can be performed and the heart may start beating again.

8. A **blood clot or foreign material, such as air or fat, that enters the bloodstream and moves until it lodges at another point in the circulation** is called a(n) _____. If it travels to the coronary arteries, a **surgical technique to bring a new blood supply to the heart muscle (myocardium) by detouring around blocked arteries**, or _____ _____ _____ _____, abbreviated as _____, may be necessary.

> **FYI**   Do you remember that thrombosis is an abnormal condition of a blood clot? A **thrombus** is attached to the interior wall of a vessel. If it breaks away and circulates in the bloodstream, it becomes known as an **embolus**. The condition of an embolus blocking an artery is referred to as an **embolism**.

9. **Distended or tortuous veins usually found in the lower extremities**, or _____ _____, usually occur in the superficial veins of the legs. One-way valves in veins help move blood upward. When these valves fail or veins lose their elasticity because of heredity, obesity, pregnancy, or illness, the blood flows backwards, pools, and then forms varicose veins. A varicose vein in the rectal area is called a hemorrhoid.

EXERCISE G   Pronounce and Spell Terms NOT Built from Word Parts

Practice pronunciation and spelling on paper and online.

1. **Practice on Paper**
   a. **Pronounce:** Read the phonetic spelling and say aloud the terms listed in the previous Medical Terms NOT Built from Word Parts Table.
   b. **Spell:** Have a study partner read the terms aloud. Write the spelling of the terms on a separate sheet of paper.

2. **Practice Online** ⊕

   a. **Access** online learning resources. Go to evolve.elsevier.com > Evolve Resources > Practice Student Resources.

   b. **Pronounce:** Select Audio Glossary > Lesson 7 > Exercise G. Select a term to hear its pronunciation and repeat aloud.

   c. **Spell:** Select Activities > Lesson 7 > Spell Terms > Exercise G. Select the audio icon and type the correct spelling of the term.

❑   Check the box when complete.

OBJECTIVE 3

Write abbreviations.

ABBREVIATIONS RELATED TO THE CARDIOVASCULAR AND LYMPHATIC SYSTEMS

Use the online **flashcards** to familiarize yourself with the following abbreviations.

ABBREVIATION	TERM	ABBREVIATION	TERM
BP	blood pressure	HF	heart failure
CABG	coronary artery bypass graft	HHD	hypertensive heart disease
CAD	coronary artery disease	HTN	hypertension
CBC	complete blood count	IV	intravenous
CPR	cardiopulmonary resuscitation	MI	myocardial infarction
DSA	digital subtraction angiography	P	pulse
DVT	deep vein thrombosis	PAD	peripheral artery disease
ECHO	echocardiogram	PTCA	percutaneous transluminal coronary angioplasty
ECG, EKG	electrocardiogram	VS	vital signs

EXERCISE H   Abbreviate Medical Terms

Write the correct abbreviation next to its medical term. Check your responses with the answer key in Appendix C.

1. Diseases and Disorders:

  a. _____ coronary artery disease

  b. _____ heart failure

  c. _____ myocardial infarction

  d. _____ hypertension

  e. _____ peripheral artery disease

  f. _____ hypertensive heart disease

  g. _____ deep vein thrombosis

2. Diagnostic Tests and Equipment:

  a. _____ blood pressure

  b. _____ complete blood count

  c. _____ echocardiogram

  d. _____ electrocardiogram

       _____

  e. _____ vital signs

  f. _____ pulse

  g. _____ digital subtraction angiography

3. Surgical Procedures:

    a. _____   coronary artery bypass graft

    b. _____   percutaneous transluminal coronary angioplasty

4. Related Terms:

    a. _____   cardiopulmonary resuscitation

    b. _____   intravenous

OBJECTIVE 4

Identify medical terms by clinical category.

Now that you have worked through the cardiovascular and lymphatic systems lesson, review and practice medical terms grouped by clinical category. Categories include signs and symptoms, diseases and disorders, diagnostic tests and equipment, surgical procedures, specialties and professions, and other terms related to the cardiovascular and lymphatic systems.

EXERCISE I   Signs and Symptoms

Write the medical terms for signs and symptoms next to their definitions.

1. _____   slow heart rate

2. _____   enlargement of the heart

3. _____   rapid loss of blood, as in bleeding

4. _____   blood pressure that is above normal (generally greater than 130/80 mm Hg in adults)

5. _____   blood pressure that is below normal (generally less than 90/60 mm Hg in adults)

6. _____   enlargement of the spleen

7. _____   rapid heart rate

8. _____   rapid breathing

EXERCISE J   Diseases and Disorders

Write the medical terms for diseases and disorders next to their definitions.

1. _____   condition in which there is a reduction in the number of erythrocytes (RBC)

2. _____   condition in which there is a ballooning of a weakened portion of the arterial wall

3. _____   hardening of the arteries

4. _____ disease of the heart muscle

5. _____ condition that reduces the flow of blood through the coronary arteries to the heart muscle (myocardium) that may progress to depriving the heart tissue of sufficient oxygen and nutrients to function normally

6. _____ blood clot or foreign material, such as air or fat, that enters the bloodstream and moves until it lodges at another point in the circulation

7. _____ condition in which there is an inability of the heart to pump enough blood through the body to supply the tissues and organs with nutrients and oxygen

8. _____ tumor of blood (collection of blood that has leaked out of a broken vessel into the surrounding tissue)

9. _____ dissolution of (red) blood (cells)

10. _____ malignant disease characterized by excessive increase in abnormal leukocytes formed in the bone marrow

11. _____ abnormal reduction of white (blood) cells

12. _____ inflammation of the lymph nodes

13. _____ disease of the lymph nodes

14. _____ tumor of the lymphatic tissue

15. _____ death (necrosis) of a portion of the heart muscle caused by lack of oxygen resulting from an interrupted blood supply (also called **heart attack**)

16. _____ inflammation of the veins

17. _____ abnormal reduction in number of blood clotting cells

18. _____ inflammation of the veins associated with blood clots

19. _____ abnormal condition of a blood clot

20. _____ condition demonstrated by distended or tortuous veins usually found in the lower extremities

EXERCISE K   Diagnostic Tests and Equipment

Write the medical terms for diagnostic tests and equipment next to their definitions.

1. _____ radiographic imaging of the blood vessels

2. _____ radiographic image of the arteries (after an injection of contrast media)

3. _____ pressure exerted by the blood against the blood vessel walls

4. _____   diagnostic procedure performed by passing a catheter into the heart from a blood vessel in the groin or arm to examine the condition of the heart and surrounding blood vessels

5. _____   laboratory test for basic blood screening that measures various aspects of erythrocytes, leukocytes, and thrombocytes (platelets)

6. _____   record of the heart using sound

7. _____   record of electrical activity of the heart

8. _____   instrument used to record electrical activity of the heart

9. _____   process of recording electrical activity of the heart

10. _____   contraction of the heart, which can be felt with a fingertip

11. _____   device used for measuring blood pressure

12. _____   instrument used to hear internal body sounds; used for performing auscultation and blood pressure measurement

13. _____   radiographic image of the veins (after an injection of contrast media)

EXERCISE L   Surgical Procedures

Write the medical terms for surgical procedures next to their definitions.

1. _____   surgical repair of a blood vessel

2. _____   surgical technique to bring a new blood supply to the heart muscle (myocardium) by detouring around blocked arteries

3. _____   excision within the artery (excision of plaque from the arterial wall)

4. _____   incision into the vein (with a needle to remove blood or instill fluid); (also called **venipuncture**)

5. _____   excision of the spleen

EXERCISE M   Specialties and Professions

Write the medical terms for specialties and professions next to their definitions.

1. _____   physician who studies and treats diseases of the heart

2. _____   study of the heart

3. _____   physician who studies and treats diseases of the blood

4. _____   study of blood

EXERCISE N   Medical Terms related to Cardiovascular and Lymphatic Systems

Write the medical terms related to the cardiovascular and lymphatic systems next to their definitions

1. _____   pertaining to the arteries

2. _____   pertaining to the heart

3. _____   emergency procedure consisting of artificial ventilation and
   _____   external cardiac compressions

4. _____   stopping (the flow of) blood

5. _____   pertaining to within a vein

6. _____   pertaining to the muscle of the heart

7. _____   blood clotting cell (also called **platelet**)

OBJECTIVE 5

Use medical language in clinical statements, the case study, and a medical record.

EXERCISE O   Use Medical Terms in Clinical Statements

Circle the medical terms and abbreviations defined in the bolded phrases. Answers are listed in Appendix C. For pronunciation practice, read the answers aloud.

1. Mr. Lauer went to his doctor for follow up on his **condition in which there is an inability of the heart to pump enough blood through the body to supply the tissues and organs with nutrients and oxygen** (hemostasis, hypertension, heart failure). He had **process of recording the electrical activity of the heart** (electrocardiography, echocardiogram, angiography) performed to help evaluate his **pertaining to the heart** (arterial, myocardial, cardiac) status.

2. Following a transpacific airline flight, Kenji Makoto developed **inflammation of the vein associated with a blood clot** (tachypnea, thrombophlebitis, lymphadenitis). After evaluation by Doppler ultrasound, anticoagulant therapy was ordered for treatment. The goal was prevention of a(n) **blood clot or foreign material, such as air or fat, that enters the bloodstream and moves until it lodges at another point in the circulation** (embolus, thrombosis, myocardial infarction).

3. **Abnormal reduction of blood clotting cells** (Leukocytopenia, Leukemia, Thrombocytopenia) can contribute to **a rapid loss of blood** (hemorrhage, aneurysm, thrombosis). If **stopping the flow of blood** (hematoma, hemostasis, hematology) can be achieved quickly, **condition in which there is a reduction in the number of erythrocytes** (anemia, leukemia, hypotension) may be avoided.

4. **Rapid heart rate** (Tachypnea, Hypertension, Tachycardia) may be noted by measuring the **contraction of the heart, which can be felt with a fingertip** (blood pressure, hemostasis, pulse) and may also be accompanied **by blood pressure that is below normal** (hypertension, heart failure, hypotension).

5. **Hardening of the arteries** (Heart failure, Cardiomyopathy, Arteriosclerosis) is a common disorder characterized by thickening, calcification, and loss of elasticity of the **pertaining to the artery** (cardiac, arterial, myocardial) walls.

6. Utilizing a **basic blood screening that measures aspects of erythrocytes, leukocytes, and thrombocytes (platelets)** (stethoscope, venogram, complete blood count), and a bone marrow biopsy, it was determined that Sophia Tompkins had **malignant disease characterized by excessive increase in abnormal leukocytes formed in the bone marrow** (lymphoma, leukemia, hematoma). She was referred to a **physician who studies and treats diseases of the blood** (hematologist, cardiologist, phlebotomist) for consultation and treatment.

7. **Condition that reduces the flow of blood through the coronary arteries to the heart muscle (myocardium)** (Thrombosis, Arteriosclerosis, Coronary artery disease) may eventually lead to an MI. Treatment includes restoring blood supply to the heart. **Surgical repair of the blood vessel** (Angiography, Arteriogram, Angioplasty) is used in some cases, and for more severe blockage, the cardiac surgeon will perform a **surgical technique to bring a new blood supply to the heart muscle (myocardium) by detouring around blocked arteries** (coronary artery bypass graft, cardiac catheterization, cardiopulmonary resuscitation).

EXERCISE P   Apply Medical Terms to the Case Study

Think back to Natalia who was introduced in the case study at the beginning of the lesson. After working through Lesson 7 on the cardiovascular and lymphatic systems, consider the medical terms that might be used to describe her experience. List two terms relevant to the case study and their meaning. ◼

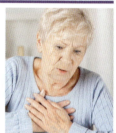

Medical Term	Definition
1. _____	_____
2. _____	_____

EXERCISE Q   Use Medical Terms in a Document

Natalia was brought to the emergency department and was admitted to the cardiology unit of the hospital. Her care is documented in the medical record below.

Use the definitions in numbers 1-9 to write medical terms within the document.

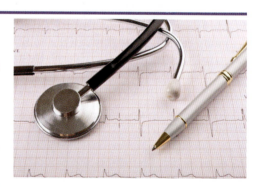

1. blood pressure that is above normal (generally greater than 130/80 mm Hg in adults)

2. distended or tortuous veins usually found in the lower extremities

3. physician who studies and treats diseases of the heart

4. surgical technique to bring a new blood supply to the heart muscle (myocardium) by detouring around blocked arteries

5. ballooning of a weakened portion of the arterial wall

6. incision into the vein (with a needle to remove blood or instill fluid)

7. record of the electrical activity of the heart

8. death (necrosis) of a portion of the heart muscle caused by lack of oxygen resulting from an interrupted blood supply

9. diagnostic procedure performed by passing a catheter into the heart from a blood vessel in the groin or arm to examine the condition of the heart and surrounding blood vessels

Refer to the medical record to answer questions 10-13.

10. The term **atherogenic** is used in the medical record to describe her risk factors for coronary artery disease. Ather/o means a fatty plaque deposited on a vessel wall. Use your knowledge of other word parts to review this term.

ather/o means _____ _____ deposited on a _____ _____.

-genic means _____, _____, _____.

Thus, **ather/o/genic** means _____ a _____ _____ deposit on a _____ _____.

31733 KROUSE, Natalia

File   Patient   Navigate   Custom Fields   Help

Chart Review   Encounters   Notes   Labs   Imaging   Procedures   Rx   Documents   Referrals   Scheduling   Billing

Name: **KROUSE, Natalia**   MR#: **31733**   Sex: F   **Allergies:** None known
DOB: 2/21/19XX   Age: 76   PCP: Lopez, Angelica DO

Cardiology Admission Report
Encounter Date: 05 March 20XX

Chief Complaint: Natalia Krouse is a 76-year-old woman who was admitted to the hospital for chest pain.

History of Present Illness: The patient has an extensive history of chronic cardiovascular issues. Atherogenic risk factors include (1.)_____, and hypercholesterolemia. She also has extensive (2.)_____ of the lower extremities bilaterally. Her family physician referred her to a (3.)_____ in 2011 for medical management of these complications. She smokes one pack of cigarettes a day and has previously declined participation in a smoking cessation program. She is not diabetic. Family history reveals a brother who has had (4.)_____ and a mother deceased from abdominal aortic (5.)_____ rupture.

Over the last 5 days, the patient reports that she has felt "very wiped out," with episodes of nausea and indigestion. This evening while taking a short walk she experienced severe chest pressure, pain radiating to left arm and jaw and dizziness that lasted 5 minutes. Neighbors called 911 and she was admitted to this hospital for evaluation through the emergency department.

Physical Exam: On exam, blood pressure is 139/86 mm Hg with a pulse of 120. Oxygen saturation is 94% on room air. Lungs are clear to auscultation. She has a regular heart rhythm without murmur. She appears fatigued, but in no acute distress.

Plan:
(6.)_____ to withdraw blood for CPK and troponin values. (7.)_____ will be obtained to rule out (8.)_____.
(9.) _____ with possible coronary stent if necessary.

Electronically signed: DeRouge, Marguerite MD on 05 March 20XX 21:27

Start   Log On/Off   Print   Edit

11. _____ is the abbreviation for heart failure, which is also sometimes referred to as congestive heart failure, or CHF.

12. **Coronary** is derived from the Latin **coronalis**, meaning crown or wreath. It describes the arteries encircling the heart. A stent is a supportive tubular device placed in the _____ (**referring to the arteries circling the heart**) artery; it is used to prevent closure of the artery after angioplasty (Figure 7.18).

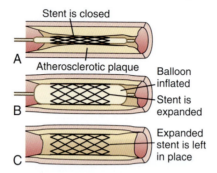

Stent is closed

A
Atherosclerotic plaque

Balloon inflated

Stent is expanded

B

Expanded stent is left in place

C

Figure 7.18 Coronary Stent. **A,** Stent at the site of plaque formation. **B,** Inflated balloon and expanded stent. **C,** Expanded stent with balloon removed.

13. Identify two new medical terms in the medical record you would like to investigate. Use your medical dictionary or an online reference to look up the definition.

Medical Term   **Definition**

a. _____   _____

b. _____   _____

EXERCISE R   **Use Medical Language in Electronic Health Records Online**

Select the correct medical terms to complete three medical records in one patient's electronic file.

⊕ Access online resources at evolve.elsevier.com > Evolve Resources > Practice Student Resources > Activities > Lesson 7 > Electronic Health Records

Topic: Coronary Artery Disease
Record 1: Echocardiogram Report
Record 2: Cardiovascular Operative Report
Record 3: Discharge Summary

❏ Check the box when complete.

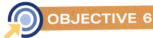

OBJECTIVE 6

Recall and assess knowledge of word parts, medical terms, and abbreviations.

EXERCISE S   **Online Review of Lesson Content**

Recall and assess your learning from working through the lesson by completing online learning activities. at evolve. elsevier.com > Evolve Resources > Practice Student Resources. Keep track of your progress by placing a check mark next to completed activities.

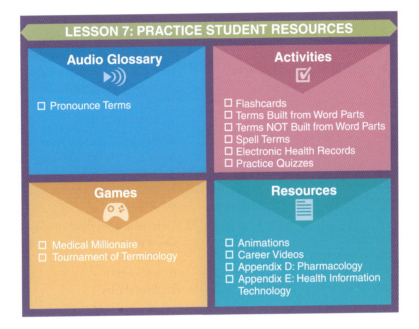

EXERCISE T Lesson Content Quiz

Test your knowledge of the terms and abbreviations introduced in this lesson. Circle the letter for the medical term or abbreviation related to the words in italics.

1. The *record of the heart using sound* showed evidence for moderately severe mitral regurgitation.
   a. echocardiogram
   b. electrocardiogram
   c. angiography

2. A patient with hypothyroidism may present with *slow heart rate.*
   a. hypotension
   b. cardiomegaly
   c. bradycardia

3. *Rapid breathing* was noted in the patient suffering from acute heart failure.
   a. tachycardia
   b. tachypnea
   c. hypertension

4. A *blood clot that has entered the bloodstream and lodged* in a pulmonary artery can cause chest pain and shortness of breath.
   a. thrombosis
   b. phlebitis
   c. embolus

5. *Emergency procedure consisting of artificial ventilation and external cardiac compressions* can be lifesaving in a patient with acute cardiac arrest.
   a. CBC
   b. CAGB
   c. CPR

6. A *pressure exerted by blood against the blood vessel walls* of 120/80 mm Hg is normal.
   a. pulse
   b. blood pressure
   c. stethoscope

7. A patient with strep throat can present with cervical *disease of the lymph nodes.*
   a. lymphadenopathy
   b. lymphadentits
   c. lymphoma

8. A right carotid *excision within the artery* was performed following a transient ischemic attack.
   a. angiography
   b. angioplasty
   c. endarterectomy

9. A chest radiograph showed *enlargement of the heart* in a patient with heart failure.
   a. cardiomegaly
   b. cardiopathy
   c. cardiology

10. Deep vein *abnormal condition of blood clots* can cause pain and swelling of the lower extremities.
    a. phlebitis
    b. embolus
    c. thrombosis

LESSON AT A GLANCE — CARDIOVASCULAR AND LYMPHATIC SYSTEMS WORD PARTS

COMBINING FORMS
aden/o   electr/o
angi/o   lymph/o
arteri/o   phleb/o, ven/o
cardi/o   splen/o
ech/o   thromb/o

SUFFIXES
-ac
-graph
-megaly
-penia
-sclerosis

PREFIXES
brady-
tachy-

LESSON AT A GLANCE — CARDIOVASCULAR AND LYMPHATIC SYSTEMS MEDICAL TERMS AND ABBREVIATIONS

SIGNS AND SYMPTOMS
bradycardia
cardiomegaly
hemorrhage
hypertension (HTN)
hypotension
splenomegaly
tachycardia
tachypnea

DISEASES AND DISORDERS
anemia
aneurysm
arteriosclerosis
cardiomyopathy
coronary artery disease (CAD)
embolus *pl.* emboli
heart failure (HF)
hematoma
hemolysis
leukemia
leukocytopenia
lymphadenitis
lymphadenopathy
lymphoma
myocardial infarction (MI)
phlebitis

thrombocytopenia
thrombophlebitis
thrombosis
varicose veins

DIAGNOSTIC TESTS AND EQUIPMENT
angiography
arteriogram
blood pressure (BP)
cardiac catheterization
complete blood count (CBC)
echocardiogram (ECHO)
electrocardiogram (ECG, EKG)
electrocardiograph
electrocardiography
pulse (P)
sphygmomanometer
stethoscope
venogram

SURGICAL PROCEDURES
angioplasty
coronary artery bypass graft (CABG)
endarterectomy
phlebotomy
splenectomy

SPECIALTIES AND PROFESSIONS
cardiologist
cardiology
hematologist
hematology

RELATED TERMS
arterial
cardiac
cardiopulmonary resuscitation (CPR)
hemostasis
intravenous (IV)
myocardial
thrombocyte

ABBREVIATIONS

BP	ECHO	MI
CABG	ECG	P
CAD	EKG	PAD
CBC	HF	PTCA
CPR	HHD	VS
DSA	HTN	
DVT	IV	

CASE STUDY   **Ruth Clifton**

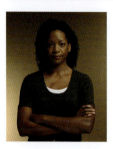

Ruth is worried about her stomach. She has been having pain on and off for about 3 months. At first it was just once in a while but now it seems to be every day. Her pain seems to be worse when she hasn't eaten for a while and after she eats something bland it usually gets a bit better. She bought some antacids at the pharmacy and chewing those also seems to help. Lately the pain in her stomach has been waking her up at night. A glass of milk usually helps with that. The last few days, though, she has had nausea and vomiting and is finding it difficult to eat. Her friend recommends that she see a stomach doctor, who helped her when she had similar problems.

■ *Consider Ruth's situation as you work through the lesson on the digestive system. At the end of the lesson, we will return to this case study and identify medical terms used to document Ruth's experience and the care she receives.*

OBJECTIVES

1	■	Build, translate, pronounce, and spell medical terms built from word parts (p. 221).
2	■	Define, pronounce, and spell medical terms NOT built from word parts (p. 241).
3	■	Write abbreviations (p. 246).
4	■	Identify medical terms by clinical category (p. 247).
5	■	Use medical language in clinical statements, the case study, and a medical record (p. 251).
6	■	Recall and assess knowledge of word parts, medical terms, and abbreviations (p. 254).

INTRODUCTION TO THE DIGESTIVE SYSTEM

Anatomic Structures of the Digestive System

abdomen (AB-duh-men)	portion of the body between the thorax and the pelvis
anus (Ā-nus)	sphincter muscle (ringlike band of muscle fiber that keeps an opening tight) at the end of the digestive tract, connected to the rectum
appendix (a-PEN-diks)	small, wormlike pouch attached to the cecum (the beginning of the large intestine)
colon (KŌ-lun)	major component of the large intestine, which is divided into four parts: ascending colon, transverse colon, descending colon, and sigmoid colon
esophagus (e-SOF-a-gus)	tube that transports food from the pharynx to the stomach

Anatomic Structures of the Digestive System—cont'd

gallbladder (GAWL-blad-er)	small, saclike structure that stores bile produced by the liver
gums (gumz)	pale pink tissue that is attached to jaw bones and teeth; provides supporting structure for the mouth
large intestine (larj) (in-TES-tin)	approximately 5-foot canal extending from the ileum to the anus
liver (LIV-er)	organ that produces bile for the digestion of fats; performs many other functions that support digestion and metabolism
mouth (mouth)	opening through which food passes into the body; breaks food into small particles by mastication (chewing) and mixing with saliva; (also called the **oral cavity**)
pancreas (PAN-kre-us)	organ that secretes multiple enzymes necessary for digestion; also secretes insulin for carbohydrate metabolism.
pharynx (FAR-inks)	performs swallowing action that passes food from the mouth into the esophagus
rectum (REK-tum)	last part of the large intestine connecting to the anus
sigmoid colon (SIG-moyd) (KŌ-lun)	S-shaped section of the large intestine leading into the rectum
small intestine (smal) (in-TES-tin)	20-foot tube extending from the stomach to the large intestine, where most of the nutrients are absorbed; has three sections: duodenum, jejunum, ileum
stomach (STUM-ek)	J-shaped sac that mixes and stores food; secretes substances that aid digestion
tongue (tung)	organ in mouth composed of skeletal muscle; responsible for movement of food from mouth to pharynx, and is also important for taste and speech

Functions of the Digestive System

- **Ingestion:** taking in nutrients through the mouth
- **Digestion:** mechanical and chemical breakdown of food for use by body cells
- **Absorption:** transfer of digested food from the small intestine to the blood stream
- **Elimination:** removal of solid waste from the body

How the Digestive System Works

The digestive tract, also known as the **alimentary canal** or **gastrointestinal (GI) tract**, is a continuous passageway from the mouth to the anus (Figure 8.1). The lips, cheeks, tongue, gums, teeth, and palate form the **oral cavity (mouth)**, where food is ingested and masticated (chewed), and enzymes are released to help break it down. Swallowing occurs in the **pharynx**, then masticated food and liquid are moved into the **esophagus**, which transports its contents to the **stomach**. The stomach secretes chemicals for digestion and also churns food, then passes it into the **small intestine**. Absorption, the passage of nutrients into the bloodstream, occurs here. Remaining materials are then emptied into the **large intestine** for the formation of feces, which are then stored in the **rectum** and eliminated through the **anus**. Accessory organs of the digestive system include the salivary glands, pancreas, liver, and gallbladder, which produce various chemicals that assist in various aspects of the digestive process.

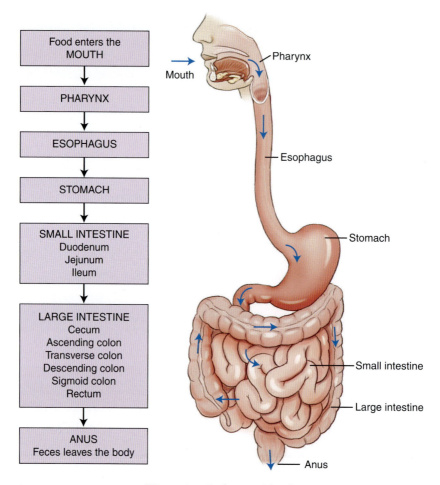

Food enters the
MOUTH

↓

PHARYNX

↓

ESOPHAGUS

↓

STOMACH

↓

SMALL INTESTINE
Duodenum
Jejunum
Ileum

↓

LARGE INTESTINE
Cecum
Ascending colon
Transverse colon
Descending colon
Sigmoid colon
Rectum

↓

ANUS
Feces leaves the body

Mouth — Pharynx

Esophagus

Stomach

Small intestine

Large intestine

Anus

Figure 8.1 Pathway of food.

CAREER FOCUS   **Professionals Who Work with the Digestive System**

- **Dental Hygienists** work with dentists to meet the oral health needs of patients. They clean teeth by removing plaque deposits and apply sealants and fluoride for preventative care. They also teach patients about appropriate oral hygiene including tooth brushing, flossing, and nutritional counseling.

- **Dental Assistants** assist dentists during many different treatment procedures (Figure 8.2). They may also take dental radiographs (x-rays) and help obtain impressions of patients' teeth for plaster casts. They also provide instructions to patients after their treatment. In addition, they prepare and sterilize equipment and assist with infection control.

CAREER FOCUS   **Professionals Who Work with the Digestive System—cont'd**

- **Registered Dietitians** (RD) are food and nutrition experts who have earned a bachelor's degree and met professional requirements to qualify for the credential RD. They may work in hospitals or other healthcare facilities, in the community, or in public health settings.

- **Dietetic Technicians** assist in providing food service and nutritional programs under the supervision of a dietitian. They may plan and produce meals based on established guidelines, teach principles of food and nutrition, or counsel patients.

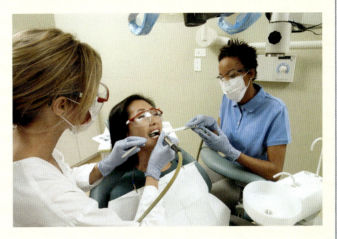

Figure 8.2 A dentist and a dental assistant work on a patient.

 FOR MORE INFORMATION

- Access online resources at evolve.elsevier.com > Practice Student Resources > Other Resources > Career Videos to watch interviews with a **Dental Hygienist** and a **Clinical Dietitian**.

 OBJECTIVE 1

Build, translate, pronounce, and spell medical terms built from word parts.

WORD PARTS   Use the paper or online **flashcards** to familiarize yourself with the following word parts.

COMBINING FORM (WR + CV)	DEFINITION	COMBINING FORM (WR + CV)	DEFINITION
abdomin/o, lapar/o	abdomen, abdominal cavity	enter/o	intestines (the small intestine)
an/o	anus	esophag/o	esophagus
append/o, appendic/o	appendix	gastr/o	stomach
chol/e	gall, bile	gingiv/o	gums
col/o, colon/o	colon	gloss/o, lingu/o	tongue
duoden/o	duodenum	hepat/o	liver

WORD PARTS	Presented with the Digestive System—cont'd		
COMBINING FORM (WR + CV)	**DEFINITION**	**COMBINING FORM (WR + CV)**	**DEFINITION**
ile/o	ileum	**peps/o**	digestion
jejun/o	jejunum	**phag/o**	swallowing, eating
or/o	mouth	**proct/o, rect/o**	rectum
pancreat/o	pancreas	**sigmoid/o**	sigmoid colon
SUFFIX	**DEFINITION**		
-algia	pain		

WORD PARTS PRESENTED IN PREVIOUS LESSONS	Used to Build Terms for the Digestive System		
COMBINING FORM (WR+CV)	**DEFINITION**	**COMBINING FORM (WR + CV)**	**DEFINITION**
cyst/o	bladder, sac	**lith/o**	stone(s), calculus (*pl.* calculi)
SUFFIX	**DEFINITION**	**SUFFIX (S)**	**DEFINITION**
-al, -eal, -ic	pertaining to	**-logy**	study of
-cele	hernia, protrusion	**-megaly**	enlargement
-centesis	surgical puncture to remove fluid	**-oma**	tumor
		-osis	abnormal condition
-ectomy	surgical removal, excision	**-plasty**	surgical repair
-graphy	process of recording, radiographic imaging	**-scope**	instrument used for visual examination
-ia	diseased state, condition of	**-scopic**	pertaining to visual examination
		-scopy	visual examination
-iasis	condition	**-stomy**	creation of an artificial opening
-itis	inflammation	**-tomy**	cut into, incision
-logist	one who studies and treats (specialist, physician)	**-y**	no meaning
PREFIX (P)	**DEFINITION**	**PREFIX (P)**	**DEFINITION**
a-, an-	absence of, without	**sub-**	below, under
dys-	difficult, painful, abnormal		

Refer to Appendix A, Word Parts Used in *Basic Medical Language*, for alphabetical lists of word parts and their meanings.

EXERCISE A   Build and Translate Medical Terms Built from Word Parts

*Use the **Word Parts Tables** to complete the following questions. Check your responses with the Answer Key in Appendix C.*

1. LABEL: *Write the combining forms for anatomical structures of the digestive system on Figure 8.3. These anatomical combining forms will be used to build and translate medical terms in Exercise A.*

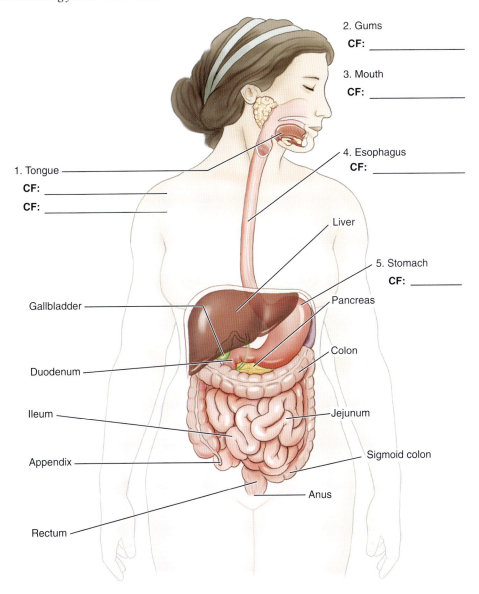

2. Gums
CF: _____

3. Mouth
CF: _____

4. Esophagus
CF: _____

1. Tongue
CF: _____
CF: _____

Liver

5. Stomach
CF: _____

Pancreas

Gallbladder

Colon

Duodenum

Ileum

Jejunum

Appendix

Sigmoid colon

Anus

Rectum

Figure 8.3 The digestive system and related combining forms.

2. MATCH: *Draw a line to match the word part with its definition.*

    a. -algia   inflammation
    b. -itis   pain

---

3. BUILD: *Using the combining form **gingiv/o** and the word parts reviewed in the previous exercise, build the following terms related to the gums. Remember, the definition usually starts with the meaning of the suffix.*

    a. pain in the gums   _____ / _____
                                                    wr   s

    b. inflammation of the gums   _____ / _____
                                                  wr   s

---

4. READ: Gingivitis (jin-ji-VĪ-tis) is frequently caused by poor oral hygiene that allows plaque to form. Plaque is a sticky substance that occurs when mouth bacteria combine with sugars and starches in food. Tooth brushing prevents the build-up of plaque. If plaque is allowed to remain, it causes tartar at the gum line which is not easily removed. This irritates the gums, causing them to become swollen and bleed easily. Other symptoms of gingivitis include **gingivalgia** (jin-ji-VAL-jē-a), bad breath, and a change in color of the gums from pink to dusky red.

---

5. LABEL: *Write word parts to complete Figure 8.4.*

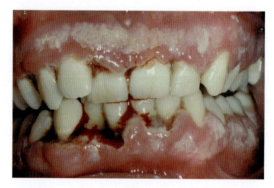

Figure 8.4 Severe _____ / _____ .
                              gums   inflammation

---

6. MATCH: *Draw a line to match the word part with its definition.*

    a. -itis   below, under
    b. -al   inflammation
    c. sub-   pertaining to

7. TRANSLATE: *Complete the definitions of the following terms built from the combining form **gloss/o**, or **lingu/o**, meaning tongue. Use the meaning of word parts to fill in the blanks. Remember, the definition usually starts with the meaning of the suffix.*

a. gloss/itis   _____ of the tongue

b. sub/lingu/al   pertaining to _____ the _____

8. BUILD: *Using the combining form **or/o**, meaning mouth, and the word parts reviewed in the matching exercise, build the following term:*

pertaining to the mouth   _____/_____
                                   wr   **s**

9. READ: Glossitis (glos-Ī-tis) may be caused by a variety of conditions including infections, allergic reactions, dry mouth, trauma, or low iron levels. **Oral** (OR-al) examination usually reveals swelling of the tongue, with color and texture changes. It is important to inspect the **sublingual** (sub-LING-gwal) surface to look for leukoplakia (white patches) that could indicate cancer or other diseases.

10. LABEL: *Write word parts to complete Figure 8.5.*

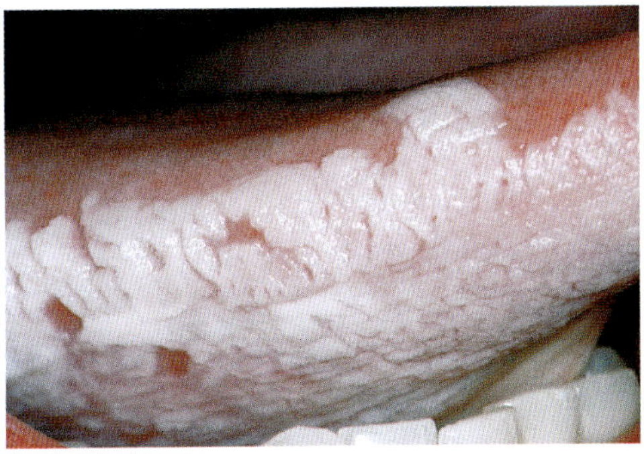

Figure 8.5 _____/_____/_____ leukoplakia.
              below   tongue   pertaining to

11. MATCH: *Draw a line to match the word part with its definition.*

a. peps/o   swallowing, eating
b. phag/o   no meaning
c. enter/o   intestines (the small intestine)
d. -ia   digestion
e. -y   diseased state, condition of
f. a-   without

12. BUILD: *Use the prefix* **dys-**, *meaning difficult, painful, abnormal, and the word parts reviewed in the previous exercise to build the following terms:*

a. painful intestines   _____/_____/_____y_____
                                    p   wr   s

b. condition of difficult digestion   _____/_____/_____
                                              p   wr   s

c. condition of difficult swallowing _____/_____/_____
                                              p   wr   s

---

13. TRANSLATE: *Complete the definition.*

a/phag/ia   _____ of without _____

---

14. READ: **Dyspepsia** (dis-PEP-sē-a) is also referred to as indigestion or upset stomach, and refers to a discomfort in the upper abdomen or chest that may be accompanied by burping, bloating, or feeling full. **Dysentery** (DIS-en-ter-ē) symptoms often include fever, abdominal pain, and bloody diarrhea. In the United States it is frequently caused by *Shigella* and *E. coli* bacteria in contaminated food or water. **Dysphagia** (dis-FĀ-ja) is often caused by problems with the esophagus, while **aphagia** (a-FĀ-ja), the loss of the ability to swallow, can be caused by either anatomic or psychological factors.

---

15. MATCH: *Draw a line to match the word part with its definition.*

a. -eal   inflammation
b. -itis   pertaining to

---

16. BUILD: *Using the combining form* **esophag/o** *meaning esophagus,* and the word parts reviewed in the previous *exercise, build the following terms:*

a. pertaining to the esophagus   _____/_____
                                            wr   s

b. inflammation of the esophagus   _____/_____
                                            wr   s

---

17. READ: **Esophagitis** (e-sof-a-JĪ-tis) is frequently caused by acid reflux, a condition which occurs when the **esophageal** (e-sof-a-JĒ-al) sphincter (a valve-like structure between the esophagus and stomach) doesn't close properly. This allows stomach contents to back up into the esophagus, causing irritation to the esophageal lining.

18. **LABEL:** *Write word parts to complete Figure 8.6.*

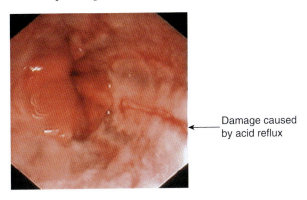

Damage caused
by acid reflux

Figure 8.6 Linear streaks visible by endoscopy in _____/_____.
esophagus   inflammation

19. **MATCH:** *Draw a line to match the word part with its definition.*

a. enter/o   one who studies and treats (specialist, physician)
b. -itis   study of
c. -logist   intestines (the small intestine)
d. -logy   inflammation

20. **BUILD:** *Using the combining form **gastr/o** and the word parts reviewed in the previous exercise, build the following terms related to the stomach.*

a. physician who studies and treats diseases   _____/ o /_____/ o /_____
   of the stomach and intestines   wr   cv   wr   cv   s

b. study of the stomach and intestines   _____/ o /_____/ o /_____
                                                        wr   cv   wr   cv   s

c. inflammation of the stomach and intestines   _____/ o /_____/_____
                                                        wr   cv   wr   s

21. **MATCH:** *Draw a line to match the word part with its definition.*

a. -ectomy   pertaining to
b. -itis   esophagus
c. -eal, -ic   excision
d. esophag/o   inflammation

22. TRANSLATE: *Complete the definitions of the following terms using the combining form* **gastr/o.**

a. gastr/itis _____ of the stomach

b. gastr/ic pertaining to the _____

c. gastr/ectomy _____ of the stomach

d. gastr/o/esophag/eal _____ to the _____ and _____

23. READ: Gastroenteritis (gas-trō-en-te-RĪ-tis) is often caused by a virus and will resolve on its own. **Gastritis** (gas-TRĪ-tis) can be caused by bacteria, certain medications (like aspirin and ibuprofen), or excessive alcohol use. A **gastroenterologist** (gas-trō-en-ter-OL-o-jist) often treats this condition. If left untreated, it may lead to stomach ulcers and bleeding. In severe cases, a partial **gastrectomy** (gas-TREK-to-mē) may be required. A complete gastrectomy may be required with certain types of **gastric** (GAS-trik) cancer, in which case the stomach is removed at the **gastroesophageal** (gas-trō-e-sof-a-JĒ-al) junction and the esophagus is connected directly to the jejunum.

24. LABEL: *Write word parts to complete Figure 8.7.*

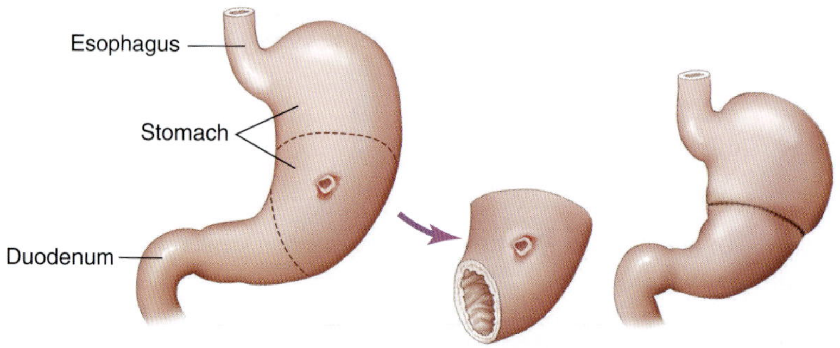

Esophagus
Stomach
Duodenum

Figure 8.7 A partial _____/_____ may be performed to remove chronic gastric ulcers.
stomach   excision

25. MATCH: *Draw a line to match the word part with its definition.*

a. -scope   creation of an artificial opening
b. -stomy   visual examination
c. -scopy   instrument used for visual examination

26. BUILD: *Using the combining form* **gastr/o** *and the word parts reviewed in the previous exercise, build the following terms.*

a. instrument used for visual examination of the stomach   _____/ o /_____
                                                            wr   cv   s

b. visual examination of the stomach   _____/ o /_____
                                       wr   cv   s

c. creation of an artificial opening into the stomach   _____/ o /_____
                                                        wr   cv   s

27. **READ**: Percutaneous endoscopic **gastrostomy** (gas-TROS-to-mē) or **PEG**, is one of the most common endo-scopic procedures performed. During **gastroscopy** (gas-TROS-ko-pē), the gastroenterologist inserts the **gas-troscope** (GAS-trō-skōp) into the mouth, through the esophagus, and into the stomach. The gastroscope is then directed anteriorly so that the light can be seen through the skin. A small incision is made and then the gastroscope is advanced through this hole, allowing it to grab the gastrostomy tube and bring it into the stomach. This tube is secured to the skin and the gastroscope is removed.

28. **LABEL**: *Write word parts to complete Figure 8.8.*

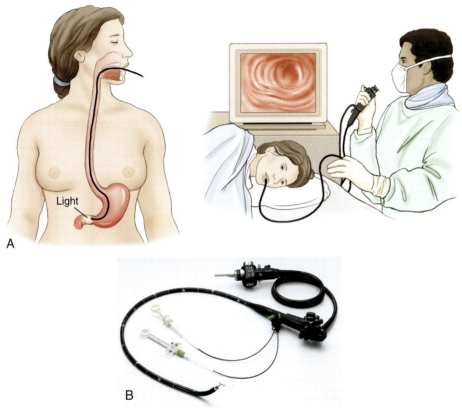

Figure 8.8 A. _____/o/_____.
                  stomach   visual examination

      B. Fiberoptic _____/o/_____, which has glass fibers
                      stomach   instrument used for visual examination
      in a flexible tube, allowing light and images to be transmitted back to the examiner.

29. **MATCH**: *Draw a line to match the word part with its definition.*

    a. -scope   pertaining to visual examination
    b. -scopic   instrument used for visual examination
    c. -scopy   abdomen, abdominal cavity
    d. abdomin/o, lapar/o   visual examination

30. TRANSLATE: *Use the combining form **lapar/o,** meaning abdominal cavity, to complete the definitions of the following terms.*

    a. lapar/o/scope   _____ used for visual examination of the _____ _____

    b. lapar/o/scopic   pertaining to _____ _____ of the abdominal cavity

    c. lapar/o/scopy   _____ _____ of the _____ _____

---

31. READ: Laparoscopic (lap-ar-ō-SKOP-ik) surgery can be performed through small incisions in the abdomen, rather than a large, open incision. It is sometimes referred to as videoscopic surgery because the surgeon performs the surgery by viewing a video screen that is connected to the **laparoscope** (LAP-a-rō-skōp). **Laparoscopy** (lap-a-ROS-ko-pē) reduces cost and trauma to the patient.

---

32. LABEL: *Write word parts to complete Figure 8.9.*

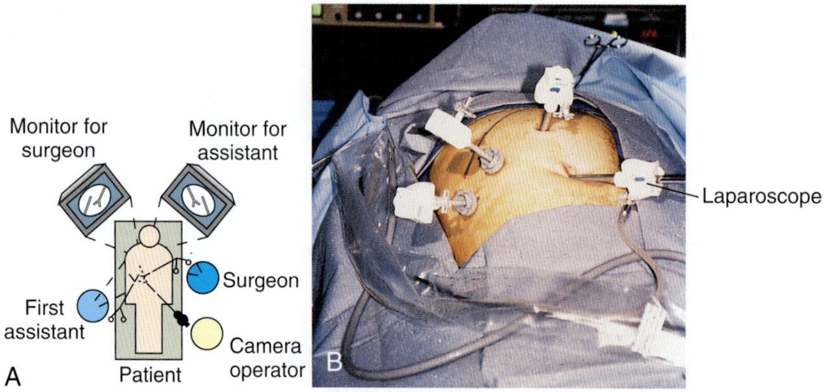

Figure 8.9 A. _____/o/_____ surgical set-up. B. Laparoscopic surgery.
                  abdominal cavity   pertaining to visual examination

---

33. MATCH: *Draw a line to match the word part with its definition.*

    a. -centesis   incision

    b. -tomy   surgical puncture to remove fluid

---

34. TRANSLATE: *Complete the definitions of the following terms.*

    a. abdomin/o/centesis   surgical _____ to remove _____ from

                            the abdominal _____

    b. lapar/o/tomy   _____ into the _____ cavity

35. READ: In an emergency, a general surgeon will often choose to perform a **laparotomy** (lap-a-ROT-o-mē) rather than a laparoscopy because the long, open incision provides a much larger view of the area in question and can be performed much more quickly. **Abdominocentesis** (ab-dom-i-nō-sen-TĒ-sis) is also known as **abdominal paracentesis**, and is often performed in people with excesses of fluid in their abdominal cavities due to liver disease, cancer, or other disorders.

36. REVIEW OF DIGESTIVE SYSTEM TERMS BUILT FROM WORD PARTS: *The following is an alphabetical list of terms built and translated in the previous exercises.*

MEDICAL TERMS BUILT FROM WORD PARTS

TERM	DEFINITION	TERM	DEFINITION
1. abdominocentesis (ab-dom-i-nō-sen-TĒ-sis)	surgical puncture to remove fluid from the abdominal cavity (also called **abdominal paracentesis**)	14. gastroesophageal (gas-trō-e-sof-a-JĒ-al)	pertaining to the stomach and esophagus
2. aphagia (a-FĀ-ja)	condition of without swallowing	15. gastroscope (GAS-trō-skōp)	instrument used for visual examination of the stomach (Figure 8.8, *B*)
3. dysentery (DIS-en-ter-ē)	painful intestines	16. gastroscopy (gas-TROS-ko-pē)	visual examination of the stomach (Figure 8.8, *A*)
4. dyspepsia (dis-PEP-sē-a)	condition of difficult digestion	17. gastrostomy (gas-TROS-to-mē)	creation of an artificial opening into the stomach
5. dysphagia (dis-FĀ-ja)	condition of difficulty swallowing	18. gingivalgia (jin-ji-VAL-jē-a)	pain in the gums
6. esophageal (e-sof-a-JĒ-al)	pertaining to the esophagus	19. gingivitis (jin-ji-VĪ-tis)	inflammation of the gums (Figure 8.4)
7. esophagitis (e-sof-a-JĪ-tis)	inflammation of the esophagus (Figure 8.6)	20. glossitis (glos-Ī-tis)	inflammation of the tongue
8. gastrectomy (gas-TREK-to-mē)	excision of the stomach (Figure 8.7)	21. laparoscope (LAP-a-rō-skōp)	instrument used for visual examination of the abdominal cavity
9. gastric (GAS-trik)	pertaining to the stomach	22. laparoscopic (lap-ar-ō-SKOP-ik)	pertaining to visual examination of the abdominal cavity (Figure 8.9)
10. gastritis (gas-TRĪ-tis)	inflammation of the stomach	23. laparoscopy (lap-a-ROS-ko-pē)	visual examination of the abdominal cavity
11. gastroenteritis (gas-trō-en-te-RĪ-tis)	inflammation of the stomach and intestines	24. laparotomy (lap-a-ROT-o-mē)	incision into the abdominal cavity
12. gastroenterologist (gas-trō-en-ter-OL-o-jist)	physician who studies and treats diseases of the stomach and intestines	25. oral (OR-al)	pertaining to the mouth
13. gastroenterology (gas-trō-en-ter-OL-o-jē)	study of the stomach and intestines	26. sublingual (sub-LING-gwal)	pertaining to under the tongue (Figure 8.5)

EXERCISE B   Pronounce and Spell Terms Built from Word Parts

Practice pronunciation and spelling on paper and online.

1. **Practice on Paper**
   a. **Pronounce**: Read the phonetic spelling and say aloud the terms listed in the previous table, Review Terms Built from Word Parts.
   b. **Spell**: Have a study partner read the terms aloud. Write the spelling of the terms on a separate sheet of paper.

2. **Practice Online** 🌐
   a. **Access** online learning resources. Go to evolve.elsevier.com > Evolve Resources > Practice Student Resources.
   b. **Pronounce**: Select Audio Glossary > Lesson 8 > Exercise B. Select a term to hear its pronunciation and repeat aloud.
   c. **Spell**: Select Activities > Lesson 8 > Spell Terms > Exercise B. Select the audio icon and type the correct spelling of the term.
   ❏ Check the box when complete.

EXERCISE C   Build and Translate MORE Medical Terms Built from Word Parts

*Use the **Word Parts Tables** to complete the following questions. Check your responses with the Answer Key in Appendix C.*

1. **LABEL**: *Write the combining forms for anatomical structures of the digestive system on Figure 8.10. These anatomical combining forms will be used to build and translate medical terms in Exercise C.*

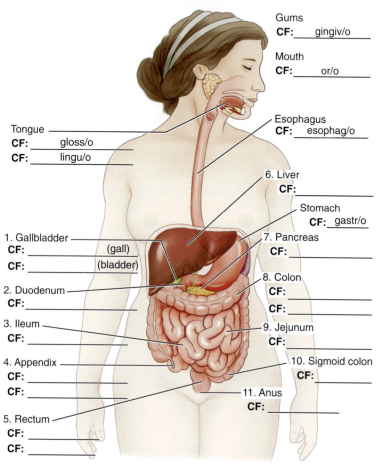

Figure 8.10 The digestive system and related combining forms.

2. **MATCH:** *Draw a line to match the word part with its definition.*

   a. duoden/o   visual examination
   b. -al   stomach
   c. esophag/o   esophagus
   d. gastr/o   pertaining to
   e. -scopy   duodenum

3. **TRANSLATE:** *Complete the definitions of the following terms by using the meaning of the word parts to fill in the blanks.*

   a. esophag/o/gastr/o/duoden/o/scopy _____ _____ of the esophagus, _____, and duodenum

   b. duoden/al   pertaining to the _____

4. **READ: Esophagogastroduodenoscopy** (e-sof-a-gō-gas-trō-dū-od-e-NOS-ko-pē) or **EGD**, is used to diagnose peptic ulcers and other conditions of the esophagus, stomach, and duodenum. Peptic ulcers may be found in the stomach and duodenum. They are called **gastric** ulcers and **duodenal** (dū-o-DĒ-nal) ulcers, respectively.

5. **MATCH:** *Draw a line to match the word part with its definition.*

   a. -stomy   creation of an artificial opening
   b. jejun/o   jejunum
   c. ile/o   ileum

6. **BUILD:** *Using the combining form and the word parts reviewed in the previous exercise, build the following terms.*

   a. creation of an artificial opening into the ileum   _____ / o / _____
                                   wr   cv   s

   b. creation of an artificial opening into the jejunum   _____ / o / _____
                                   wr   cv   s

7. **READ:** While gastrostomy is the preferred method for those who cannot ingest food by mouth, a patient who is at risk of aspiration (stomach contents refluxing up the esophagus and then entering the lungs through the bronchi) may have a **jejunostomy** (je-jū-NOS-te-mē) instead. G-tubes and J-tubes (gastrostomy and jejunostomy, respectively) provide nutrients for patients, while **ileostomy** (il-lē-OS-to-mē) outlets are used for the elimination of waste.

FYI **Duodenum** is derived from the Latin **duodeni**, meaning **12 each**, a reference to its length. It was named in 240 BC by a Greek physician. **Jejunum** is derived from the Latin **jejunus**, meaning **empty**; it was so named because the early anatomists always found it empty. **Ileum** is derived from the Greek **eilein**, meaning **to roll**, a reference to the peristaltic waves that move food along the digestive tract. This term was first used in the early part of the seventeenth century.

8. **MATCH:** *Draw a line to match the word part with its definition.*

    a. -oma   enlargement
    b. -itis   tumor
    c. -megaly   inflammation

9. **TRANSLATE:** *Complete the definitions of the following terms built from the combining form* **hepat/o,** *meaning liver.*

    a. hepat/itis   inflammation of the _____

    b. hepat/oma   _____ of the liver

    c. hepat/o/megaly   _____ of the _____

10. **READ:** One highly contagious form of **hepatitis** (hep-a-TĪ-tis) is hepatitis A, which is found worldwide but is more common in areas with poor sanitation and low socioeconomic status. **Hepatoma** (hep-a-TŌ-ma) is usually a malignant tumor of the liver; risk factors include hepatitis B and hepatitis C. All forms of hepatitis can cause **hepatomegaly** (hep-a-tō-MEG-a-lē); other causes include alcohol use, metastases from cancer, and heart failure.

11. **LABEL:** *Write word parts to complete Figure 8.11.*

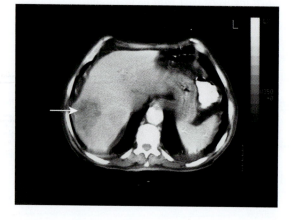

Figure 8.11 CT scan revealing a _____/_____.
                                           liver   tumor

12. **MATCH:** *Draw a line to match the word part with its definition.*

    a. -itis   bladder, sac
    b. -ectomy   stone(s), calculus (*pl.* calculi)
    c. cyst/o   excision
    d. lith/o   inflammation

13. **TRANSLATE:** *Complete the definitions of the following terms built from the combining form* **chol/e**, *meaning gall and bile. Hint: The* **e** *in chol/e/cyst is a combining vowel, and in this textbook it will only be used with the word root* **chol**.

a. chol/e/cyst/itis   _____ of the gallbladder

b. chol/e/cyst/ectomy   excision of the _____

c. chol/e/lith/iasis   condition of gall _____ (s)

> **FYI**   The combining form for gall and bile, **chol/e**, and the combining form for bladder, **cyst/o**, together mean **gallbladder**.

14. **READ:** The liver, bile ducts, and gallbladder comprise the biliary system, which creates, transports, stores, and releases bile into the small intestine to facilitate the absorption of fat. **Cholelithiasis** (kō-le-li-THĪ-a-sis) may occur when the composition of bile becomes unbalanced or when there is blockage in the bile ducts, trapping the bile and causing it to thicken. Many people have no symptoms with gallstones, but some go on to develop **cholecystitis** (kō-le-sis-TI-tis), which can be very painful and can occasionally lead to rupture of the gallbladder if left untreated. A **cholecystectomy** (kō-le-sis-TEK-to-mē) is the most common treatment for this disease.

> **FYI**   **Cholecystectomy** was first performed in 1882 by a German surgeon. Laparoscopic cholecystectomy was first performed in 1987 in France.

15. **LABEL:** *Write word parts to complete Figure 8.12.*

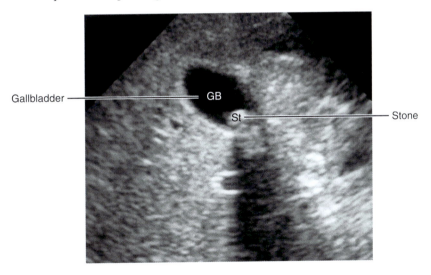

Gallbladder ————— GB

St ————— Stone

Figure 8.12 Abdominal ultrasound showing _____/e/_____/_____.
gall   stone   condition

16. MATCH: *Draw a line to match the word part with its definition.*

a. -ic   inflammation
b. -itis   pertaining to

17. BUILD: *Use the combining form **pancreat/o**, meaning pancreas, along with the word parts reviewed in the previous exercise to build the following terms.*

a. pertaining to the pancreas

_____/_____
                                 wr   s

b. inflammation of the pancreas

_____/_____
                                 wr   s

> **FYI**   **Pancreas** is derived from the Greek **pan**, meaning **all**, and **krea**, meaning **flesh**. The pancreas was first described in 300 BC. It was so named because of its fleshy appearance.

18. READ: The pancreas secretes enzymes necessary for digestion, and also produces insulin, which regulates glucose (sugar) levels in the body. In diabetes mellitus type 1, **pancreatic** (pan-krē-AT-ik) production of insulin is greatly decreased, leading to high glucose levels. **Pancreatitis** (pan-krē-a-TĪ-tis) may be caused by blockage of the common bile duct, or by excessive alcohol use, cigarette smoking, and many other diseases.

19. MATCH: *Draw a line to match the word part with its definition.*

a. -itis   excision
b. -ectomy   inflammation

20. TRANSLATE: *Complete the definitions of the following terms built from the combining forms **append/o** and **appendic/o**, meaning appendix.*

a. append/ectomy   excision of the _____
b. appendic/itis   _____ of the _____

21. READ: The appendix is a small pouch attached to the cecum (the first part of the large intestine); its function remains unknown. It is susceptible to inflammation and infection, resulting in **appendicitis** (a-pen-di-SĪ-tis). Acute appendicitis is a surgical emergency requiring immediate **appendectomy** (ap-en-DEK-to-mē).

22. LABEL: *Write word parts to complete Figure 8.13.*

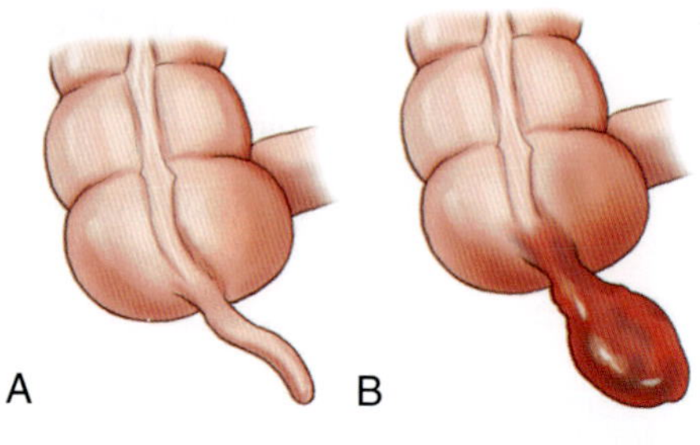

Figure 8.13 A. Normal Appendix.
       B. _____/_____.
                  appendix   inflammation

A   B

23. MATCH: *Draw a line to match the word part with its definition.*

a. -itis   visual examination
b. -stomy   process of recording, radiographic imaging
c. -ectomy   creation of an artificial opening
d. -graphy   inflammation
e. -scopy   excision

---

24. BUILD: *Use the combining form **colon/o**, along with the word parts reviewed in the previous exercise, to build terms related to the colon.*

a. visual examination of the colon   _____ / o / _____
                                                       wr   cv   s

b. radiographic imaging of the colon   CT _____ / o / _____
    (using a CT scanner and software)   wr   cv   s

---

25. READ: A common screening method for colon cancer is **colonoscopy** (kō-lon-OS-kō-pē), which allows the gastroenterologist to see lesions directly and biopsy or remove them as indicated. **CT colonography** (C-T) (kō-lon-OG-ra-fē), also called **virtual colonoscopy**, is especially useful in cases where a mass is present that will not allow a colonoscope to pass through; the radiologist can visualize the colon beyond the lesion.

---

26. LABEL: *Write word parts to complete Figure 8.14.*

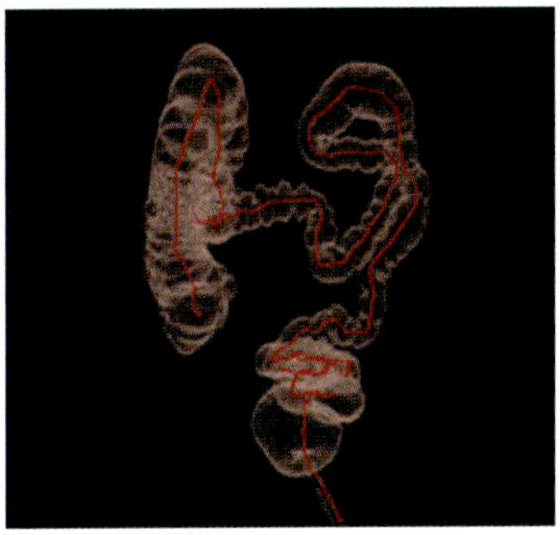

Figure 8.14 Image of the large intestine produced by
        CT _____ / o / _____.
               colon   radiographic imaging

---

27. BUILD: *Now use the combining form **col/o**, along with the word parts reviewed in the previous matching exercise, to build more terms related to the colon.*

a. inflammation of the colon   _____ / _____
                                            wr   s

b. creation of an artificial opening into the colon   _____ / o / _____
                                          wr   cv   s

c. excision of the colon   _____ / _____
                                        wr   s

28. **READ:** Antibiotic-associated **colitis** (kō-LĪ-tis), which is caused by a bacterium called *Clostridium difficile* (*C. difficile*), was traditionally found in hospitalized patients; however, it is also now occurring more frequently in the general community. It is usually treated with medicines, but in severe cases, a partial **colectomy** (kō-LEK-to-mē) may be required. If needed, a **colostomy** (ko-LOS-to-mē) may be created to allow the passage of stool.

29. **LABEL:** *Write word parts to complete Figure 8.15.*

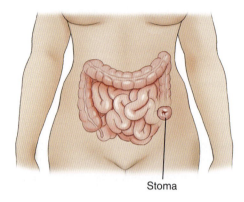

Stoma

Figure 8.15 _____/o/_____ following a partial colectomy.

                        colon   creation of an artifical opening

30. **MATCH:** *Draw a line to match the word part with its definition.*

   a. -scopy   instrument used for visual examination
   b. sigmoid/o   visual examination
   c. proct/o   sigmoid colon
   d. -scope   rectum

31. **TRANSLATE:** *Complete the definitions of the following terms.*

   a. sigmoid/o/scopy   visual _____ of the sigmoid _____
   b. proct/o/scope   _____ used for visual examination of the rectum
   c. proct/o/scopy   visual examination of the _____

32. **READ: Sigmoidoscopy** (sig-moy-DOS-ko-pē) visualizes the rectum and sigmoid colon and stops at the transverse colon. Because it is less involved than colonoscopy, less anesthesia is required for this procedure. In cases of rectal bleeding, a **proctoscope** (PROK-tō-skōp) may be used to examine the rectum just inside the anus. **Proctoscopy** (prok-TOS-ko-pē) is a useful method for diagnosing internal hemorrhoids and anal fissures.

33. LABEL: *Write word parts to complete Figure 8.16.*

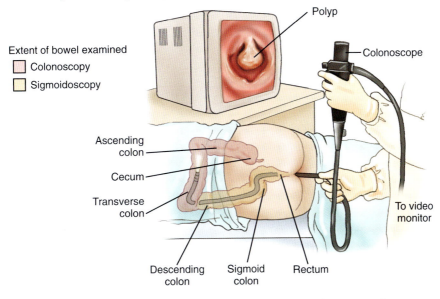

Polyp

Extent of bowel examined
- Colonoscopy
- Sigmoidoscopy

Colonoscope

Ascending colon

Cecum

Transverse colon

To video monitor

Descending colon   Sigmoid colon   Rectum

Figure 8.16 _____/o/_____ and colonoscopy showing a polyp in
        sigmoid colon   visual examination
the transverse colon.

---

34. MATCH: *Draw a line to match the word part with its definition.*

a. an/o   rectum
b. rect/o   pertaining to
c. -cele   anus
d. -al   hernia, protrusion

---

35. BUILD: *using the combining form* **rect/o,** *along with the word parts reviewed in the previous exercise, to build terms related to the rectum.*

a. hernia of the rectum   _____/ o /_____
                                    wr   cv   s

b. pertaining to the rectum   _____/_____
                                      wr   s

---

36. TRANSLATE: *Complete the definition.*

an/al   _____ to the _____

---

37. READ: Rectocele (REK-tō-sēl), also called **posterior prolapse**, occurs when the thin layer of tissue between the vagina and the anterior **rectal** (REK-tal) wall weakens (such as after childbirth or with chronic constipation), causing the rectum to bulge into the vagina. Chronic constipation can also cause **anal** (Ā-nal) fissures, which are tiny tears that are often accompanied by pain and bleeding with bowel movements.

38. REVIEW OF MORE DIGESTIVE SYSTEM TERMS BUILT FROM WORD PARTS: *the following is an alphabetical list of terms built and translated in the previous exercises.*

MEDICAL TERMS BUILT FROM WORD PARTS

TERM	DEFINITION	TERM	DEFINITION
1. anal (Ā-nal)	pertaining to the anus	14. hepatitis (hep-a-TĪ-tis)	inflammation of the liver
2. appendectomy (ap-en-DEK-to-mē)	excision of the appendix	15. hepatoma (hep-a-TŌ-ma)	tumor of the liver (Figure 8.11)
3. appendicitis (a-pen-di-SĪ-tis)	inflammation of the appendix (Figure 8.13, B)	16. hepatomegaly (hep-a-tō-MEG-a-lē)	enlargement of the liver
4. cholecystectomy (kō-le-sis-TEK-to-mē)	excision of the gallbladder	17. ileostomy (il-lē-OS-to-mē)	creation of an artificial opening into the ileum
5. cholecystitis (kō-le-sis-TI-tis)	inflammation of the gallbladder	18. jejunostomy (je-jū-NOS-te-mē)	creation of an artificial opening into the jejunum
6. cholelithiasis (kō-le-li-THĪ-a-sis)	condition of gallstone(s) (Figure 8.12)	19. pancreatic (pan-krē-AT-ik)	pertaining to the pancreas
7. colectomy (kō-LEK-to-mē)	excision of the colon	20. pancreatitis (pan-krē-a-TĪ-tis)	inflammation of the pancreas
8. colitis (kō-LĪ-tis)	inflammation of the colon	21. proctoscope (PROK-tō-skōp)	instrument used for visual examination of the rectum
9. colonoscopy (kō-lon-OS-kō-pē)	visual examination of the colon	22. proctoscopy (prok-TOS-ko-pē)	visual examination of the rectum
10. colostomy (ko-LOS-to-mē)	creation of an artificial opening into the colon (Figure 8.15)	23. rectal (REK-tal)	pertaining to the rectum
11. CT colonography (C-T) (kō-lon-OG-ra-fē)	radiographic imaging of the colon (using a CT scanner and software) (Figure 8.14)	24. rectocele (REK-tō-sēl)	hernia of the rectum (also called posterior prolapse)
12. duodenal (dū-o-DĒ-nal)	pertaining to the duodenum	25. sigmoidoscopy (sig-moy-DOS-ko-pē)	visual examination of the sigmoid colon (Figure 8.16)
13. esophagogastroduo-denoscopy (EGD) (e-sof-a-gō-gas-trō-dū-od-e-NOS- ko-pē)	visual examination of the esophagus, stomach, and duodenum		

EXERCISE D   Pronounce and Spell MORE Terms Built from Word Parts

Practice pronunciation and spelling on paper and online.

1. Practice on Paper

  a. Pronounce: Read the phonetic spelling and say aloud the terms listed in the previous table, Review of MORE Terms Built from Word Parts.

  b. Spell: Have a study partner read the terms aloud. Write the spelling of the terms on a separate sheet of paper.

2. **Practice Online** 🌐
    a. **Access** online learning resources. Go to evolve.elsevier.com > Evolve Resources > Practice Student Resources.
    b. **Pronounce:** Select Audio Glossary > Lesson 8 > Exercise D. Select a term to hear its pronunciation and repeat aloud.
    c. **Spell:** Select Activities > Lesson 8 > Spell Terms > Exercise D. Select the audio icon and type the correct spelling of the term.

❏ Check the box when complete.

OBJECTIVE 2

Define, pronounce, and spell medical terms NOT built from word parts.

The terms listed below may contain word parts, but are difficult to translate literally.

MEDICAL TERMS NOT BUILT FROM WORD PARTS

TERM	DEFINITION
bariatric surgery (bar-ē-AT-trik) (SUR-jer-ē)	surgical reduction of gastric capacity to treat morbid obesity, a condition that can cause serious illness
barium enema (BE) (BAR-ē-um) (EN-e-ma)	diagnostic procedure in which a series of radiographic images are taken of the large intestine after the rectal administration of the contrast agent barium; (also called **lower GI series**)
celiac disease (SĒ-lē-ak) (di-ZĒZ)	malabsorption syndrome caused by an immune reaction to gluten (a protein in wheat, rye, and barley), which may damage the lining of the small intestine that is responsible for absorption of food into the bloodstream; (also called **gluten enteropathy**)
cirrhosis (sir-RŌ-sis)	chronic disease of the liver with gradual destruction of cells and formation of scar tissue; commonly caused by alcoholism and certain types of viral hepatitis
constipation (kon-sti-PĀ-shun)	infrequent or difficult evacuation of stool
Crohn disease (krōn) (di-ZĒZ)	chronic inflammation of the intestinal tract usually affecting the ileum and colon; characterized by cobblestone ulcerations and the formation of scar tissue that may lead to intestinal obstruction

FYI **Bariatric** contains the word roots **bar**, meaning **weight**, and **iatr**, meaning **treatment**.

MEDICAL TERMS NOT BUILT FROM WORD PARTS—cont'd

TERM	DEFINITION
diarrhea (dī-a-RĒ-a)	frequent discharge of liquid stool
endoscopic retrograde cholangiopancreatography (ERCP) (en-dō-SKOP-ic) (RET-rō-grād) (kō-lan-jē-ō-pan-krē-a-TOG-rah-fē)	endoscopic procedure involving radiographic imaging of the biliary ducts and pancreatic ducts
gastroesophageal reflux disease (GERD) (gas-trō-e-sof-a-JĒ-al) (RĒ-fluks) (di-ZĒZ)	disorder characterized by the abnormal backward flow of the gastrointestinal contents into the esophagus
hemorrhoids (HEM-o-roydz)	swollen or distended veins in the rectal area, which may be internal or external and can be a source of rectal bleeding and pain
irritable bowel syndrome (IBS) (IR-i-ta-bl) (BOW-el) (SIN-drōm)	periodic disturbances of bowel function, such as diarrhea and/or constipation, usually associated with abdominal pain
parenteral (pah-REN-ter-al)	pertaining to treatment other than through the digestive system.
peptic ulcer (PEP-tik) (UL-ser)	erosion of the mucous membrane of the stomach or duodenum associated with increased secretion of acid from the stomach, bacterial infection (*Helicobacter pylori*), or use of nonsteroidal antiinflammatory drugs (often referred to as **gastric** or **duodenal ulcer** depending on its location)
polyp (POL-ip)	tumorlike growth extending outward from a mucous membrane
stoma (STŌ-ma)	surgical opening between an organ and the surface of the body, such as the opening established in the abdominal wall by colostomy, ileostomy, or a similar operation
ulcerative colitis (UC) (UL-ser-a-tiv) (kō-LĪ-tis)	disease characterized by inflammation of the colon with the formation of ulcers, which can cause bloody diarrhea
upper GI series (UGI series) (UP-er) (G-Ī) (SĒR-ēz)	diagnostic procedure in which a series of radiographic images are taken of the pharynx, esophagus, stomach, and duodenum after oral administration of the contrast agent barium

FYI The **angi/o** in cholangiopancreatography refers not to blood vessels, but to bile ducts.

EXERCISE E Label

Write the medical terms pictured and defined using the previous table of Medical Terms NOT Built from Word Parts. Check your work with the Answer Key in Appendix C.

1. _____
endoscopic procedure involving radiographic imaging of the biliary ducts and pancreatic ducts

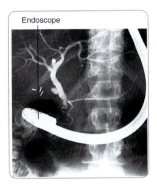

2. _____
erosion of the mucous membrane of the stomach or duodenum

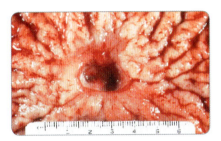

3. _____
disorder characterized by the abnormal backward flow of the gastrointestinal contents into the esophagus

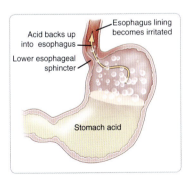

4. _____
diagnostic procedure in which a series of radiographic images are taken of the large intestine after the rectal administration of the contrast agent barium

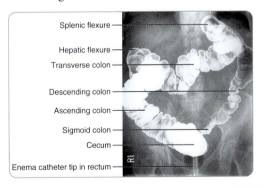

5. _____

tumorlike growth extending outward from a mucous membrane

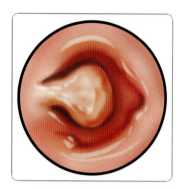

6. _____

surgical opening between an organ and the surface of the body.

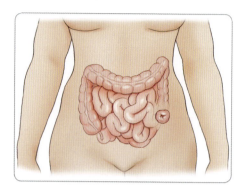

7. _____

surgical reduction of gastric capacity to treat morbid obesity, a condition that can cause serious illness

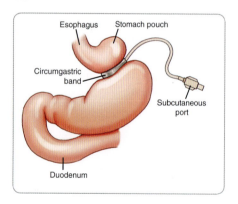

8. _____

swollen or distended veins in the rectal area

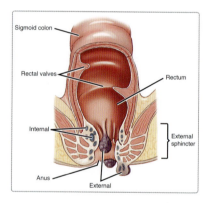

EXERCISE F   Learn Medical Terms NOT Built from Word Parts

Fill in the blanks with medical terms defined in bold using the Medical Terms NOT Built from Word Parts table. Answers are listed in Appendix C.

1. The **disorder characterized by the abnormal backward flow of the gastrointestinal contents into the esopha-gus,** or _____ abbreviated as _____, causes heart-burn and the gradual breakdown of the mucous barrier of the esophagus.

2. Periodic disturbances of bowel function, usually associated with abdominal pain, or _____ _____ abbreviated as _____, can be of three different types: **infrequent or difficult evacuation of stool** _____ type (IBS-C), **frequent discharge of liquid stool** _____ type (IBS-D), or mixed-type IBS with alternating constipation and diarrhea.

3. A **tumorlike growth extending outward from a mucous membrane**, or _____, may be diagnosed from the results of a **series of radiographic images taken after the rectal administration of a contrast agent** _____. Polyps are usually benign and are commonly found in the intestines as well as in the nose and throat.

4. Abdominal sonography is commonly used to visualize organs such as the liver, gallbladder, bile ducts, and pancreas. While not as frequently used for diagnosis, **endoscopic procedure involving radiographic imaging of the biliary ducts and pancreatic ducts**, or _____ _____, abbreviated ERCP, is an excellent method for treating abnormalities of the biliary and pancreatic ducts, including the removal of stones.

5. Bloody diarrhea is the main symptom of **inflammation of the colon with the formation of ulcers** _____ abbreviated UC. UC is usually resolved with a colectomy and with the creation of a **surgical opening between an organ and the surface of the body** or _____. **Chronic inflammation of the intestinal tract usually affecting the ileum and colon characterized by cobblestone ulcerations and the formation of scar tissue that may lead to intestinal obstruction**, or _____, can actually occur anywhere in the gastrointestinal tract and can only be controlled, not cured.

6. Chronic alcoholism is the leading cause of **chronic disease of the liver with gradual destruction of cells and formation of scar tissue** or _____. The amount of alcohol that causes this disease is different for every person.

7. A(n) **erosion of the mucous membrane of the stomach or duodenum**, or _____, may be diagnosed by a **series of radiographic images taken of the pharynx, esophagus, stomach, and duodenum after the oral administration of the contrast agent barium** _____.

8. Malabsorption syndrome caused by an **immune reaction to gluten, which may damage the lining of the small intestine that is responsible for absorption of food into the bloodstream**, or _____, is caused by an interaction between genes, gluten intake, and environment. In very severe cases, patients may require **pertaining to treatment other than through the digestive system**, or _____, fluid replacement and nutritional support.

EXERCISE G   Pronounce and Spell Terms NOT Built from Word Parts

Practice pronunciation and spelling on paper and online.

1. **Practice on Paper**
   a. **Pronounce**: Read the phonetic spelling and say aloud the terms listed in the previous Medical Terms NOT Built from Word Parts Table.
   b. **Spell**: Have a study partner read the terms aloud. Write the spelling of the terms on a separate sheet of paper.

2. **Practice Online** 🌐
   a. **Access** online learning resources. Go to evolve.elsevier.com > Evolve Resources > Practice Student Resources.
   b. **Pronounce**: Select Audio Glossary > Lesson 8 > Exercise G. Select a term to hear its pronunciation and repeat aloud.
   c. **Spell**: Select Activities > Lesson 8 > Spell Terms > Exercise G. Select the audio icon and type the correct spelling of the term.

❑ Check the box when complete.

OBJECTIVE 3

Write abbreviations.

ABBREVIATIONS RELATED TO THE DIGESTIVE SYSTEM

Use the online **flashcards** to familiarize yourself with the following abbreviations.

ABBREVIATION	TERM	ABBREVIATION	TERM
BE	barium enema	IBS	irritable bowel syndrome
BM	bowel movement	PEG	percutaneous endoscopic gastrostomy
EGD	esophagogastroduodenoscopy	TPN	total parenteral nutrition
ERCP	endoscopic retrograde cholangiopancreatography	UC	ulcerative colitis
GERD	gastroesophageal reflux disease	UGI series	upper GI series
GI	gastrointestinal		

EXERCISE H   Abbreviate Medical Terms

Write the correct abbreviation next to its medical term.

1. Diseases and disorders:

   a. _____   gastroesophageal reflux disease

   b. _____   irritable bowel syndrome

   c. _____   ulcerative colitis

2. Diagnostic tests and equipment:

    a. _____ barium enema

    b. _____ esophagogastroduodenoscopy

    c. _____ endoscopic retrograde cholangiopancreatography

    d. _____ series upper GI series

3. Surgical procedures:

_____ percutaneous endoscopic gastrostomy

4. Related terms:

    a. _____ bowel movement

    b. _____ gastrointestinal

    c. _____ total parenteral nutrition

OBJECTIVE 4

Identify medical terms by clinical category.

Now that you have worked through the digestive system lesson, review and practice medical terms grouped by clinical category. Categories include signs and symptoms, diseases and disorders, diagnostic tests and equipment, surgical procedures, specialties and professions, and other terms related to the digestive system.

EXERCISE I   Signs and Symptoms

Write the medical terms for signs and symptoms next to their definitions.

1. _____ condition of without swallowing

2. _____ infrequent or difficult evacuation of stool

3. _____ frequent discharge of liquid stool

4. _____ condition of difficult digestion

5. _____ condition of difficult swallowing

6. _____ pain in the gums

7. _____ enlargement of the liver

EXERCISE J   Diseases and Disorders

Write the medical terms for diseases and disorders next to their definitions.

1. _____ inflammation of the appendix

2. _____ inflammation of the gallbladder

3. _____ condition of gallstone(s)

4. _____ inflammation of the colon

5. _____ chronic inflammation of the intestinal tract usually affecting the ileum and colon; characterized by cobblestone ulcerations and the formation of scar tissue that may lead to intestinal obstruction

6. _____ painful intestines

7. _____ inflammation of the esophagus

8. _____ inflammation of the stomach

9. _____ inflammation of the stomach and intestines

10. _____ disorder characterized by the abnormal backward flow of the gastrointestinal contents into the esophagus
    _____

11. _____ inflammation of the gums

12. _____ inflammation of the tongue

13. _____ swollen or distended veins in the rectal area, which may be internal or external and can be a source of rectal bleeding and pain

14. _____ inflammation of the liver

15. _____ tumor of the liver

16. _____ malabsorption syndrome caused by an immune reaction to gluten, which may damage the lining of the small intestine that is responsible for absorption of food into the bloodstream

17. _____ periodic disturbances of bowel function, such as diarrhea and/or constipation, usually associated with abdominal pain

18. _____ inflammation of the pancreas

19. _____ erosion of the mucous membrane of the stomach or duodenum associated with increased secretion of acid from the stomach, bacterial infection (*Helicobacter pylori*), or use of nonsteroidal antiinflammatory drugs

20. _____ tumorlike growth extending outward from a mucous membrane

21. _____ hernia of the rectum

22. _____ disease characterized by inflammation of the colon with the formation of ulcers, which can cause bloody diarrhea

23. _____ chronic disease of the liver with gradual destruction of cells and formation of scar tissue; commonly caused by alcoholism and certain types of viral hepatitis

EXERCISE K   Diagnostic Tests and Equipment

Write the medical terms for diagnostic tests and equipment next to their definitions.

1. _____ diagnostic procedure in which a series of radiographic images are taken of the large intestine after the rectal administration of the contrast agent

2. _____ visual examination of the colon

3. CT _____ radiographic imaging of the colon (using a CT scanner and software)

4. _____ endoscopic procedure involving radiographic imaging of the biliary ducts and pancreatic ducts

5. _____ visual examination of the esophagus, stomach, and duodenum

6. _____ instrument used for visual examination of the stomach

7. _____ visual examination of the stomach

8. _____ instrument used for visual examination of the abdominal cavity

9. _____ pertaining to visual examination of the abdominal cavity

10. _____ visual examination of the abdominal cavity

11. _____ instrument used for visual examination of the rectum

12. _____ visual examination of the rectum

13. _____ visual examination of the sigmoid colon

14. _____ diagnostic procedure in which a series of radiographic images are taken of the pharynx, esophagus, stomach, and duodenum after oral administration of the contrast agent barium

EXERCISE L   Surgical Procedures

Write the medical terms for surgical procedures next to their definitions.

1. _____ surgical puncture to remove fluid from the abdominal cavity

2. _____ excision of the appendix

3. _____ surgical reduction of gastric capacity to treat morbid obesity, a condition that can cause serious illness

4. _____ excision of the gallbladder

5. _____ excision of the colon

6. _____ creation of an artificial opening into the colon

7. _____ excision of the stomach

8. _____ creation of an artificial opening into the stomach

9. _____ creation of an artificial opening into the ileum

10. _____ creation of an artificial opening into the jejunum

11. _____ incision into the abdominal cavity

EXERCISE M Specialties and Professions

Write the medical terms for specialties and professions next to their definitions.

1. _____ physician who studies and treats diseases of the stomach and intestines

2. _____ study of the stomach and intestines

EXERCISE N Medical Terms Related to the Digestive System

Write the medical terms related to the digestive system next to their definitions.

1. _____ pertaining to the anus

2. _____ pertaining to the duodenum

3. _____ pertaining to the esophagus

4. _____ pertaining to the stomach

5. _____ pertaining to the stomach and esophagus

6. _____ pertaining to the mouth

7. _____ pertaining to the pancreas

8. _____ pertaining to the rectum

9. _____ pertaining to under the tongue

10. _____ pertaining to treatment other than through the digestive system

11. _____ surgical opening between an organ and the surface of the body

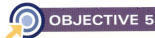

OBJECTIVE 5

Use medical language in clinical statements, the case study, and a medical record.

EXERCISE O   **Use Medical Terms in Clinical Statements**

Circle the medical terms and abbreviations defined in the bolded phrases. Answers are listed in Appendix C. For pronunciation practice, read the answers aloud.

1. The patient came to the hospital with epigastric pain, fat intolerance, and jaundice. The physician ordered abdominal sonography, which confirmed a diagnosis of **inflammation of the gallbladder** (cholecystitis, cholelithiasis, hepatitis). The patient was scheduled for **pertaining to visual examination of the abdominal cavity** (sigmoidoscopy, laparoscopy, colonoscopy), and **excision of the gallbladder** (gastrectomy, abdominocentesis, cholecystectomy).

2. A(n) **creation of an artificial opening into the stomach** (jejunostomy, ileostomy, gastrostomy) was performed to feed a patient diagnosed with a cancerous **pertaining to the esophagus** (esophageal, gastroesophageal, duodenal) tumor.

3. A(n) **visual examination of the esophagus, stomach, and duodenum** (endoscopic retrograde cholangiopancreatography, esophagogastroduodenoscopy, abdominal ultrasonography) is performed by a **physician who studies and treats diseases of the stomach and intestines** (gastroenterologist, hepatologist, urologist) to diagnose **erosion of the mucous membrane of the stomach or duodenum** (ulcerative colitis, dysentery, peptic ulcer).

4. **Enlarged liver** (Hepatitis, Hepatomegaly, Hepatoma) may be associated with **inflammation of the liver** (hepatitis, hepatomegaly, hepatoma), **tumor of the liver** (hepatitis, hepatomegaly, hepatoma), **chronic disease of the liver with gradual destruction of cells and formation of scar tissue** (celiac disease, cirrhosis, Crohn disease), fatty liver, or even normal pregnancy.

5. Symptoms of chronic **disorder characterized by the abnormal backward flow of the gastrointestinal contents into the esophagus** (GERD, ERCP, EGD) is often caused by dysfunction of the **pertaining to the stomach and esophagus** (esophageal, gastroesophageal, ileocecal) sphincter. Symptoms may include condition of **difficult swallowing** (dyspepsia, dysentery, dysphagia), **inflammation of the esophagus** (gastritis, esophagitis, pancreatitis), and bleeding.

6. Dentists and dental hygienists treat disorders related to the **pertaining to the mouth** (oral, rectal, anal) cavity. They check for **inflammation of the gums** (gingivitis, gingivalgia, stomatitis), **inflammation of the tongue** (gingivitis, glossitis, gastroenteritis) and check the **pertaining to under the tongue** (subcostal, sublingual, subcutaneous) surface, looking for oral cancer or other abnormalities.

7. **Disease characterized by inflammation of the colon with the formation of ulcers** (Crohn disease, Peptic ulcers, Ulcerative colitis) does not affect the small intestine. For those with severe disease a **total excision of the colon** (appendectomy, colectomy, cholecystectomy), with the **creation of an artificial opening into the ileum** (ileostomy, jejunostomy, colostomy), is a permanent cure.

EXERCISE P   Apply Medical Terms to the Case Study

Think back to Ruth Clifton, who was introduced in the case study at the beginning of the lesson. After working through Lesson 8 on the digestive system, consider the medical terms that might be used to describe her experience. List two terms relevant to the case study and their meanings. ■

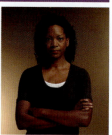

Medical Term   **Definition**

1. _____   _____

2. _____   _____

EXERCISE Q   Use Medical Terms in a Document

Ms. Clifton made an appointment with a gastroenterologist. He recommended an endoscopic procedure; the report is documented in the following medical record.

Use the definitions in numbers 1-9 to write medical terms within the document on the next page.

1. difficult digestion

2. visual examination of the esophagus, stomach, and duodenum

3. pertaining to within a vein

4. pertaining to a side

5. instrument used for visual examination of the stomach

6. pertaining to the stomach

7. pertaining to away

8. inflammation of the stomach

9. pertaining to the duodenum

Refer to the medical record to answer questions 10-12.

10. In the history section of the medical document, there are some terms that you may not have seen before. One of them is **hematemesis**. The suffix -**emesis** means **vomiting**. Use your knowledge of word parts to translate **hemat/emesis.**

    hemat/o means: _____

    -**emesis** means: _____

    Remembering that the definition usually starts with the meaning of the suffix, **hematemesis** is defined as

    _____.

```
038721 CLIFTON, Ruth                                                    _ □ X
File    Patient    Navigate    Custom Fields    Help
```

| Chart Review | Encounters | Notes | Labs | Imaging | **Procedures** | Rx | Documents | Referrals | Scheduling | Billing |

Name: **CLIFTON, Ruth**   MR#: **038721**   Sex: F   **Allergies:** None Known
                          DOB: **9/15/19XX**   Age: 40   **PCP:** Steinburge, Daniel DO

Endoscopy Report:
Date: 12 December 20XX 10:15

History of Present Illness: A 40-year-old woman was referred to the endoscopy unit clinic for evaluation. Patient reports nausea and vomiting with upper abdominal pain. She complains of (1.)_____ but denies hematemesis. She denies using alcohol or salicylates. The medications she states she is taking are not known for ulcerogenic side effects.

Procedure: (2.)_____: The patient was given 2 mg of (3.)_____ Versed along with lidocaine spray to the pharynx. After the patient was placed in the left (4.)_____ decubitus position, the (5.)_____was passed into the pharynx without difficulty. No evidence of reflux. The stomach was entered and some (6.)_____ juices were aspirated. The esophagus, cardia, and body of the stomach were free of abnormalities. A biopsy of the gastric mucosa was taken for *H. pylori*. In the (7.)_____ antral area some mild erythematous changes were noted. The pylorus had normal peristaltic activity. In the first part of the duodenum, however, a single 1 cm ulceration of the proximal duodenum was observed. The second part of the duodenum was free of mucosal abnormalities. Withdrawing the scope confirmed the findings upon entry. The patient tolerated the procedure quite well and recovered uneventfully.

Vital signs will be taken every half hour for the next 2 hours.

Postprocedural Diagnosis:

(8.) _____

(9.)_____ ulcer

Electronically signed: Garcia, Jesus MD on 12 December 20XX 11:02

```
Start   Log On/Off   Print   Edit
```

> **FYI**   **-emesis** can be used as a suffix, as noted above in hematemesis, or as in hyperemesis (excessive vomiting). **Emesis** can also be used as a stand-alone term, such as "the patient complained of nausea and emesis." In each case, the term **emesis** comes from the Greek **emein** meaning **to vomit**.

11. Another term in the history is ulcer/o/genic. Ulcerogenic means _____ ulcers.

12. Identify two new medical terms in the medical record you would like to investigate. Use your medical dictionary or an online resource to look up the definition.

Medical Term	Definition
1. _____	_____
2. _____	_____

EXERCISE R   Use Medical Language in Electronic Health Records Online

Select the correct medical terms to complete three medical records in one patient's electronic file.

 Access online resources at evolve.elsevier.com > Evolve Resources > Practice Student Resources > Activities > Lesson 8 > Electronic Health Records

Topic: Partial Bowel Obstruction
Record 1: Office Visit
Record 2: Radiology Report
Record 3: Colonoscopy Report

❏   Check the box when complete.

OBJECTIVE 6

Recall and assess knowledge of word parts, medical terms, and abbreviations.

EXERCISE S   Online Review of Lesson Content

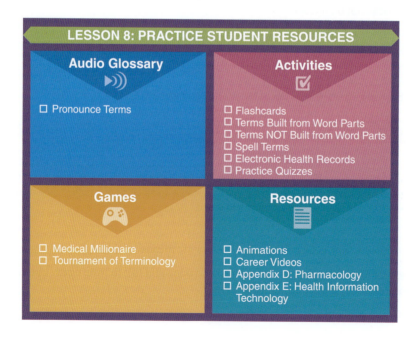

Recall and assess your learning from working through the lesson by completing online learning activities at evolve. elsevier.com > Evolve Resources > Practice Student Resources. Keep track of your progress by placing a check mark next to completed activities.

LESSON 8: PRACTICE STUDENT RESOURCES

Audio Glossary

☐ Pronounce Terms

Activities

☐ Flashcards
☐ Terms Built from Word Parts
☐ Terms NOT Built from Word Parts
☐ Spell Terms
☐ Electronic Health Records
☐ Practice Quizzes

Games

☐ Medical Millionaire
☐ Tournament of Terminology

Resources

☐ Animations
☐ Career Videos
☐ Appendix D: Pharmacology
☐ Appendix E: Health Information
   Technology

EXERCISE T Lesson Content Quiz

Test your knowledge of the terms and abbreviations introduced in this lesson. Circle the letter for the medical term or abbreviation related to the words in italics.

1. A patient diagnosed with *gallstones* has:
   a. cholelithiasis
   b. cholecystitis
   c. colitis

2. Symptoms of bloody diarrhea, abdominal pain and cramping, and fatigue may be associated with *disease characterized by inflammation of the colon with the formation of ulcers, which can cause bloody diarrhea.*
   a. UC
   b. IBS
   c. GERD

3. *Surgical reduction of gastric capacity to treat morbid obesity, a condition which can cause serious illness* may be necessary in some patients with morbid obesity, especially if it is associated with hypertension or diabetes.
   a. abdominocentesis
   b. bariatric surgery
   c. laparoscopy

4. *Difficult swallowing* may be a complication of Parkinson disease.
   a. dysphagia
   b. aphagia
   c. dyspepsia

5. Eating very spicy food may lead to *inflammation of the tongue.*
   a. gingivitis
   b. pancreatitis
   c. glossitis

6. *Inflammation of the stomach* may have some symptoms that are similar to peptic ulcers; a(n) *instrument used for visual examination of the stomach* may help differentiate between the two diseases.
   a. gastroesophageal reflux disease; laparoscope
   b. gastritis; gastroscope
   c. gastroenteritis; proctoscope

7. A *creation of an artificial opening into the colon* may be necessary if there is blockage proximal to the *pertaining to the rectum* portion of the colon.
   a. colonoscopy; oral
   b. colostomy; rectal
   c. colectomy; anal

8. *Malabsorption syndrome caused by an immune reaction to gluten* is considered a multisystem disorder with varying signs and symptoms, including abdominal bloating and pain, chronic diarrhea or constipation, steatorrhea (excessive fat in the stool), vomiting, weight loss, fatigue, and iron deficiency anemia.
   a. Crohn disease
   b. dysentery
   c. celiac disease

9. *Visual examination of the esophagus, stomach, and duodenum* may be performed to diagnose *disorder characterized by the abnormal backward flow of the gastrointestinal contents into the esophagus.*
   a. EGD; GERD
   b. ERCP; IBS
   c. BE: PEG

10. *Enlargement of the liver* may be due to hepatitis, fatty liver, or biliary disease.
    a. hemorrhoids
    b. hepatoma
    c. hepatomegaly

LESSON AT A GLANCE | DIGESTIVE SYSTEM WORD PARTS

COMBINING FORMS

abdomin/o, lapar/o	gastr/o	peps/o	**SUFFIX**
an/o	gingiv/o	phag/o	-algia
append/o, appendic/o	gloss/o, lingu/o	proct/o, rect/o	
chol/e	hepat/o	sigmoid/o	
col/o, colon/o	ile/o		
duoden/o	jejun/o		
enter/o	or/o		
esophag/o	pancreat/o		

LESSON AT A GLANCE | DIGESTIVE SYSTEM MEDICAL TERMS AND ABBREVIATIONS

SIGNS AND SYMPTOMS
aphagia
constipation
diarrhea
dyspepsia
dysphagia
gingivalgia
hepatomegaly

DISEASES AND DISORDERS
appendicitis
celiac disease
cholecystitis
cholelithiasis
cirrhosis
colitis
Crohn disease
dysentery
esophagitis
gastritis
gastroenteritis
gastroesophageal reflux disease
  (GERD)
gingivitis
glossitis
hemorrhoids
hepatitis
hepatoma
irritable bowel syndrome (IBS)
pancreatitis

peptic ulcer
polyp
rectocele
ulcerative colitis (UC)

DIAGNOSTIC TESTS AND EQUIPMENT
barium enema (BE)
colonoscopy
CT colonography
endoscopic retrograde
  cholangiopancreatography (ERCP)
esophagogastroduodenoscopy (EGD)
gastroscope
gastroscopy
laparoscope
laparoscopic
laparoscopy
proctoscope
proctoscopy
sigmoidoscopy
upper GI series (UGI series)

SURGICAL PROCEDURES
abdominocentesis
appendectomy
bariatric surgery
cholecystectomy
colectomy
colostomy

gastrectomy
gastrostomy
ileostomy
jejunostomy
laparotomy

SPECIALTIES AND PROFESSIONS
gastroenterologist
gastroenterology

RELATED TERMS
anal
duodenal
esophageal
gastric
gastroesophageal
oral
pancreatic
parenteral
rectal
stoma
sublingual

ABBREVIATIONS

BE	GERD	TPN
BM	GI	UC
EGD	IBS	UGI series
ERCP	PEG	

Eye and Ear

CASE STUDY | **Javier Berjarano**

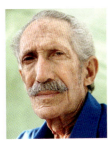

Javier moved into an assisted living community six months ago. He is doing well, but lately he notices that he can't see or hear as well as he used to. He isn't really sure when it started, but now he can't see details on the TV, even when he wears his glasses. Everything looks kind of cloudy. He also keeps trying to turn up the volume, but his neighbors get mad because it is too loud even though he can barely hear it. His right ear is really itchy, like when he was a kid with all those ear infections. He wonders if all these eye and ear problems are just from getting older. His daughter comes to visit and decides he needs to get this checked out. She schedules appointments for him with an eye doctor and an ear doctor.

■ *Consider Javier's situation as you work through the lesson on the eye and ear. We will return to this case study and identify medical terms used to describe and document his experiences.*

OBJECTIVES

1 ■ Build, translate, pronounce, and spell medical terms built from word parts (p. 261).

2 ■ Define, pronounce, and spell medical terms NOT built from word parts (p. 273).

3 ■ Write abbreviations (p. 277).

4 ■ Identify medical terms by clinical category (p. 278).

5 ■ Use medical language in clinical statements, the case study, and a medical record (p. 280).

6 ■ Recall and assess knowledge of word parts, medical terms, and abbreviations (p. 284).

INTRODUCTION TO THE EYE AND THE EAR

Anatomic Structures of the Eye

choroid (KŌR-oid)	middle layer of the eye containing many blood vessels
cornea (KŌR-nē-a)	transparent anterior part of the sclera that lies over the iris and pupil
iris (Ī-ris)	pigmented muscular structure that regulates the amount of light entering the eye by controlling the size of the pupil
lens (lenz)	lies directly behind the pupil; focuses and bends light
optic nerve (OP-tik) (nurv)	carries visual images from the retina to the brain
pupil (PŪ-pil)	opening through which light passes in the center of the iris

Anatomic Structures of the Eye—cont'd

retina
(RET-i-nah)

innermost layer of the eye; contains the vision receptors

sclera
(SKLER-ah)

outer protective layer of the eye (also called **white of the eye**)

Function of the Eye

• Vision

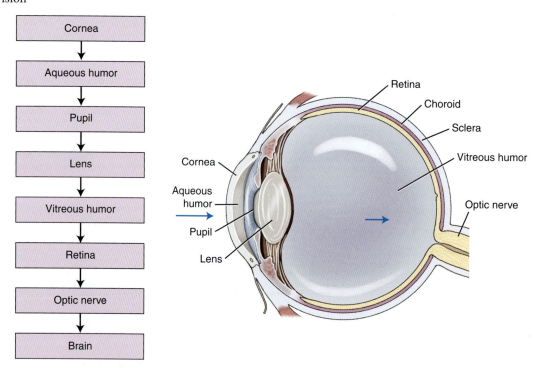

Cornea
↓
Aqueous humor
↓
Pupil
↓
Lens
↓
Vitreous humor
↓
Retina
↓
Optic nerve
↓
Brain

Figure 9.1 Pathway of light.

Anatomic Structures of the Ear

auricle (pinna) (AW-ri-kl), (PIN-a)	external, visible part of the ear located on both sides of the head; directs sound waves to the external auditory canal
cochlea (KŌK-lē-ah)	coiled portion of the inner ear that contains the organ for hearing
eustachian tube (yū-STĀ-shan) (toob)	passage between the middle ear and the pharynx; equalizes air pressure on both sides of the tympanic membrane
external auditory canal (meatus) (ek-STER-nal) (AW-di-tor-ē) (kah-NAL) (mē-Ā-tas)	short tube ending at the tympanic membrane
external ear (ek-STER-nal) (ēr)	consists of the auricle and external auditory canal (meatus)

Anatomic Structures of the Ear—cont'd

inner ear (labyrinth) (IN-ar) (ēr), (LAB-e-rinth)	bony spaces within the temporal bone of the skull that contain the cochlea, the semicircular canals, and vestibule. The cochlea facilitates hearing. The semicircular canals and vestibule facilitate equilibrium and balance.
middle ear (MID-l) (ēr)	consists of the tympanic membrane, eustachian tube, and ossicles
ossicles (OS-i-kalz)	bones of the middle ear (stapes, incus, and malleus) that carry sound vibrations
tympanic membrane (eardrum) (tim-PAN-ik) (MEM-brăn), (ĔR-drum)	semitransparent membrane that separates the external auditory canal (meatus) and the middle ear cavity; transmits sound vibrations to the ossicles

Functions of the Ear

- Hearing
- Sense of balance

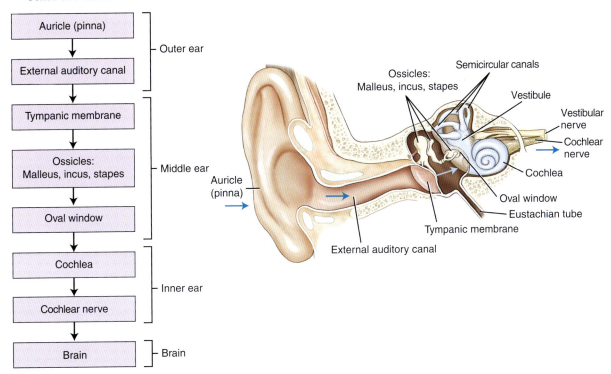

Figure 9.2 Perception of sound.

How the Eye and the Ear Work

The eye and the ear are organs of the sensory system, which communicates outside stimuli to the brain for interpretation. In addition to vision and hearing, the sensory system communicates information regarding pain, touch, pressure, taste, and other sensations.

The eye is the organ of vision. Light first passes through the **cornea.** The **iris** regulates the amount of light entering the eye by controlling **pupil** size. The **lens** lies behind the pupil and focuses the light projected onto the **retina**. The **optic nerve** transmits the image from the retina to the brain, where it is interpreted. The **sclera,** which appears white, forms the outer protective layer of the eye. Cavities within the eye are filled with transparent fluids, called humors, that maintain the shape of the eye. The eyebrows, eyelids, and eyelashes are accessory structures of the eye.

The ear, which is the organ of hearing and balance, is made up of three parts: the **external ear,** the **middle ear**, and the **inner ear**. The process of hearing begins as sound waves, directed by the **auricles,** enter the **external auditory canal.** As the sound waves ripple through the external ear, the **tympanic membrane** vibrates. The **ossicles** in the middle ear carry the vibration to the inner ear, where the stimulus is transmitted by the cochlear nerve to the brain where it is interpreted as sound. Balance is a function of the **inner ear** and is maintained through a series of complex processes. The vestibular nerve transmits information about motion and body position from the semicircular canals and the vestibule to the brain for interpretation.

CAREER FOCUS   **Professionals Who Work with the Eye and Ear**

- **Ophthalmic Medical Technicians** are supervised by ophthalmologists and perform a variety of clinical and administrative duties, including taking patient medical histories, providing patient instruction, performing vision and diagnostic tests, scheduling appointments, and other clerical tasks.

- **Opticians** are specialists who generally work closely with optometrists to fill prescriptions for lenses. They provide fitting for glasses and contact lenses and often have administrative duties, including answering phones, scheduling appointments, and processing payments.

- **Audiology Technicians** are supervised by audiologists and perform a variety of clinical and administrative duties, including performing hearing tests, fitting hearing aids, providing patient instruction, scheduling appointments, and other clerical tasks.

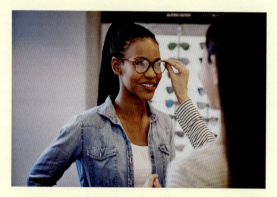

Figure 9.3 An optician fitting glasses.

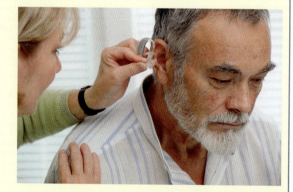

Figure 9.4 An audiology technician fits a hearing aid for a patient.

🌐 **FOR MORE INFORMATION**

- To learn more about careers in eye care visit the website hosted by the Joint Commission on Allied Health Personnel in Ophthalmology at www.jcahpo.org.

- Access online resources at evolve.elsevier.com > Practice Student Resources > Other Resources > Career Videos to watch an interview with an Audiologist.

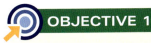

OBJECTIVE 1

Build, translate, pronounce, and spell medical terms built from word parts.

WORD PARTS   Use the paper or online **flashcards** to familiarize yourself with the following word parts.

COMBINING FORM (WR + CV)	DEFINITION	COMBINING FORM (WR + CV)	DEFINITION
EYE		**EAR**	
blephar/o	eyelid	**audi/o**	hearing
ir/o, irid/o	iris	**myring/o**	eardrum (tympanic membrane)
kerat/o	cornea (also means hard, horny tissue)	**ot/o**	ear
		tympan/o	middle ear
ophthalm/o	eye		
opt/o	vision		
retin/o	retina		
scler/o	sclera		

SUFFIX (S)	DEFINITION	SUFFIX (S)	DEFINITION
-metry	measurement	**-ptosis**	drooping, sagging, prolapse
-plegia	paralysis		

> **FYI**   In Greek mythology, **Iris** was the special messenger of the queen of heaven. She passed from heaven to earth over the rainbow while dressed in rainbow hues. Her name was applied to the circular eye muscle because of its varied colors.

WORD PARTS PRESENTED IN PREVIOUS LESSONS   Used to Build Terms for the Eye and Ear

COMBINING FORM (WR + CV)	DEFINITION	COMBINING FORM (WR + CV)	DEFINITION
laryng/o	larynx (voice box)		

SUFFIX (S)	DEFINITION	SUFFIX (S)	DEFINITION
-al, -ic	pertaining to	**-meter**	instrument used to measure
-ectomy	surgical removal, excision	**-plasty**	surgical repair
-itis	inflammation	**-scope**	instrument used for visual examination
-logist	one who studies and treats (specialist, physician)		
-logy	study of	**-tomy**	cut into, incision

Refer to Appendix A, Word Parts Used in *Basic Medical Language,* for alphabetical lists of word parts and their meanings.

EXERCISE A   Build and Translate Terms Built from Word Parts

*Use the **Word Parts Tables** to complete the following questions. Check your responses with the Answer Key in Appendix C.*

1. **LABEL:** *Write the combining forms for anatomical structures of the eye on Figure 9.5. These anatomical combining forms will be used to build and translate medical terms in Exercise A.*

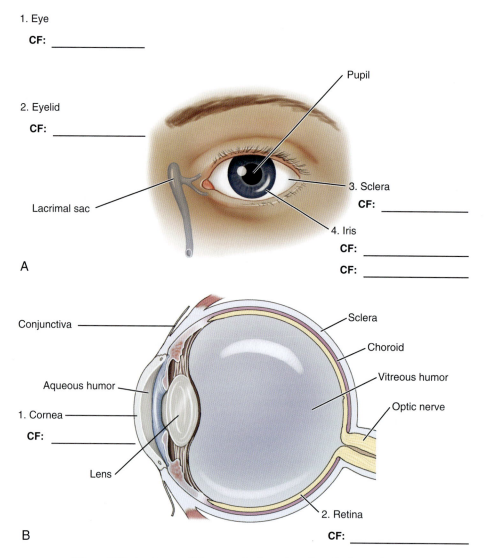

1. Eye
   CF: _____

2. Eyelid
   CF: _____

Pupil

Lacrimal sac

3. Sclera
   CF: _____

4. Iris
   CF: _____
   CF: _____

A

Conjunctiva

Aqueous humor

1. Cornea
   CF: _____

Lens

Sclera

Choroid

Vitreous humor

Optic nerve

2. Retina
   CF: _____

B

Figure 9.5 Anatomy of the eye. **A.** Anterior view. **B.** Lateral view.

2. MATCH: *Draw a line to match the suffix with its definition.*

a. -logy   instrument used for visual examination
b. -scope   instrument used to measure
c. -logist   study of
d. -meter   inflammation
e. -itis   one who studies and treats (specialist, physician)

3. BUILD: *Using the combining form **ophthalm/o**, build the following terms. Remember, the definition usually starts with the meaning of the suffix.*

a. study of the eye   _____/_o_/_____
                                                          wr   cv   s

b. physician who studies and treats diseases of the eye   _____/_o_/_____
                                                          wr   cv   s

4. TRANSLATE: *Complete the definitions of the following diagnostic terms. Remember, the definition usually starts with the meaning of the suffix.*

a. ophthalm/o/scope   _____ used for visual examination of the _____

b. kerat/o/meter   instrument used to _____ (the curvature of) the _____

> **FYI**   Look carefully at the spelling of **ophthalm**. Note that it is **o-ph-thalm**. Often this word is misspelled by omitting the first *h*. Think of the pronunciation of the word part beginning with **o-ph**, which sounds like the word **off**, followed by the **th** sound of **thalm**.

5. READ: Ophthalmology (of-thal-MOL-o-jē), abbreviated **Ophth**, is the branch of medicine specializing in the study of diseases and disorders of the eye. An **ophthalmologist** (of-thal-MOL-o-jist) is a medical doctor specializing in eye and vision care. In addition to diagnosing and treating diseases and disorders of the eye, ophthalmologists provide a wide range of services, including performing eye surgery and prescribing corrective lenses. An **ophthalmoscope** (of-THAL-mō-skōp) is used to direct light into the eye and examine the retina, blood vessels, and other structures. A **keratometer** (ker-a-TOM-e-ter), also called an ophthalmometer, gives information about the curvature of the cornea and is used in the fitting of contact lenses.

6. LABEL: *Write word parts to complete Figure 9.6.*

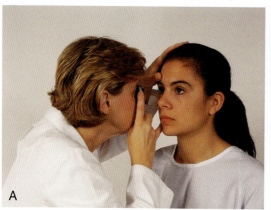 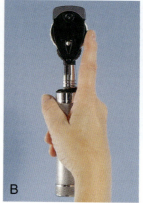 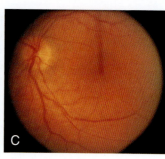

Figure 9.6 **A.** Visual examination of the eye. **B.** _____ /o/ _____.
                                                   eye   instrument used for visual examination
          C. Ophthalmoscopic view of the retina.

7. TRANSLATE: *Complete the definitions of the following terms describing inflammation of structures of the eye.*

   a. blephar/itis   _____ of the _____

   b. ir/itis   inflammation of the _____

   c. retin/itis   inflammation of the _____

   d. scler/itis   inflammation of the _____

8. Blepharitis (blef-a-RĬ-tis), often caused by bacteria, is an irritating condition accompanied by erythema (redness), crusted eyelashes, itchiness, and a burning sensation. **Iritis** (ī-RĪ-tis), **retinitis** (ret-i-NĪ-tis), and **scleritis** (skle-RĪ-tis) are more serious conditions that can lead to vision loss. Iritis has several causes, including injury, bacterial and fungal infections, and underlying autoimmune disorders. Cytomegalovirus (CMV) retinitis can lead to the destruction of the retina, resulting in blindness. Scleritis, a painful inflammatory disease, may be associated with other systemic conditions such as rheumatoid arthritis.

9. LABEL: *Write word parts to complete Figure 9.7.*

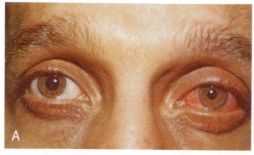 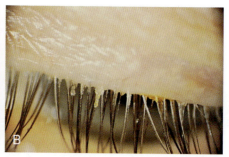

Figure 9.7 Types of inflammation. **A.** _____ / _____. **B.** _____ / _____.
                                     sclera   inflammation   eyelid   inflammation

10. MATCH: *Draw a line to match the suffix with its definition.*

a. -ptosis   excision
b. -plegia   surgical repair
c. -ectomy   drooping, sagging, prolapse
d. -plasty   paralysis

---

11. BUILD: *Build the following terms using suffixes indicating surgical procedures.*

a. excision of (a portion of) the iris (*Hint: use the combining form for iris with a "d" in it*)

_____/_____
wr   s

b. surgical repair of the eyelid

_____/_o_/_____
wr   cv   s

c. surgical repair of the cornea

_____/_o_/_____
wr   cv   s

---

12. TRANSLATE: *Complete the definitions of the following terms by using the meaning of word parts to fill in the blanks.*

a. irid/o/plegia   _____ of the _____

b. blephar/o/ptosis (*Hint: use the definition for the suffix beginning with a "d"*)   _____ of the _____

---

13. LABEL: *Write word parts to complete Figure 9.8.*

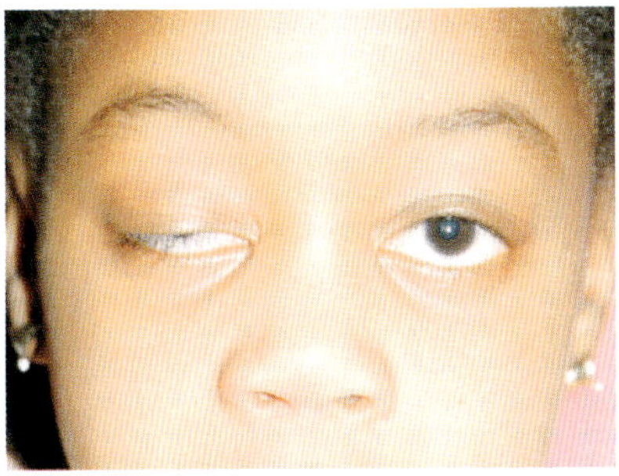

Figure 9.8 Congenital _____/o/_____.
                        eyelid   drooping

---

14. READ: Blepharoptosis (blef-ar-op-TŌ-sis), also called **ptosis**, may be unilateral, affecting one eyelid, or bilateral, affecting both eyelids. Blepharoptosis is most often seen in older adults, though it may be congenital (present at birth) and impair normal vision development in children. **Blepharoplasty** (BLEF-a-rō-plas-tē) may be performed to correct blepharoptosis and to restore vision. In **iridoplegia** (ir-i-dō-PLĒ-ja), the pupil size does not change in response to a change in light. Paralysis of the iris may be due to injury, inflammation, or use of pupil-dilating drops used for an eye exam. **Iridectomy** (ir-i-DEK-to-mē) is a surgical procedure used to treat closed-angle glaucoma and melanoma of the iris. **Keratoplasty** (KER-a-tō-plas-tē) is a surgical procedure performed for several reasons, including corneal transplants, excision of corneal lesions, and repair of refraction errors such as myopia (nearsightedness) and hyperopia (farsightedness).

> **FYI**   **Refraction** refers to how the anterior surface of the eye and the lens bend light to focus on the retina for visual perception. **Refraction errors,** which primarily cause blurry vision, may occur as a result of the shape of the eye, curvature of the cornea, and shape or age of the lens. Common refraction errors include **myopia**, **hyperopia**, **astigmatism**, and **presbyopia**. Corrective lenses and surgery are used to treat visual impairments.

---

15. MATCH: *Draw a line to match the combining form or suffix with its definition.*

a. -al, -ic   measurement
b. -metry   vision
c. opt/o   pertaining to

---

16. BUILD: *Write word parts to build the following terms. (Hint: use the suffix ending in "c" for pertaining to.)*

a. measurement of vision   _____/_o_/_____
                                                     wr   cv   s

b. pertaining to vision   _____/_____
                                                     wr   s

c. pertaining to the eye   _____/_____
                                                     wr   s

---

17. TRANSLATE: *Complete the definitions of the following terms built with the suffix –al.*

a. scler/al   _____ to the _____
b. retin/al   _____ to the _____

---

18. READ: **Optometry** (op-TOM-e-trē) is a healthcare profession which provides primary vision care. **Optic** (OP-tik) and **ophthalmic** (of-THAL-mik) are adjectives used to describe nouns related to vision and to the eye, respectively. Examples include optic nerve and ophthalmic exam. **Scleral** (SKLE-ral) buckling is a surgical procedure used to repair **retinal** (RET-i-nal) detachment.

---

19. REVIEW OF EYE TERMS BUILT FROM WORD PARTS: *the following is an alphabetical list of terms built and translated in the previous exercises.*

MEDICAL TERMS BUILT FROM WORD PARTS

TERM	DEFINITION	TERM	DEFINITION
1. **blepharitis** (blef-a-RĪ-tis)	inflammation of the eyelid (Figure 9.7, *B*)	4. **iridectomy** (ir-i-DEK-to-mē)	excision of (a portion of) the iris
2. **blepharoplasty** (BLEF-a-rō-plas-tē)	surgical repair of the eyelid	5. **iridoplegia** (ir-i-dō-PLĒ-ja)	paralysis of the iris
3. **blepharoptosis** (blef-ar-op-TŌ-sis)	drooping of the eyelid (also called **ptosis**) (Figure 9.8)	6. **iritis** (ī-RĪ-tis)	inflammation of the iris

MEDICAL TERMS BUILT FROM WORD PARTS—cont'd

TERM	DEFINITION	TERM	DEFINITION
7. **keratometer** (ker-a-TOM-e-ter)	instrument used to measure (the curvature of) the cornea; (also called **ophthalmometer**)	13. **optic** (OP-tik)	pertaining to vision
8. **keratoplasty** (KER-a-tō-plas-tē)	surgical repair of the cornea	14. **optometry** (op-TOM-e-trē)	measurement of vision
9. **ophthalmic** (of-THAL-mik)	pertaining to the eye	15. **retinal** (RET-i-nal)	pertaining to the retina
10. **ophthalmologist** (of-thal-MOL-o-jist)	physician who studies and treats diseases of the eye	16. **retinitis** (ret-i-NĪ-tis)	inflammation of the retina
11. **ophthalmology (Ophth)** (of-thal-MOL-o-jē)	study of the eye	17. **scleral** (SKLE-ral)	pertaining to the sclera
12. **ophthalmoscope** (of-THAL-mō-skōp)	instrument used for visual examination of the eye (Figure 9.6, *B*)	18. **scleritis** (skle-RĪ-tis)	inflammation of the sclera (Figure 9.7, *A*)

EXERCISE B   Pronounce and Spell Terms Built from Word Parts

Practice pronunciation and spelling on paper and online.

1. **Practice on Paper**
   a. **Pronounce**: Read the phonetic spelling and say aloud the terms listed in the previous table, Review of Eye Terms Built from Word Parts.
   b. **Spell**: Have a study partner read the terms aloud. Write the spelling of the terms on a separate sheet of paper.

2. **Practice Online** ⊕
   a. **Access** online learning resources. Go to evolve.elsevier.com > Evolve Resources > Practice Student Resources.
   b. **Pronounce**: Select Audio Glossary > Lesson 9 > Exercise B. Select a term to hear its pronunciation and repeat aloud.
   c. **Spell**: Select Activities > Lesson 9 > Spell Terms > Exercise B. Select the audio icon and type the correct spelling of the term.

❏   Check the box when complete.

EXERCISE C   Build and Translate MORE Medical Terms Built from Word Parts

1. **LABEL**: *Write the combining forms for anatomical structures of the ear on Figure 9.9. These anatomical combining forms will be used to build and translate medical terms in Exercise C.*

1. Ear CF: _____

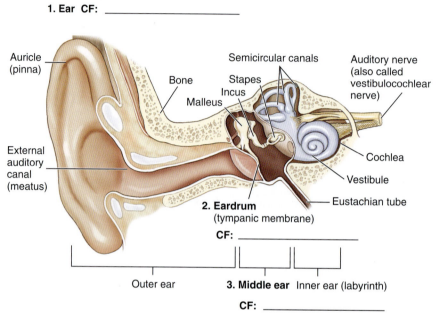

Auricle (pinna)

Bone

Semicircular canals

Stapes
Incus
Malleus

Auditory nerve (also called vestibulocochlear nerve)

External auditory canal (meatus)

Cochlea

Vestibule

Eustachian tube

2. Eardrum (tympanic membrane)

CF: _____

Outer ear

3. Middle ear Inner ear (labyrinth)

CF: _____

Figure 9.9 Anatomy of the ear.

2. **MATCH**: *Draw a line to match the suffix with its definition.*

   a. -rrhea   instrument used for visual examination
   b. -plasty   flow, discharge
   c. -scope   inflammation
   d. -itis   surgical repair

3. **TRANSLATE**: *Complete the definitions of the following terms built from the combining form **ot/o**, meaning ear.*

   a. ot/o/rrhea *(Hint: use the*   _____ from the _____
        definition that starts with
        a "d" for the suffix)

   b. ot/o/scope   _____ used for visual _____

                                          of the _____

   c. ot/o/plasty   _____ _____ of the (outer) ear

4. LABEL: *Write word parts to complete Figure 9.10.*

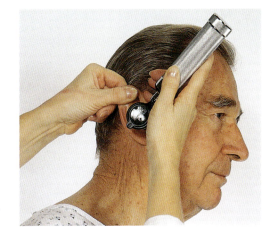

Figure 9.10 Visual examination of the ear with

an _____ /o/ _____.

      ear   instrument used for visual examination

---

5. BUILD: *Using word parts, build the following terms describing inflammation of structures of the ear.*

a. inflammation of the ear   _____/_____

                                                           wr   s

b. inflammation of the eardrum   _____/_____

                                                           wr   s

---

6. READ: Otorrhea (ō-tō-RĒ-a) refers to discharge from the ear as seen with **otitis** (ō-TĪ-tis) media, an infection of the middle ear. **Myringitis** (mir-in-JĪ-tis) is associated with acute otitis media and refers to the inflammation of the eardrum. An **otoscope** (Ō-tō-skōp) is useful for detecting inflammation of the eardrum and auditory canal. **Otoplasty** (Ō-tō-plas-tē) is a surgical procedure to reshape the outer ear (auricle).

---

7. LABEL: *Write word parts to complete Figure 9.11.*

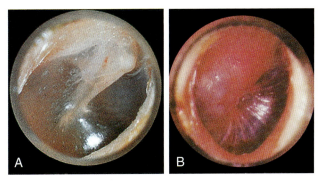

Figure 9.11 A. Healthy eardrum (tympanic membrane).

                 B. Eardrum with acute _____/_____ media.

                                              ear   inflammation

8. **MATCH:** *Draw a line to match the word part with its definition.*

   a. -ic   surgical repair
   b. -tomy   incision
   c. -plasty   pertaining to
   d. -logy   larynx (voice box)
   e. -logist   study of
   f. laryng/o   one who studies and treats (specialist, physician)

9. **BUILD:** *Write word parts to build the following terms using the combining form **tympan/o**, meaning middle ear.*

   a. pertaining to the middle ear   _____/_____
                                            wr   s

   b. surgical repair of the middle ear   _____/ o /_____
                                          wr   cv   s

10. **TRANSLATE:** *Complete the definitions of the following terms built from the combining form **myring/o**, meaning eardrum.*

    a. myring/o/tomy   _____ of the _____
    b. myring/o/plasty   surgical _____ of the _____

11. **READ:** **Tympanic** (tim-PAN-ik) is an adjective used to describe a noun, as in tympanic membrane (a membrane of the middle ear called the eardrum). **Tympanoplasty** (TIM-pa-nō-plas-tē) refers to surgical procedures performed on the middle ear, including repair of the ossicles and repair of the eardrum. **Myringoplasty** (mi-RING-gō-plas-tē) is a less complicated surgical procedure used to repair a perforated eardrum. **Myringotomy** (mir-ing-GOT-o-mē) is a surgical procedure which can be used to place a tube through the eardrum to help drain fluid from the middle ear with the goal of reducing ear infections.

12. **LABEL:** *Write word parts to complete Figure 9.12.*

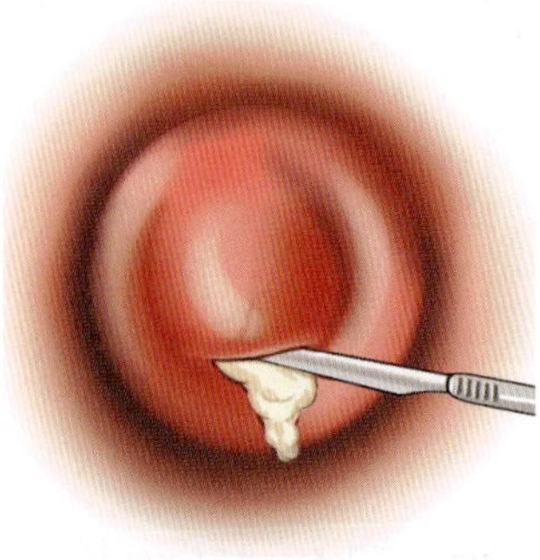

Figure 9.12 _____/o/_____
                   eardrum   incision
is performed to release pus from the middle ear through the tympanic membrane to treat acute otitis media.

13. BUILD: *Write word parts to build the following terms using **ot/o**, meaning ear.*

a. study of the ear, (nose), and the larynx (throat)

_____ / o / _____ / o / _____
  wr   cv   wr   cv   s

b. physician who studies and treats diseases of
the ear, (nose), and the larynx (throat)

_____ / o / _____ / o / _____
  wr   cv   wr   cv   s

14. Otolaryngology (ō-tō-lar-ing-GOL-o-jē) is the medical specialty dedicated to medical and surgical treatment of the head and neck, including the ear, nose, and throat (**ENT**). Surgical procedures on structures of the ear are performed by an **otolaryngologist** (ō-tō-lar-ing-GOL-o-jist). Otolaryngologists are referred to as ENT physicians or more simply ENTs.

> **FYI** The terms **otolaryngology** and **otolaryngologist** are shortened versions of the terms **otorhinolaryngology** and **otorhinolaryngologist**. In the longer versions, reference to the ear, nose, and throat can be more clearly seen with the inclusion of the corresponding combining forms: **ot/o** (ear), **rhin/o** (nose), and **laryng/o** (larynx/throat).

15. MATCH: *Draw a line to match the word part with its definition.*

a. audi/o   measurement
b. -logy   one who studies and treats (specialist, physician)
c. -logist   instrument used to measure
d. -meter   hearing
e. -metry   study of

16. TRANSLATE: *Complete the definitions of the following terms using the combining form **audi/o**.*

a. audi/o/logy   _____ of _____

b. audi/o/logist   specialist who _____ and _____ (impaired) _____

c. audi/o/meter   _____ used to _____ _____

d. audi/o/metry   _____ of _____

17. READ: Audiology (aw-dē-OL-o-jē) is a healthcare profession dedicated to diagnosing and treating hearing disorders. An **audiologist** (aw-dē-OL-o-jist) measures hearing using an **audiometer** (aw-dē-OM-e-ter) and other equipment. **Audiometry** (aw-dē-OM-e-trē) exam results are graphed, showing hearing deficits according to loudness and tonal frequency.

18. **LABEL:** *Write word parts to complete Figure 9.13.*

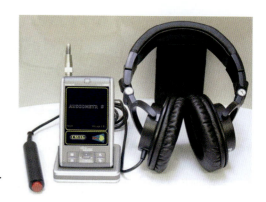

Figure 9.13 _____ /o/ _____.
               hearing   instrument used to measure

19. **REVIEW OF EAR TERMS BUILT FROM WORD PARTS:** *the following is an alphabetical list of terms built and translated in the previous exercises.*

MEDICAL TERMS BUILT FROM WORD PARTS

TERM	DEFINITION	TERM	DEFINITION
1. **audiologist** (aw-dē-OL-o-jist)	specialist who studies and treats (impaired) hearing	9. **otoplasty** (Ō-tō-plas-tē)	surgical repair of the (outer) ear
2. **audiology** (aw-dē-OL-o-jē)	study of hearing	10. **otolaryngologist (ENT)** (ō-tō-lar-ing-GOL-o-jist)	physician who studies and treats diseases of the ear, (nose), and the larynx (throat)
3. **audiometer** (aw-dē-OM-e-ter)	instrument used to measure hearing (Figure 9.13)	11. **otolaryngology** (ō-tō-lar-ing-GOL-o-jē)	study of the ear, (nose), and larynx (throat)
4. **audiometry** (aw-dē-OM-e-trē)	measurement of hearing	12. **otorrhea** (ō-tō-RĒ-a)	discharge from the ear
5. **myringitis** (mir-in-JĪ-tis)	inflammation of the eardrum	13. **otoscope** (Ō-tō-skōp)	instrument used for visual examination of the ear (Figure 9.10)
6. **myringoplasty** (mi-RING-gō-plas-tē)	surgical repair of the eardrum	14. **tympanic** (tim-PAN-ik)	pertaining to the middle ear
7. **myringotomy** (mir-ing-GOT-o-mē)	incision into the eardrum (Figure 9.12)	15. **tympanoplasty** (TIM-pa-nō-plas-tē)	surgical repair of the middle ear
8. **otitis** (ō-TĪ-tis)	inflammation of the ear (Figure 9.11, *B*)		

EXERCISE D Pronounce and Spell MORE Terms Built from Word Parts

Practice pronunciation and spelling on paper and online.

1. **Practice on Paper**
    a. **Pronounce**: Read the phonetic spelling and say aloud the terms listed in the previous table, Review of Ear Terms Built from Word Parts.
    b. **Spell**: Have a study partner read the terms aloud. Write the spelling of the terms on a separate sheet of paper.

2. **Practice Online** ⊕
    a. **Access** online learning resources. Go to evolve.elsevier.com > Evolve Resources > Practice Student Resources.
    b. **Pronounce**: Select Audio Glossary > Lesson 9 > Exercise D. Select a term to hear its pronunciation and repeat aloud.
    c. **Spell**: Select Activities > Lesson 9 > Spell Terms > Exercise D. Select the audio icon and type the correct spelling of the term.

❑ Check the box when complete.

OBJECTIVE 2

Define, pronounce, and spell medical terms NOT built from word parts.

The terms listed below may contain word parts, but are difficult to translate literally.

MEDICAL TERMS **NOT** BUILT FROM WORD PARTS	
TERM	**DEFINITION**
astigmatism (AST) (a-STIG-ma-tizm)	irregular curvature of the refractive surfaces of the eye (cornea or lens); causes blurry vision (Figure 9.14, *C*)
cataract (KAT-a-rakt)	clouding of the lens of the eye
glaucoma (glaw-KŌ-ma)	eye disorder characterized by optic nerve damage usually caused by the abnormal increase of intraocular pressure
hyperopia (hī-per-Ō-pē-a)	farsightedness (Figure 9.14, *B*)
LASIK (LĀ-sik)	laser procedure that reshapes the corneal tissue beneath the surface of the cornea; LASIK is an acronym composed of the first letters of words in the term laser-assisted in situ keratomileusis.
macular degeneration (MAC-ū-lar) (dē-gen-e-RĀ-shun)	progressive deterioration of the central portion of the retina resulting in a loss of central vision; when caused by the aging process it is referred to as age-related macular degeneration and is abbreviated as **ARMD**
myopia (mī-Ō-pē-a)	nearsightedness (Figure 9.14, *A*)

MEDICAL TERMS NOT BUILT FROM WORD PARTS—cont'd

TERM	DEFINITION
optometrist (op-TOM-e-trist)	healthcare professional who performs eye exams, administers vision tests, and prescribes corrective lenses. Optometrists are state-licensed healthcare professionals who have earned doctorate degrees (OD).
otitis media (OM) (ō-TĪ-tis) (MĒ-dē-a)	inflammation of the middle ear
presbycusis (pres-bē-KŪ-sis)	hearing impairment occurring with age
presbyopia (pres-bē-Ō-pē-a)	vision impairment occurring with age
retinal detachment (RET-in-al) (dē-TACH-ment)	separation of the retina from the choroid in the posterior portion of the eye resulting in a disruption of vision that may be permanent if treatment is delayed; onset may be gradual or sudden and is not painful
tinnitus (tin-NĪ-tus)	ringing in the ears

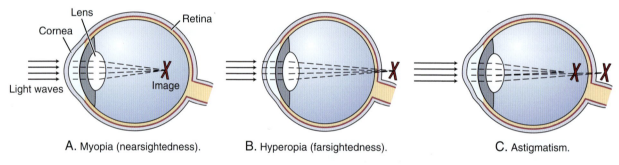

A. Myopia (nearsightedness).   B. Hyperopia (farsightedness).   C. Astigmatism.

Figure 9.14 Refractive errors.

EXERCISE E   Label

Write the medical terms pictured and defined using the previous table of Medical Terms NOT Built from Word Parts. Check your work with the Answer Key in Appendix C.

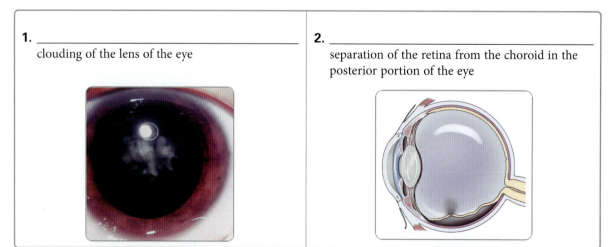

1. _____
   clouding of the lens of the eye

2. _____
   separation of the retina from the choroid in the posterior portion of the eye

3. _____

progressive deterioration of the central portion of the retina resulting in loss of central vision

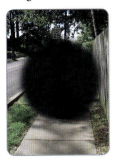

4. _____

laser procedure that reshapes the corneal tissue beneath the surface of the cornea

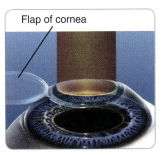

Flap of cornea

5. _____

healthcare professional who performs eye exams, administers vision tests, and prescribes corrective lenses

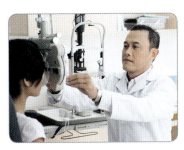

6. _____

ringing in the ears

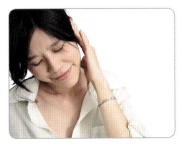

7. a. _____

vision impairment occurring with age

b. _____

hearing impairment occurring with age

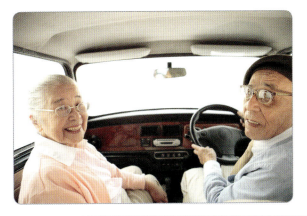

EXERCISE F   **Learn Medical Terms NOT Built from Word Parts**

Fill in the blanks with medical terms defined in bold using the Medical Terms NOT Built from Word Parts table. Check responses in Appendix C.

1. A **laser procedure that reshapes corneal tissue**, or _____, is used to correct **irregular curvature of the refractive surfaces of the eye**, or _____. **Farsightedness**, or _____; and **nearsightedness**, or _____, can also be corrected using this technique.

2. **Eye disorder usually caused by abnormally increased intraocular pressure,** or _____, leads to atrophy of the optic nerve and results in blindness. Early treatment is essential because loss of vision from this condition cannot be regained.

3. **Clouding of the lens of the eye,** or a(n) _____, is most commonly caused by the deterioration of the lens as a result of the aging process. Surgery may be advised if visual impairment is significant. A **healthcare professional who performs eye exams, administers vision tests, and prescribes corrective lenses,** or a(n) _____, may assist after surgery with a change in eyeglass prescription for the patient.

> **FYI**   **Cataracts** are the gradual development of cloudiness within the lenses of the eyes, not a film over the eye as commonly thought. They usually occur in both eyes. Most cataracts develop in persons aged 50 years or older and are caused by degenerative changes.

4. A distortion of central vision may be an early symptom of a **progressive deterioration of the central portion of the retina resulting in a loss of central vision,** or _____. Although there is no known cure, **ARMD,** or _____macular degeneration, may be treated with anti-VEGF injections, photodynamic therapy, and laser surgery.

5. **Separation of the retina from the choroid,** or _____, is a medical emergency that can result in permanent vision loss if not treated quickly. Usually, a tear in the retina causes fluid to leak, pulling it pull away from supporting tissue.

6. A myringotomy may be performed in a severe case of **inflammation of the middle ear,** or _____ _____, to release pus accumulated behind the tympanic membrane.

7. A common symptom of diseases and conditions of the ear is **ringing in the ears,** or _____, and warrants further examination by a healthcare professional.

8. **Vision impairment occurring with age** _____ usually becomes noticeable as a person reaches the mid to late 40s. **Hearing impairment occurring with age** _____ _____ usually presents as bilateral hearing loss after the age of 50.

EXERCISE G   **Pronounce and Spell Terms NOT Built from Word Parts**

Practice pronunciation and spelling on paper and online.

1. **Practice on Paper**

    a. **Pronounce**: Read the phonetic spelling and say aloud the terms listed in the previous Medical Terms NOT Built from Word Parts table.

    b. **Spell**: Have a study partner read the terms aloud. Write the spelling of the terms on a separate sheet of paper.

2. **Practice Online** ⊕

    a. **Access** online learning resources. Go to evolve.elsevier.com > Evolve Resources > Practice Student Resources.

    b. **Pronounce**: Select Audio Glossary > Lesson 9 > Exercise G. Select a term to hear its pronunciation and repeat aloud.

    c. **Spell**: Select Activities > Lesson 9 > Spell Terms > Exercise G. Select the audio icon and type the correct spelling of the term.

❏ Check the box when complete.

OBJECTIVE 3

Write abbreviations.

ABBREVIATIONS RELATED TO THE EYE AND EAR

Use the online **flashcards** to familiarize yourself with the following abbreviations.

ABBREVIATION	TERM	ABBREVIATION	TERM
ARMD	age-related macular degeneration	IOP	intraocular pressure
AST	astigmatism	OM	otitis media
ENT	ear, nose, and throat; otolaryngologist	Ophth	ophthalmology
HOH	hard of hearing	VA	visual acuity

EXERCISE H   **Abbreviate Medical Terms**

Write the correct abbreviation next to its medical term. Abbreviations may be used twice.

1. Signs and Symptoms:

    a. _____ intraocular pressure

    b. _____ hard of hearing

2. Diseases and Disorders:

    a. _____ otitis media

    b. _____ astigmatism

    c. _____ age-related macular degeneration

3. Diagnostic Test:

_____ visual acuity

4. Specialties and Professions:

a. _____ ophthalmology

b. _____ otolaryngologist

5. Related:

_____ ears, nose, and throat

OBJECTIVE 4

Identify medical terms by clinical category.

Now that you have worked through the lesson on the eye and the ear, review and practice medical terms grouped by clinical category. Categories include signs and symptoms, diseases and disorders, diagnostic tests and equipment, surgical procedures, specialties and professions, and other terms related to the eye and ear. Check your responses with the Answer Key in Appendix C.

EXERCISE I   Signs and Symptoms

Write the medical terms for signs and symptoms next to their definitions.

1. _____ discharge from the ear

2. _____ ringing in the ears

EXERCISE J   Diseases and Disorders

Write the medical terms for diseases and disorders next to their definitions.

1. _____ irregular curvature of the refractive surfaces of the eye (cornea or lens)

2. _____ inflammation of the middle ear

3. _____ nearsightedness

4. _____ farsightedness

5. _____ clouding of the lens of the eye

6. _____ progressive deterioration of the central portion of the retina resulting in loss of central vision

7. _____ separation of the retina from the choroid in the posterior portion of the eye resulting in a disruption of vision

8. _____   eye disorder characterized by optic nerve damage usually
                                caused by the increase of intraocular pressure

9. _____   hearing impairment occurring with age

10. _____   vision impairment occurring with age

11. _____   inflammation of the eyelid

12. _____   drooping of the eyelid

13. _____   paralysis of the iris

14. _____   inflammation of the iris

15. _____   inflammation of the sclera

16. _____   inflammation of the retina

17. _____   inflammation of the eardrum

18. _____   inflammation of the ear

EXERCISE K   Diagnostic Tests and Equipment

Write the medical terms for diagnostic tests and equipment next to their definitions.

1. _____   instrument used for visual examination of the eye

2. _____   instrument used to measure (the curvature of) the cornea

3. _____   instrument used to measure hearing

4. _____   instrument used for visual examination of the ear

5. _____   measurement of hearing

EXERCISE L   Surgical Procedures

Write the medical terms for surgical procedures next to their definitions.

1. _____   surgical repair of the eyelid

2. _____   excision of (a portion of) the iris

3. _____   surgical repair of the cornea

4. _____   laser procedure that reshapes the corneal tissue beneath the
                                surface of the cornea

5. _____   surgical repair of the eardrum

6. _____   incision into the eardrum

7. _____   surgical repair of the (outer) ear

8. _____   surgical repair of the middle ear

Specialties and Professions

Write the medical terms for specialties and professions next to their definitions.

1. _____   physician who studies and treats diseases of the eye

2. _____   study of the eye

3. _____   measurement of vision

4. _____   healthcare professional who performs eye exams, administers vision tests, and prescribes corrective lenses

5. _____   specialist who studies and treats impaired hearing

6. _____   study of hearing

7. _____   physician who studies and treats diseases of the ear, (nose), and the larynx (throat)

8. _____   study of the ear, (nose), and larynx (throat)

EXERCISE N   **Medical Terms Related to the Eye and Ear**

Write the medical terms related to the eye and ear sensory systems to their definitions.

1. _____   pertaining to the eye

2. _____   pertaining to vision

3. _____   pertaining to the retina

4. _____   pertaining to the sclera

5. _____   pertaining to the middle ear

OBJECTIVE 5

Use medical language in clinical statements, the case study, and a medical record.

Check responses for the following exercises in Appendix C.

EXERCISE O   **Use Medical Terms in Clinical Statements**

Circle the medical terms defined in the bolded phrases. For pronunciation practice read the answers aloud.

1. The **physician who studies and treats diseases of the eye** (ophthalmologist, optometrist, optician) is trained in surgery and specializes in eye and vision care, including the diagnosis and treatment of diseases and disorders of the eye, performing eye surgery, and prescribing lenses.

2. A **procedure using a laser to reshape corneal tissue** (iridectomy, LASIK, blepharoplasty) was performed to correct **farsightedness** (astigmatism, hyperopia, myopia).

3. **Excision of a portion of the iris**, called an (iritis, iridectomy, iridoplegia), may be performed to treat some forms of an **eye disorder characterized by optic nerve damage, usually caused by the abnormal increase of intraocular pressure** (glaucoma, cataracts, macular degeneration).

4. The goal of **surgical repair of the eyelids** (blepharoptosis, blepharoplasty, blepharitis) is to correct impaired peripheral vision caused by **drooping eyelids** (blepharoptosis, blepharoplasty, blepharitis).

5. The optometrist used an **instrument used to measure (the curvature) of the cornea** (keratoplasty, keratometer, ophthalmoscope) to collect data for the fitting of the patient's contact lenses.

6. **Vision loss occurring with age** (ARMD, Presbyopia, Presbycusis) may be diagnosed and treated by a **healthcare professional who performs eye exams, administers vision tests, and prescribes corrective lenses** (ophthalmologist, optometrist, audiologist).

7. The **instrument used to visually examine the ear** is called an (otoscope, ophthalmoscope, audiometer). The **instrument used to measure hearing** is called an (otoscope, ophthalmoscope, audiometer).

8. The pediatric **ENT** (audiologist, otolaryngologist, ophthalmologist) is planning to release pus from a child's middle ear by performing a(n) **incision into the eardrum** (tympanoplasty, myringoplasty, myringotomy).

9. **Surgical repair of the eardrum** (Myringotomy, Myringitis, Myringoplasty) is one form of **surgical repair of the middle ear** (keratoplasty, tympanoplasty, otoplasty).

10. **Hearing loss occurring with age** (Tinnitus, Presbyopia, Presbycusis) may be diagnosed and treated by a(n) **specialist who studies and treats impaired hearing** (otolaryngologist, optometrist, audiologist).

EXERCISE P Apply Medical Terms to the Case Study

Think back to Javier introduced in the case study at the beginning of the lesson. After working through Lesson 9 on the eye and the ear, consider the medical terms that might be used to describe his experiences. List three terms relevant to the case study and their meanings. ■

Medical Term   **Definition**

1. _____   _____

2. _____   _____

3. _____   _____

EXERCISE Q Use Medical Terms in a Document

With the help of his daughter, Javier is able to visit the ophthalmologist and otolaryngologist. His experiences are documented in the following consultation report.

Use the definitions in numbers 1-14 to write abbreviations and medical terms within the consultation report.

1. abbreviation for ear, nose, and throat

2. ringing in the ears

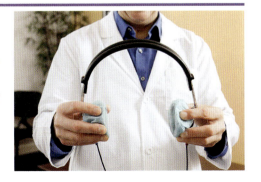

3. inflammation of the middle ear

4. surgical repair of the middle ear

5. eye disorder characterized by optic nerve damage usually caused by the abnormal increase of intraocular pressure

6. physician who studies and treats diseases of the eye

7. healthcare professional who performs eye exams, administers vision tests, and prescribes corrective lenses

8. instrument used for visual examination of the ear

9. pertaining to the middle ear

10. discharge from the ear

11. specialist who studies and treats impaired hearing

12. inflammation of the ear

13. study of hearing

14. physician who studies and treats diseases of the ear, (nose), and the larynx (throat)

Refer to the ENT Consultation to answer questions 15-17.

15. The term **ocular**, used in the medical record to describe the movement observed, is built from word parts. Use your medical dictionary or a reliable online source to define the word parts, and then use your skills to build the term.

    ocul/o means _____

    -ar means _____

    Remember, most definitions begin with the suffix.

    ocul/ar means _____

16. The term **lesion** was presented in the integumentary system lesson. Can you recall its meaning?

    lesion _____

17. Identify two new medical terms in the medical record you would like to investigate. Use your medical dictionary or an online reference to look up the definition.

    Medical Term   **Definition**

    1. _____   _____

    2. _____   _____

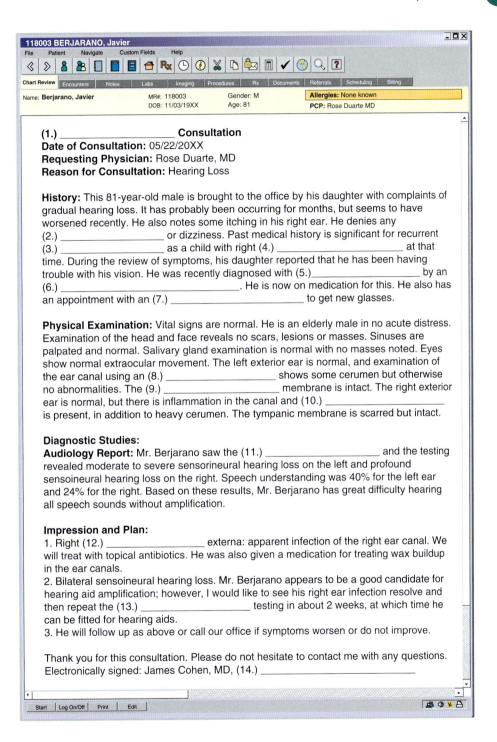

118003 BERJARANO, Javier

File   Patient   Navigate   Custom Fields   Help

Chart Review | Encounters | Notes | Labs | Imaging | Procedures | Rx | Documents | Referrals | Scheduling | Billing

Name: **Berjarano, Javier**   MR#: 118003   Gender: M   **Allergies:** None known
DOB: 11/03/19XX   Age: 81   **PCP:** Rose Duarte MD

(1.) _____ Consultation
Date of Consultation: 05/22/20XX
Requesting Physician: Rose Duarte, MD
Reason for Consultation: Hearing Loss

History: This 81-year-old male is brought to the office by his daughter with complaints of gradual hearing loss. It has probably been occurring for months, but seems to have worsened recently. He also notes some itching in his right ear. He denies any (2.) _____ or dizziness. Past medical history is significant for recurrent (3.) _____ as a child with right (4.) _____ at that time. During the review of symptoms, his daughter reported that he has been having trouble with his vision. He was recently diagnosed with (5.)_____ by an (6.) _____. He is now on medication for this. He also has an appointment with an (7.) _____ to get new glasses.

Physical Examination: Vital signs are normal. He is an elderly male in no acute distress. Examination of the head and face reveals no scars, lesions or masses. Sinuses are palpated and normal. Salivary gland examination is normal with no masses noted. Eyes show normal extraocular movement. The left exterior ear is normal, and examination of the ear canal using an (8.) _____ shows some cerumen but otherwise no abnormalities. The (9.) _____ membrane is intact. The right exterior ear is normal, but there is inflammation in the canal and (10.) _____ is present, in addition to heavy cerumen. The tympanic membrane is scarred but intact.

Diagnostic Studies:
Audiology Report: Mr. Berjarano saw the (11.) _____ and the testing revealed moderate to severe sensorineural hearing loss on the left and profound sensoineural hearing loss on the right. Speech understanding was 40% for the left ear and 24% for the right. Based on these results, Mr. Berjarano has great difficulty hearing all speech sounds without amplification.

Impression and Plan:
1. Right (12.) _____ externa: apparent infection of the right ear canal. We will treat with topical antibiotics. He was also given a medication for treating wax buildup in the ear canals.
2. Bilateral sensorineural hearing loss. Mr. Berjarano appears to be a good candidate for hearing aid amplification; however, I would like to see his right ear infection resolve and then repeat the (13.) _____ testing in about 2 weeks, at which time he can be fitted for hearing aids.
3. He will follow up as above or call our office if symptoms worsen or do not improve.

Thank you for this consultation. Please do not hesitate to contact me with any questions.
Electronically signed: James Cohen, MD, (14.) _____

Start | Log On/Off | Print | Edit

EXERCISE R   **Use Medical Language in Electronic Health Records Online**

Select the correct medical terms to complete three medical records in one patient's electronic file.

 Access online resources at evolve.elsevier.com > Evolve Resources > Practice Student Resources > Activities > Lesson 9 > Electronic Health Records

Topic: Glaucoma
Record 1: New Patient Evaluation
Record 2: Consultation Letter to PCP
Record 3: Operative Note

❏   Check the box when complete.

OBJECTIVE 6

Recall and assess knowledge of word parts, medical terms, and abbreviations.

EXERCISE S   **Online Review of Lesson Content**

Recall and assess your learning from working through the lesson by completing online learning activities at evolve. elsevier.com > Evolve Resources > Practice Student Resources. Keep track of your progress by placing a check mark next to completed activities.

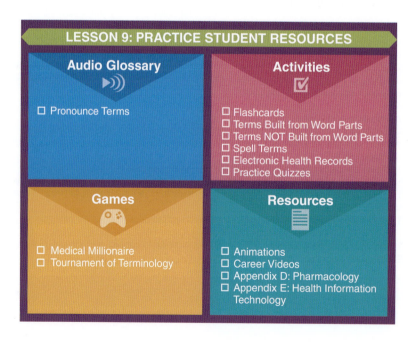

LESSON 9: PRACTICE STUDENT RESOURCES

Audio Glossary
▶))
☐ Pronounce Terms

Activities
☑
☐ Flashcards
☐ Terms Built from Word Parts
☐ Terms NOT Built from Word Parts
☐ Spell Terms
☐ Electronic Health Records
☐ Practice Quizzes

Games
☐ Medical Millionaire
☐ Tournament of Terminology

Resources
☐ Animations
☐ Career Videos
☐ Appendix D: Pharmacology
☐ Appendix E: Health Information Technology

EXERCISE T   Lesson Content Quiz

Test your knowledge of the terms and abbreviations introduced in this lesson. Circle the letter for the medical term or abbreviation related to the words in italics.

1. *Separation of the retina from the choroid in the posterior portion of the eye resulting in a disruption of vision* may cause a sudden increase in floaters, flashes of light, and worsening vision.
   a. retinal detachment
   b. glaucoma
   c. cataract

2. *Irregular curvature of the refractive surfaces of the eye* can produce blurred or distorted vision.
   a. myopia
   b. macular degeneration
   c. astigmatism

3. Presbycusis is an age-related condition which may cause one to be *hard of hearing.*
   a. HH
   b. HOH
   c. IOP

4. The patient was scheduled for ophthalmic surgery with intraocular lens implant to treat the *cataract* in her left eye.
   a. eye disorder caused by optic nerve damage
   b. farsightedness
   c. clouding of the lens of the eye

5. The patient presented with a painful redness in both eyes, photophobia, and diminished vision, which suggested the probability of *iritis.*
   a. inflammation of the outer protective layer of the eye
   b. inflammation of the pigmented muscular structure (colored portion) of the eye
   c. inflammation of the innermost layer of the eye

6. The child said he could read the book but had difficulty reading road signs. The ophthalmologist said he had *nearsightedness.*
   a. astigmatism
   b. hyperopia
   c. myopia

7. The patient presented with redness of the white of the eye accompanied by pain, tenderness, and tearing. He complained of diminished vison. The doctor diagnosed him with *scleritis.*
   a. inflammation of the iris
   b. inflammation of the outer protective layer of the eye
   c. inflammation of the middle layer of the eye

8. The nurse practitioner used *the instrument for visual examination of the eye* to check on the health of the patient's eyes during her annual physical exam.
   a. ophthalmoscope
   b. opthalmoscope
   c. ophthaloscope

9. The child's right outer ear became misshapen following a dog bite to the right side of his face. *Surgical repair of the (outer) ear* was performed by the plastic surgeon.
   a. otoplasty
   b. blepharoplasty
   c. tympanoplasty

10. The baby was tugging at his ears, crying more than normal, and was not sleeping. The pediatrician used an otoscope to examine the middle ear and noted *inflammation of both eardrums.*
    a. tinnitus
    b. iritis
    c. myringitis

LESSON AT A GLANCE | EYE AND EAR WORD PARTS

COMBINING FORMS

Eye	Ear
blephar/o	audi/o
ir/o	myring/o
irid/o	ot/o
kerat/o	tympan/o
ophthalm/o	
opt/o	
retin/o	
scler/o	

SUFFIXES

-metry
-plegia
-ptosis

LESSON AT A GLANCE | EYE AND EAR MEDICAL TERMS AND ABBREVIATIONS

SIGNS AND SYMPTOMS

otorrhea
tinnitus

DISEASES AND DISORDERS

astigmatism (AST)
blepharitis
blepharoptosis
cataract
glaucoma
hyperopia
iridoplegia
iritis
macular degeneration
myopia
myringitis
otitis
otitis media (OM)
presbycusis
presbyopia
retinal detachment
retinitis
scleritis

DIAGNOSTIC TESTS AND EQUIPMENT

audiometer
audiometry
keratometer
ophthalmoscope
otoscope

SURGICAL PROCEDURES

blepharoplasty
iridectomy
keratoplasty
LASIK
myringoplasty
myringotomy
otoplasty
tympanoplasty

SPECIALITIES AND PROFESSIONS

audiologist
audiology
ophthalmologist
ophthalmology (Ophth)
optometrist
optometry
otolaryngologist (ENT)
otolaryngology

RELATED TERMS

ophthalmic
optic
retinal
scleral
tympanic

ABBREVIATIONS

ARMD	HOH	Ophth
AST	IOP	VA
ENT	OM	

Musculoskeletal System

CASE STUDY **Shanti Mehra**

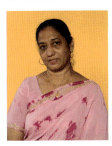

Shanti was walking to the store to buy more cigarettes. It was cold and icy and the sidewalks were slippery. She saw a pile of slush on the sidewalk in front of her and tried to scoot around it. Unfortunately, she slipped on some ice on the pavement. She tried to use her hand to brace her fall but her hand and wrist buckled under her when she fell. Now her wrist is really swollen and very painful. She also has muscle pain all over and thinks she may have bruised her hip bone.

■ *Consider Shanti's situation as you work through the lesson on the musculoskeletal system. At the end of the lesson, we will return to this case study and identify medical terms used to document Shanti's experience and the care she receives.*

OBJECTIVES

1 ■ Build, translate, pronounce, and spell medical terms built from word parts (p. 289).

2 ■ Define, pronounce, and spell medical terms NOT built from word parts (p. 312).

3 ■ Write abbreviations (p. 317).

4 ■ Identify medical terms by clinical category (p. 318).

5 ■ Use medical language in clinical statements, the case study, and a medical record (p. 322).

6 ■ Recall and assess knowledge of word parts, medical terms, and abbreviations (p. 326).

INTRODUCTION TO THE MUSCULOSKELETAL SYSTEM

Anatomic Structures of the Musculoskeletal System

bone (bōn)	organ made up of hard connective tissue with a dense outer layer and spongy inner layer
bone marrow (bōn) (MAR-ō)	material found in the cavities of bones; red marrow is responsible for blood cell formation, yellow marrow serves as a storehouse for fat
bursa (pl. bursae) (BER-sa), (BER-sē)	fluid-filled sac that allows for easy movement of one part of a joint over another
cartilage (KAR-ti-lej)	firm connective tissue primarily found in joints, covers the contacting surfaces of bones
joint (joint)	structure forming the union between bones and often allowing for movement
ligament (LIG-a-ment)	flexible, tough bands of fibrous connective tissue that attach one bone to another at a joint

Anatomic Structures of the Musculoskeletal System—cont'd

muscle (MUS-el)	tissue composed of specialized cells with the ability to contract to produce movement
tendon (TEN-den)	band of fibrous connective tissue that attaches muscle to bone

Functions of the Musculoskeletal System

- Provides body framework, support, and movement
- Protects internal organs
- Stores calcium
- Produces blood cells

How the Musculoskeletal System Works

Muscles, bones, and joints, along with other associated structures, provide the body with a flexible and protective framework. More than six hundred **muscles** cover the bones, maintain posture, and move the body through a process of contracting and relaxing. Two hundred and six **bones** form the adult human skeleton and provide structure for the body as a whole (Figure 10.2). There are several types of bones performing various functions such as bearing weight and protecting organs. Although bones are hard and seem lifeless, they are complete organs with living cells integrated into a mineral framework, which stores calcium. Bones have a dense outer layer and a spongy inner layer. Red **bone marrow,** found in some bones, generates blood cells. **Joints** form the union between bones and often allow for movement, although some do not. Most of the joints in the skeleton are freely moving and contain **cartilage** and **bursae. Cartilage** provides smooth surfaces within the joint and supports weight-bearing activities. **Bursae,** resting between the joint and tendon, allow **tendons** to slide over bones as they move. The organs and structures of the musculoskeletal system work together to protect, support, and move the body.

CAREER FOCUS | Professionals Who Work with the Musculoskeletal System

- **Surgical Technologists**, also called operating room technicians or scrub techs, work under the supervision of surgeons and are in charge of the instruments and supplies needed during surgical procedures. They are responsible for maintaining sterile techniques during operations and they help surgeons by assisting with their gowns and gloves, handing them instruments, and applying sterile dressings to the patients. They are also responsible for counting instruments and cleaning and preparing the operating room between procedures.

- **Occupational Therapy Assistants (OTAs)** work under the direction of occupational therapists to implement treatment plans that help restore or maintain a patient's ability to function independently on a daily basis. Their duties include teaching patients basic movement and mobility techniques, monitoring their progress, and alerting the therapists about any necessary changes to the prescribed regimen.

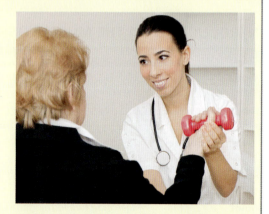

Figure 10.1 Physical therapist assistant conducting strength training with a patient.

CAREER FOCUS **Professionals Who Work with the Musculoskeletal System—cont'd**

- **Physical Therapist Assistants (PTAs)** provide physical therapy services under the direction and supervision of a licensed physical therapist. This may involve teaching patients exercises for mobility, strength and coordination, training for activities such as walking with crutches, canes, or walkers, massage, and the use of therapies such as ultrasound and electrical stimulation.

 FOR MORE INFORMATION

- To learn more about careers for **physical therapist assistants** go to the American Physical Therapy Association's website at apta.org/aboutptas/
- Access online resources at evolve.elsevier.com > Practice Student Resources > Other Resources > Career Videos to watch interviews with a **Physical Therapist**, **Physical Therapist Assistant**, and a **Surgical Technologist**.

OBJECTIVE 1

Build, translate, pronounce, and spell medical terms built from word parts.

WORD PARTS Use the paper or online **flashcards** to familiarize yourself with the following word parts.

COMBINING FORM (WR + CV)	DEFINITION	COMBINING FORM (WR + CV)	DEFINITION
arthr/o	joint(s)	**kyph/o**	hump (thoracic spine)
burs/o	bursa	**lord/o**	bent forward (lumbar spine)
carp/o	carpals, wrist (bone)	**necr/o**	death
chondr/o	cartilage	**oste/o**	bone
cost/o	rib(s)	**phalang/o**	phalanx (*pl.* phalanges) (any bone of the fingers or toes)
crani/o	skull (cranium)		
femor/o	femur (upper leg bone)	**pub/o**	pubis (anterior portion of the pelvis)
ili/o	ilium (upper, wing-shaped part on each side of the pelvis)		
		rachi/o, spondyl/o, vertebr/o	vertebra, spine, vertebral column
ischi/o	ischium (lower, posterior portion of the pelvis on which one sits)	**scoli/o**	crooked, curved (spine)
		stern/o	sternum (breast bone)
		ten/o, tendin/o	tendon
kinesi/o	movement, motion	**troph/o**	development
SUFFIX	DEFINITION	SUFFIX (S)	DEFINITION
-asthenia	weakness	**-malacia**	softening
-desis	surgical fixation, fusion	**-schisis**	split, fissure
PREFIX	DEFINITION		
inter-	between		

WORD PARTS PRESENTED IN PREVIOUS LESSONS | Used to Build Terms for the Musculoskeletal System

COMBINING FORM (WR + CV)	DEFINITION	COMBINING FORM (WR + CV)	DEFINITION
my/o	muscle(s), muscle tissue	path/o	disease
electr/o	electrical activity	sarc/o	flesh, connective tissue

SUFFIX	DEFINITION	SUFFIX (S)	DEFINITION
-a, -y	no meaning	-itis	inflammation
-ac, -al, -eal, -ic	pertaining to	-logy	study of
-algia	pain	-oma	tumor
-centesis	surgical puncture to remove fluid	-osis	abnormal condition
		-penia	abnormal reduction (in number)
-ectomy	surgical removal, excision	-plasty	surgical repair
-gram	record, radiographic image	-scopic	pertaining to visual examination
-ia	diseased state, condition of	-scopy	visual examination
-iasis	condition	-tomy	cut into, incision

PREFIX (P)	DEFINITION	PREFIX (P)	DEFINITION
a-, an-	absence of, without	hyper-	above, excessive
brady-	slow	intra-	within
dys-	difficult, painful, abnormal	sub-	below, under

Refer to Appendix A, Word Parts Used in *Basic Medical Language*, for alphabetical lists of word parts and their meanings.

EXERCISE A   **Build and Translate Medical Terms Built from Word Parts**

*Use the **Word Parts Tables** to complete the following questions. Check your responses with the Answer Key in Appendix C.*

1. **LABEL:** *Write the combining forms for anatomical structures of the musculoskeletal system on Figure 10.2. These anatomical combining forms will be used to build and translate medical terms in Exercise A.*

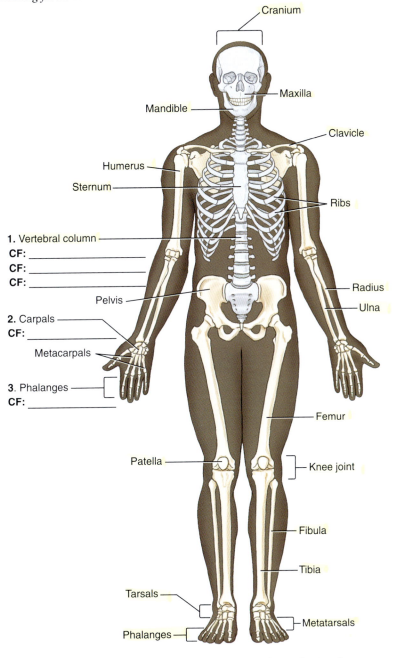

Cranium

Maxilla

Mandible

Clavicle

Humerus

Sternum

Ribs

1. Vertebral column
CF: _____
CF: _____
CF: _____

Radius

Pelvis

Ulna

2. Carpals
CF: _____

Metacarpals

3. Phalanges
CF: _____

Femur

Patella

Knee joint

Fibula

Tibia

Tarsals

Metatarsals

Phalanges

Figure 10.2 Skeletal system, anterior view, with combining forms.

2. MATCH: *Draw a line to match the word part with its definition.*

a. -al   surgical repair
b. -ectomy   between
c. -plasty   pertaining to
d. inter-   excision

---

3. BUILD: *Using the combining form **vertebr/o** and the word parts reviewed in the previous exercise, build the following terms related to the vertebra and spine. Remember, the definition usually starts with the meaning of the suffix.*

a. pertaining to the vertebra(e)

_____ / _____
wr   s

b. pertaining to between the vertebrae

_____ / _____ / _____
p   wr   s

c. excision of a vertebra

_____ / _____
wr   s

d. surgical repair of a vertebra

_____ / o / _____
wr   cv   s

---

4. LABEL: *Write word parts to complete Figure 10.3.*

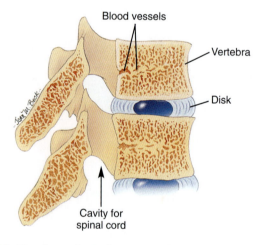

Blood vessels

Vertebra

Disk

Cavity for
spinal cord

Figure 10.3 Vertebrae. Sagittal section of vertebrae showing normal

_____ / _____ / _____ disks.
between   vertebrae   pertaining to

> **FYI**   **Disk** is sometimes spelled **disc** in names of bony structures.

---

5. READ: **The vertebral** (VER-te-bral) column is composed of three main sets of bones, called vertebrae (Figure 10.4). The cervical vertebrae are abbreviated C1-C7 and referred to as the cervical spine. The thoracic vertebrae are T1-T12, called the thoracic spine. The lumbar vertebrae are L1-L5, called the lumbar spine. The sacrum and coccyx complete the column. The **intervertebral** (in-ter-VER-te-bral) disks fill the spaces between vertebrae and are composed of a fibrous, cartilage-type tissue. A **vertebroplasty** (VER-te-brō-plas-tē) may be performed in cases where a vertebra has collapsed due to osteoporosis, while a **vertebrectomy** (ver-te-BREK-to-mē) might be performed if the vertebra cannot be repaired and must be replaced.

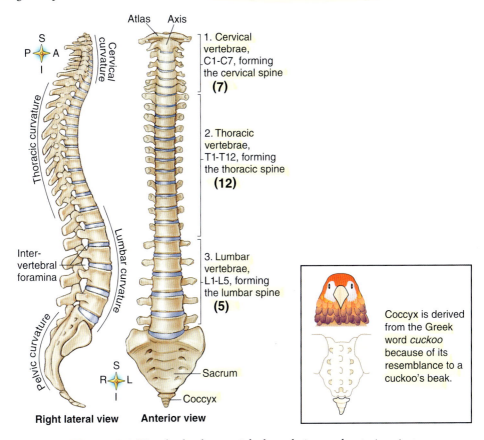

Atlas   Axis

1. Cervical vertebrae, C1-C7, forming the cervical spine **(7)**

2. Thoracic vertebrae, T1-T12, forming the thoracic spine **(12)**

3. Lumbar vertebrae, L1-L5, forming the lumbar spine **(5)**

Cervical curvature

Thoracic curvature

Lumbar curvature

Pelvic curvature

Inter-vertebral foramina

Sacrum

Coccyx

Right lateral view   Anterior view

Coccyx is derived from the Greek word *cuckoo* because of its resemblance to a cuckoo's beak.

Figure 10.4 Vertebral column, right lateral view and anterior view.

---

6. MATCH: *Draw a line to match the word part with its definition.*

a. -schisis   joint(s)
b. -tomy   inflammation
c. -itis   split, fissure
d. arthr/o   incision

---

7. TRANSLATE: *Complete the definitions of the following terms built from the combining form **rachi/o**, meaning vertebral column. Remember, the definition usually starts with the meaning of the suffix.*

a. rachi/schisis   _____ of the _____ column

b. rachi/o/tomy   _____ into the vertebral _____

8. **BUILD:** *Using the combining form* **spondyl/o,** *meaning vertebra, spine, vertebral column, and the word parts reviewed in the matching exercise, build the following term:*

inflammation of the spinal joints   _____/_____/_____
                                                                     wr   wr   s

9. **READ: Rachischisis** (rā-KIS-kis-sis) refers to a split in a vertebra, and is commonly seen in spina bifida. **Spondylarthritis** (spon-dil-ar-THRĪ-tis) may present with back pain, stiffness and inflammation of the tendons that attach to the spine. A **rachiotomy** (rā-kē-OT-o-mē) is a surgical procedure which allows access to the spinal column through a vertebra.

10. **MATCH:** *Draw a line to match the word part with its definition.*

    a. -osis   crooked, curved (spine)
    b. kyph/o   hump (thoracic spine)
    c. lord/o   abnormal condition
    d. scoli/o   bent forward (lumbar spine)

11. **TRANSLATE:** *Complete the definitions of the following terms:*

    a. scoli/osis   _____ _____ of crooked, curved (spine)
    b. kyph/osis   abnormal condition of a _____ (thoracic spine)
    c. lord/osis   _____ _____ of bent _____ (lumbar spine)

12. **LABEL:** *Write word parts to complete Figure 10.5.*

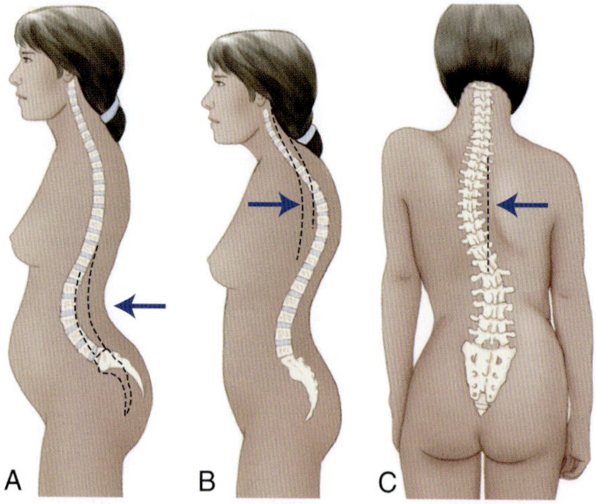

Figure 10.5 Abnormal curvatures of the vertebral column.

A. _____/_____.
        bent forward (lumbar spine)   abnormal condition
B. _____/_____.
        hump (thoracic spine)   abnormal condition
C. _____/_____.
        crooked, curved   abnormal condition

A   B   C

13. **MATCH:** *Draw a line to match the word part with its definition.*
    a. -al, -eal   excision
    b. -ectomy   pertaining to

14. **BUILD:** *Using the combining form **carp/o**, meaning wrist, and the word parts reviewed in the previous exercise, build the following term:*

a. pertaining to the wrist   _____ /_____
                                          wr   s

b. excision of a wrist (bone)   _____ /_____
                                          wr   s

15. **READ:** **Carpal** (KAR-pal) means pertaining to the wrist bones (Figure 10.6). "Meta-" is a prefix meaning "beyond." Metacarpal refers to the bones beyond (distal to) the carpals, between the wrist bones and the fingers. A **carpectomy** (kar-PEK-to-mē) refers to removal of a wrist bone, which may be performed in cases of severe arthritis.

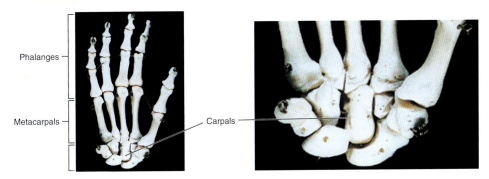

Figure 10.6 The carpal, metacarpal, and phalangeal bones.

16. **TRANSLATE:** *Complete the definitions of the following terms using the word root **phalang/o**, meaning phalanx (any bone of the fingers or toes).*

a. phalang/eal   _____ to a _____ (any bone of the fingers or toes)

b. phalang/ectomy   _____ of a _____ (any bone of the fingers or toes)

17. **READ:** When **phalangeal** (fa-LAN-jē-al) terms are used, they are accompanied by descriptive words to designate a specific finger or toe bone. For example, a physician would say "The patient had a **phalangectomy** (fal-an-JEK-to-mē) of the distal phalanx of the fifth finger, right hand." The thumb is counted as the first finger, the index finger is second, and thus the pinky is the fifth finger.

18. **MATCH:** *Draw a line to match the word part with its definition.*

a. a-   above, excessive
b. dys-   no meaning
c. hyper-   absence of, without
d. -y   pertaining to
e. -ic   difficult, painful, abnormal

19. BUILD: *Using the combining form **troph/o** and the word parts reviewed in the previous exercise, build the following terms related to growth.*

a. abnormal development

            _____ / _____ /y

                          p   wr   s

b. without development (process of wasting away)

            _____ / _____ /y

                          p   wr   s

c. excessive development

            _____ / _____ /y

                          p   wr   s

d. pertaining to excessive development

            _____ / _____ / _____

                          p   wr   s

---

20. READ: Hypertrophy (hī-PER-tro-fē) occurs when muscles are overdeveloped, which may result from weight-lifting. Almost any muscle can become **hypertrophic** (hī-per-TRŌF-ik); when the heart muscle is overdeveloped it is called **hypertrophic cardiomyopathy**. Loss of muscle mass, or **atrophy** (AT-rō-fē), occurs when muscles are not used, which may result from disability or a sedentary lifestyle. Muscular **dystrophy** (DIS-tro-fē), or **MD**, is a group of hereditary diseases characterized by abnormal muscles and weakness.

---

21. LABEL: *Write word parts to complete Figure 10.7.*

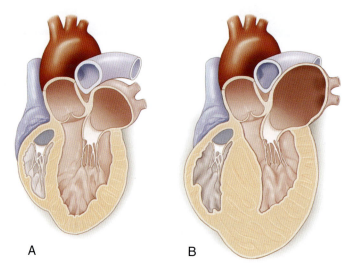

       A   B

Figure 10.7 A. Normal heart muscle.

       B. _____ / _____ / _____ heart muscle in cardiomyopathy.

             excessive   development   pertaining to

22. **LABEL:** *Write the combining forms for anatomical structures of a joint in Figure 10.8.*

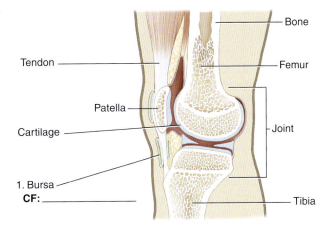

Figure 10.8 Knee joint and related combining form for bursa.

23. **MATCH:** *Draw a line to match the word part with its definition.*

    a. -itis   excision
    b. -ectomy   incision
    c. -tomy   inflammation

24. **TRANSLATE:** *Complete the definitions of the following terms using the combining form* **burs/o***, meaning bursa.*

    a. burs/ectomy   excision of a _____
    b. burs/itis   _____ of the _____
    c. burs/o/tomy   _____ into a bursa

25. **READ:** **Bursitis** (ber-SĪ-tis) refers to inflammation of the fluid-filled sac around a joint. Over time, this fluid can increase and the bursa may thicken. Sometimes a **bursotomy** (ber-SOT-o-mē) is performed and a drain is placed if the swelling becomes severe. In chronic bursitis, the bursa may become thickened or even infected and a **bursectomy** (ber-SEK-to-mē) may be performed.

26. **LABEL:** *Write word parts to complete Figure 10.9.*

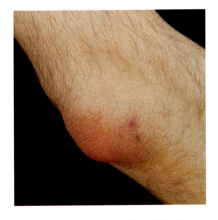

Figure 10.9 Olecranon (elbow) _____ / _____ .
                                   bursa   inflammation

27. LABEL: *Write the combining forms for anatomical structures of the pelvis on Figure 10.10.*

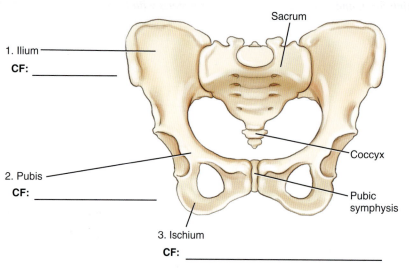

Sacrum

1. Ilium

CF: _____

2. Pubis

CF: _____

3. Ischium

CF: _____

Coccyx

Pubic symphysis

> **FYI**   Compare the combining form for ilium, **ili/o,** the portion of the pelvis, with the combining form for ileum, **ile/o,** the distal portion of the small intestine. The pronunciation is the same. Think of **il**ium with an **i** and **int**estine with an **e** to help distinguish the word roots.

Figure 10.10 Pelvis, anterior view, with combining forms.

---

28. MATCH: *Draw a line to match the word part with its definition.*

   a. -al, -ac   pertaining to
   b. femor/o   femur (see Figure 10.2)

---

29. TRANSLATE: *Complete the definitions of the following terms.*

   a. ili/ac   pertaining to the _____

   b. femor/al   _____ to the femur

   c. ili/o/femor/al   pertaining to the _____ and the _____

   d. ischi/al   _____ to the ischium

   e. ischi/o/pub/ic   pertaining to the _____ and the pubis

---

30. READ: The **ischial** (IS-kē-al) bones are referred to as the "sitting bones." The **iliofemoral** (il-lē-ō-FEM-or-al) ligament is one of the strongest in the body; it connects the pelvis to the thigh bone. At birth, the three bones of the pelvis are separate and distinct, but in childhood they fuse together. The first fusion results in the **ischiopubic** (is-kē-ō-PŪ-bik) ramus (a projection of the bones where they meet).

---

31. MATCH: *Draw a line to match the word part with its definition.*

   a. -algia   electrical activity
   b. -asthenia   pain
   c. -gram   record, radiographic image
   d. electr/o   muscle(s), muscle tissue
   e. my/o   weakness

32. BUILD: *Using the combining form* **my/o** *and the word parts reviewed in the previous exercise, build the following terms related to muscle. Hint: for a. and b. the definition of the term starts with the meaning of the combining form.*

a. muscle pain

_____/_____
wr   s

b. muscle weakness

_____/_____
wr   s

c. record of the electrical activity of a muscle

_____/ o /_____/ o /_____
wr   cv   wr   cv   s

33. READ: Myalgia (mī-AL-ja) is a symptom of many disorders. Fibromyalgia is a disorder characterized by widespread musculoskeletal pain accompanied by fatigue, sleep, memory, and mood issues. **Myasthenia** (mī-as-THĒ-nē-a) gravis, abbreviated MG, is an autoimmune neuromuscular disease leading to fluctuating muscle loss and fatigue. Symptoms may include drooping eyelids, blurred vision, or slurred speech. An **electromyogram** (ē-lek-trō-MĪ-ō-gram) may show patterns that are specific to MG.

34. LABEL: *Write word parts to complete Figure 10.11.*

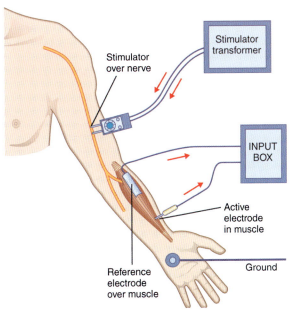

Figure 10.11 Diagram of an _____/o/_____/o/_____ (EMG) of the forearm.
electrical activity   muscle   record

35. MATCH: *Draw a line to match the word part with its definition.*

    a. brady-   no meaning

    b. dys-   slow

    c. -a   difficult, painful, abnormal

---

36. BUILD: *Using the combining form* **kinesi/o**, *and the word parts reviewed in the previous exercise, build the following terms related to movement.*

    a. slow movement   _____ / _____ /a

                                          p   wr   s

    b. painful movement   _____ / _____ /a

                                          p   wr   s

---

37. READ: Bradykinesia (brad-ē-ki-NĒ-zha) and **dyskinesia** (dis-ki-NĒ-zha) refer to abnormalities in muscle movement caused by neurological irregularities and are usually associated with Parkinson disease. Shuffling when walking and having little or no facial expressions are types of unusually slow movement seen in bradykinesia. Dyskinesias are involuntary movements, such as swaying of the body, twitching, and bobbing of the head.

---

38. REVIEW OF MUSCULOSKELETAL SYSTEM TERMS BUILT FROM WORD PARTS: *The following is an alphabetical list of terms built and translated in the previous exercises.*

MEDICAL TERMS BUILT FROM WORD PARTS

TERM	DEFINTION	TERM	DEFINTION
1. atrophy (AT-rō-fē)	without development (process of wasting away)	**8. dyskinesia** (dis-ki-NĒ-zha)	painful movement
2. bradykinesia (brad-ē-ki-NĒ-zha)	slow movement	**9. dystrophy** (DIS-tro-fē)	abnormal development
3. bursectomy (ber-SEK-to-mē)	excision of the bursa	**10. electromyogram (EMG)** (ē-lek-trō-MĪ-ō-gram)	record of the electrical activity of the muscle (Figure 10.11)
4. bursitis (ber-SĪ-tis)	inflammation of the bursa (Figure 10.9)	**11. femoral** (FEM-or-al)	pertaining to the femur
5. bursotomy (ber-SOT-o-mē)	incision into the bursa	**12. hypertrophic** (hī-per-TRŌF-ik)	pertaining to excessive development (Figure 10.7, *B*)
6. carpal (KAR-pal)	pertaining to the wrist (Figure 10.6)	**13. hypertrophy** (hī-PER-tro-fē)	excessive development
7. carpectomy (kar-PEK-to-mē)	excision of a wrist (bone)	**14. iliac** (IL-ē-ak)	pertaining to the ilium

MEDICAL TERMS BUILT FROM WORD PARTS—cont'd

TERM	DEFINTION	TERM	DEFINTION
15. **iliofemoral** (il-lē-ō-FEM-or-al)	pertaining to the ilium and femur	24. **phalangectomy** (fal-an-JEK-to-mē)	excision of a phalanx (any bone of the fingers or toes)
16. **intervertebral** (in-ter-VER-te-bral)	pertaining to between the vertebrae (Figure 10.3)	25. **rachiotomy** (rā-kē-OT-o-mē)	incision into the vertebral column
17. **ischial** (IS-kē-al)	pertaining to the ischium	26. **rachischisis** (rā-KIS-kis-sis)	fissure of the vertebral column
18. **ischiopubic** (is-kē-ō-PŪ-bik)	pertaining to the ischium and pubis	27. **scoliosis** (skō-lē-Ō-sis)	abnormal condition of crooked, curved (spine) (Figure 10.5, *C*)
19. **kyphosis** (kī-FŌ-sis)	abnormal condition of a hump (thoracic spine) (Figure 10.5, *B*)	28. **spondylarthritis** (spon-dil-ar-THRĪ-tis)	inflammation of the vertebral joints
20. **lordosis** (lōr-DŌ-sis)	abnormal condition of bent forward (lumbar spine) (Figure 10.5, *A*)	39. **vertebral** (VER-te-bral)	pertaining to the vertebra(e)
21. **myalgia** (mī-AL-ja)	muscle pain	30. **vertebrectomy** (ver-te-BREK-to-mē)	excision of the vertebra
22. **myasthenia** (mī-as-THĒ-nē-a)	muscle weakness	31. **vertebroplasty** (VER-te-brō-plas-tē)	surgical repair of the vertebra
23. **phalangeal** (fa-LAN-jē-al)	pertaining to a phalanx (any bone of the fingers or toes) (Figure 10.6)		

EXERCISE B   Pronounce and Spell Terms Built from Word Parts

Practice pronunciation and spelling on paper and online.

1. **Practice on Paper**
   a. **Pronounce**: Read the phonetic spelling and say aloud the terms listed in the previous table, Review of Terms Built from Word Parts.
   b. **Spell**: Have a study partner read the terms aloud. Write the spelling of the terms on a separate sheet of paper.

2. **Practice Online** ⊕
   a. **Access** online learning resources. Go to evolve.elsevier.com > Evolve Resources > Practice Student Resources.
   b. **Pronounce**: Select Audio Glossary > Lesson 10 > Exercise B. Select a term to hear its pronunciation and repeat aloud.
   c. **Spell**: Select Activities > Lesson 10 > Spell Terms > Exercise B. Select the audio icon and type the correct spelling of the term.

❏   Check the box when complete.

EXERCISE C   Build and Translate MORE Medical Terms Built from Word Parts

*Use the **Word Parts Tables** to complete the following questions. Check your responses with the Answer Key in Appendix C.*

1. **LABEL:** *Write the combining forms for anatomical structures of the musculoskeletal system on Figure 10.12. These anatomical combining forms will be used to build and translate medical terms in Exercise C.*

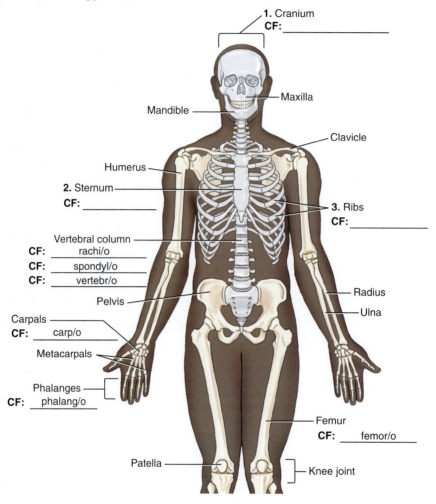

1. Cranium
CF:_____

Maxilla

Mandible

Clavicle

Humerus

2. Sternum
CF:_____

3. Ribs
CF:_____

Vertebral column
CF:_____rachi/o_____
CF:_____spondyl/o_____
CF:_____vertebr/o_____

Pelvis

Radius

Ulna

Carpals
CF:_____carp/o_____

Metacarpals

Phalanges
CF:_____phalang/o_____

Femur
CF:_____femor/o_____

Patella

Knee joint

Figure 10.12 Skeletal system, anterior view, with combining forms.

2. **MATCH:** *Draw a line to match the word part with its definition.*

a. -tomy	pertaining to
b. intra-	incision
c. -schisis	within
d. -malacia	split, fissure
e. -al	diseased state, condition of
f. -ia	softening

3. **BUILD**: *Using the combining form* **crani/o** *and the word parts reviewed in the previous exercise, build the following terms related to the skull (cranium). Remember, the definition usually starts with the meaning of the suffix.*

   a. pertaining to within the skull

   _____/_____/_____
               p   wr   s

   b. fissure of the skull

   _____/_o_/_____
             wr   cv   s

   c. incision into the skull

   _____/_o_/_____
             wr   cv   s

   d. softening of the skull

   _____/_o_/_____
             wr   cv   s

---

4. **READ**: An **intracranial** (in-tra-KRĀ-nē-al) hemorrhage may be caused by extremely high blood pressure, an aneurysm, a stroke, or by various traumatic injuries. If it is severe, a **craniotomy** (krā-nē-OT-o-mē) may be required to access the brain and evacuate the blood. **Cranioschisis** (krā-nē-OS-ki-sis) usually occurs along the midsagittal plane of the skull and may be accompanied by protrusion of the brain and its meninges (linings). **Craniomalacia** (krā-nē-ō-ma-LĀ-sha) may be discovered during examination of the newborn, in which gentle pressure on the skull produces a sudden collapse.

---

5. **LABEL**: *Write the word parts to complete Figure 10.13.*

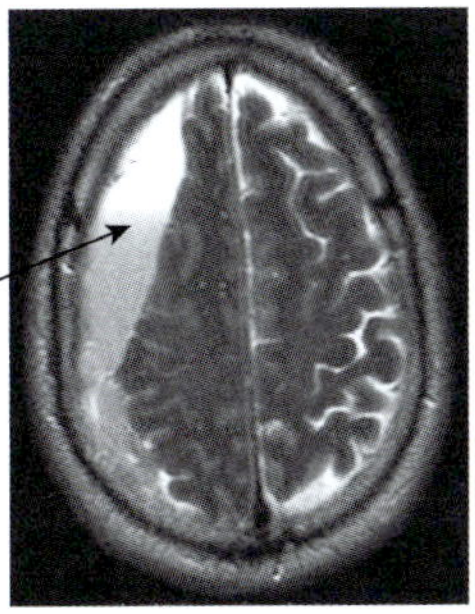

Blood
appears
white on
this MRI

Figure 10.13 Magnetic resonance imaging (MRI) of a subdural hematoma,

a type of _____/_____/_____ bleeding.
         within   cranium   pertaining to

---

6. **MATCH**: *Draw a line to match the word part with its definition.*

   a. -al   between
   b. inter-   pertaining to
   c. sub-   below, under

---

7. **TRANSLATE**: *Complete the definitions of the following terms by using the meaning of the word parts to fill in the blanks.*

   a. stern/al   pertaining to the _____
   b. stern/o/cost/al   pertaining to the sternum and the _____

8. **READ:** The sternum is a bony plate at the anterior wall of the chest. It is divided into three parts called the manubrium, the body, and the xiphoid process. The **sternal** (STER-nal) angle divides the manubrium from the sternal body. The xiphoid process is at the bottom of the sternum and can usually be felt on exam. The **sternocostal** (ster-nō-KOS-tal) joints connect the sternum to the ribs.

9. **LABEL:** *Write the word parts to complete Figure 10.14.*

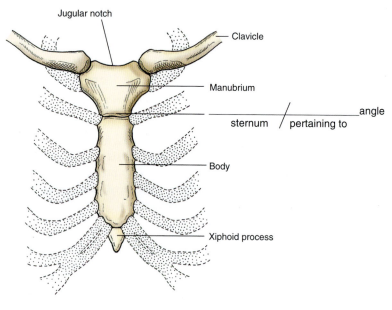

Jugular notch

Clavicle

Manubrium

_____ angle
sternum / pertaining to

Body

Xiphoid process

Figure 10.14 Sternum and rib joints.

10. **BUILD:** *Using the combining form **cost/o** and the word parts reviewed in the previous matching exercise, build the following terms related to the rib(s).*

   a. pertaining to between the ribs   _____ / _____ / _____

                                                      p   wr   s

   b. pertaining to below the rib(s)   _____ / _____ / _____

                                                      p   wr   s

11. **READ:** The **intercostal** (in-ter-KOS-tal) muscles are responsible for forced (voluntary) respiratory inspiration and expiration. **Subcostal** (sub-KOS-tal) retractions appear as the sucking in of the skin and muscles beneath the sternum (breastbone) and ribs and can be a sign of respiratory difficulty.

12. **LABEL:** *Write the combining forms for anatomical structures of the musculoskeletal system on Figure 10.15.*

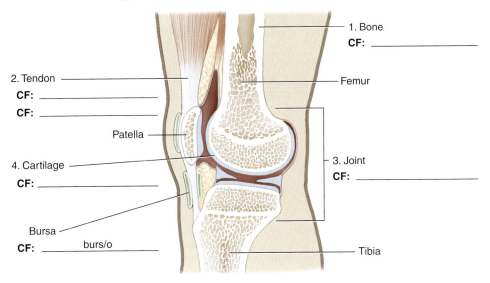

1. Bone
   CF: _____

Femur

2. Tendon
   CF: _____
   CF: _____

Patella

3. Joint
   CF: _____

4. Cartilage
   CF: _____

Bursa
   CF: _____ burs/o _____

Tibia

Figure 10.15 Knee joint and related combining forms

---

13. **MATCH:** *Draw a line to match the word part with its definition.*

a. -itis   pertaining to
b. -ectomy   excision
c. -malacia   softening
d. -al   inflammation

---

14. **TRANSLATE:** *Complete the definitions of the following terms built from the combining form **chondr/o**, meaning cartilage. Use the meaning of word parts to fill in the blanks.*

a. cost/o/chondr/al   pertaining to _____ and cartilage
b. chondr/itis   inflammation of _____
c. chondr/ectomy   _____ of _____
d. chondr/o/malacia   _____ of cartilage

> **FYI**   **Cartilage** is made up of connective tissue and covers the ends of two adjoining bones. It is also found in other semi-rigid structures such as the nose, ear, and trachea.

---

15. **READ:** **Chondromalacia** (kon-drō-ma-LĀ-sha) patella is a general term meaning damage to the cartilage under the kneecap. It is also called "runner's knee." **Chondritis** (kon-DRĪ-tis) can occur in the ear cartilage after piercing and often indicates an infection. A **chondrectomy** (kon-DREK-to-mē) may be necessary, and plastic surgery may be required to restore the appearance of the ear. Another common form of chondritis occurs at the **costochondral** (kos-tō-KON-dral) joints and can cause pain with breathing or coughing; it is referred to as costochondritis.

16. LABEL: *Write the word parts to complete Figure 10.16.*

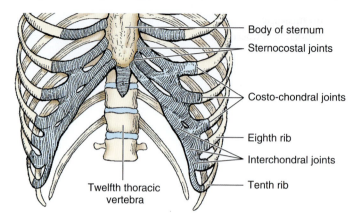

Body of sternum
Sternocostal joints

Costo-chondral joints

Eighth rib
Interchondral joints

Tenth rib

Twelfth thoracic
vertebra

Figure 10.16 Lower sternum and ribs, showing sternocostal,

_____/o/_____/_____, and interchondral joints.
   rib(s)   cartilage   pertaining to

---

17. MATCH: *Draw a line to match the word part with its definition.*

a. -osis   death
b. -itis   abnormal condition
c. necr/o   inflammation

---

18. BUILD: *Use the combining form **oste/o**, along with the word parts reviewed in the previous exercise, to build terms related to bone.*

a. abnormal condition of death   _____/_____
                                              wr   s

b. abnormal condition of death of the bone   _____/ o /_____/_____
   (tissue)   wr   cv   wr   s

c. inflammation of the bone and cartilage   _____/ o /_____/_____
                                                  wr   cv   wr   s

---

19. READ: Osteonecrosis (os-tē-ō-ne-KRŌ-sis) is the death of bone cells due to lack of blood flow. Avascular **necrosis** (ne-KRŌ-sis) is another term for this. **Osteochondritis** (os-tē-ō-kon-DRĬ-tis) dissecans is actually a type of osteonecrosis because small pieces of cartilage and bone become separated from the end of a bone and lose their blood supply.

20. **MATCH:** *Draw a line to match the word part with its definition.*

    a. path/o   no meaning
    b. -malacia   abnormal reduction
    c. -penia   softening
    d. -y   disease

21. **TRANSLATE:** *Complete the definitions of the following terms by using the meaning of the word parts to fill in the blanks.*

    a. oste/o/path/y   of the bone

    b. oste/o/penia   abnormal _____ of _____ mass

    c. oste/o/malacia   of the bone

> **FYI**   The suffix **-penia** comes from the Greek word meaning **poverty** or **need.** In Lesson 7, the suffix -penia was used to describe an **abnormal reduction in number**, such as with **leukocytopenia** (abnormal reduction in the number of white cells). Here, -penia refers to an **abnormal reduction**, not in the number of bone cells, but of the bone mass itself.

22. **READ:** **Osteomalacia** (os-tē-ō-ma-LĀ-sha) is often caused by vitamin D deficiency and is a defect in the bone building process. **Osteopenia** (os-tē-ō-PĒ-ne-a) is any reduction of the bone mass below normal, and means that existing bone cells are being reabsorbed by the body faster than new ones can be made. While **osteopathy** (os-tē-OP-a-thē) refers to disease of the bone, it also refers to a practice of medicine.

> **FYI**   **Osteopathy** practice uses the same forms of treatment and diagnosis as conventional medicine but places greater emphasis on the relationship between body organs and the musculoskeletal system. A physician who practices osteopathy is called a doctor of osteopathy, or DO (most commonly referred to as an "osteopath"). A physician who practices conventional (allopathic) medicine is a doctor of medicine or an MD.

23. **MATCH:** *Draw a line to match the word part with its definition.*

    a. sarc/o   tumor
    b. -oma   inflammation
    c. -itis   flesh, connective tissue

24. **BUILD:** *Use the combining form **oste/o**, along with the word parts reviewed in the previous exercise, to build terms related to bone.*

    a. inflammation of the bone(s) and the joint(s)   _____ / o / _____ / _____
                                                                                   wr   **cv**   **wr**   **s**

    b. tumor of the bone and connective tissue   _____ / o / _____ / _____
                                                                                   wr   **cv**   **wr**   **s**

25. **READ:** **Osteoarthritis** (os-tē-ō-ar-THRĪ-tis) is the most common form of arthritis and is the result of degeneration and loss of bone cartilage, especially of the knees and hips. **Osteosarcoma** (os-tē-ō-sar-KŌ-ma) is a malignant tumor that arises from connective tissues and most frequently involves the long bones.

26. **LABEL:** *Write the word parts to complete Figure 10.17.*

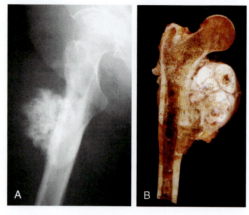

Figure 10.17 Lateral radiograph (A) and pathology specimen (B) of _____/o/_____/_____.
                                             bone   connective tissue   tumor

27. **MATCH:** *Draw a line to match the word part with its definition.*

a.	-algia	surgical repair
b.	-desis	inflammation
c.	-plasty	surgical fixation, fusion
d.	-itis	pain

28. **TRANSLATE:** *Complete the definitions of the following terms built from the combining form **arthr/o**, meaning joint(s). Use the meaning of word parts to fill in the blanks.*

a. arthr/algia   pain in the _____

b. arthr/itis   _____ of the joint(s)

c. arthr/o/desis   _____ _____ (fusion) of a joint

d. arthr/o/plasty   surgical _____ of a _____

29. **READ:** Osteoarthritis, rheumatoid arthritis, and gout are three forms of **arthritis** (ar-THRĪ-tis). While **arthralgia** (ar-THRAL-ja) is associated with all three forms, they differ in terms of other symptoms such as swelling, redness, and stiffness. In **arthrodesis** (ar-thrō-DĒ-sis), two bones on the end of a joint are fused, eliminating the joint itself. In **arthroplasty** (AR-thrō-plas-tē), the joint space is preserved, and the joint is restored to its full range of motion.

30. **MATCH:** *Draw a line to match the word part with its definition.*

    a. -centesis   visual examination
    b. -gram   record, radiographic image
    c. -scopy   pertaining to visual examination
    d. -scopic   surgical puncture to remove fluid

---

31. **BUILD:** *Continue using the combining form* **arthr/o**, *along with the word parts reviewed in the previous exercise, to build terms related to joints.*

    a. surgical puncture of a joint to remove fluid   _____ / o / _____
                                                                       wr   cv   s

    b. radiographic image of a joint   _____ / o / _____
                                                                        wr   cv   s

    c. visual examination of a joint   _____ / o / _____
                                                                        wr   cv   s

    d. pertaining to visual examination of a joint   _____ / o / _____
                                                                                wr   cv   s

---

32. **LABEL:** *Write the word parts to complete Figure 10.18.*

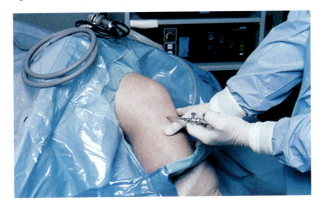

    Figure 10.18 An arthroscope is used to perform a(n) _____ / o / _____
                                                                      joint   visual examination

    for diagnostic purposes or for _____ / o / _____
                                             joint   pertaining to visual examination
    surgery to repair ligaments or to remove cartilage.

---

33. **MATCH:** *Draw a line to match the word part with its definition.*

    a. -desis   inflammation
    b. -itis   surgical repair
    c. -plasty   surgical fixation, fusion

34. **TRANSLATE:** *Complete the definitions of the following terms built from the combining forms* **ten/o** *and* **tendin/o**, *meaning tendon. Use the meaning of word parts to fill in the blanks. Note that the combining form* **tendin/o** *contains an* **i** *compared with the term itself,* **tendon**, *which is spelled with an* **o**.

a. tendin/itis _____ of the tendon(s)

b. ten/o/plasty surgical _____ of a _____

c. ten/o/desis _____ _____ (fusion) of a tendon

35. **READ:** In some patients with biceps **tendinitis** (ten-di-NĪ-tis), **tenodesis** (ten-ō-DĒ-sis) may be needed to remove the biceps at its attachment to the shoulder and to reinsert it in a different area. In cases of Achilles tendon rupture, **tenoplasty** (TEN-ō-plas-tē) may be needed to restore function of the ankle.

> **FYI**   The **Achilles tendon**, located between the calf muscle and the heel, is the thickest and strongest tendon in the body. Its name is derived from the classical tale of Achilles. To make him invulnerable, Achilles' mother dipped him into the river Styx. She held him by this tendon, which was not immersed, and later a mortal wound was inflicted on Achilles' heel.

36. **REVIEW OF MORE MUSCULOSKELETAL SYSTEM TERMS BUILT FROM WORD PARTS:** *the following is an alphabetical list of terms built and translated in the previous exercises.*

MEDICAL TERMS BUILT FROM WORD PARTS

TERM	DEFINITION	TERM	DEFINITION
1. **arthralgia** (ar-THRAL-ja)	pain in the joint	11. **chondromalacia** (kon-drō-ma-LĀ-sha)	softening of cartilage
2. **arthritis** (ar-THRĪ-tis)	inflammation of the joint(s)	12. **costochondral** (kos-tō-KON-dral)	pertaining to the ribs and cartilage (Figure 10.16)
3. **arthrocentesis** (ar-thrō-sen-TĒ-sis)	surgical puncture of a joint to remove fluid	13. **craniomalacia** (krā-nē-ō-ma-LĀ-sha)	softening of the skull
4. **arthrodesis** (ar-thrō-DĒ-sis)	surgical fixation (fusion) of a joint	14. **cranioschisis** (krā-nē-OS-ki-sis)	fissure of the skull
5. **arthrogram** (AR-thrō-gram)	radiographic image of a joint	15. **craniotomy** (krā-nē-OT-o-mē)	incision into the skull
6. **arthroplasty** (AR-thrō-plas-tē)	surgical repair of a joint	16. **intercostal** (in-ter-KOS-tal)	pertaining to between the ribs (Figure 10.16)
7. **arthroscopic** (ar-thrō-SKOP-ik)	pertaining to visual examination of a joint (Figure 10.18)	17. **intracranial** (in-tra-KRĀ-nē-al)	pertaining to within the skull (Figure 10.13)
8. **arthroscopy** (ar-THROS-ko-pē)	visual examination of a joint (Figure 10.18)	18. **necrosis** (ne-KRŌ-sis)	abnormal condition of death
9. **chondrectomy** (kon-DREK-to-mē)	excision of cartilage	19. **osteoarthritis (OA)** (os-tē-ō-ar-THRĪ-tis)	inflammation of the bone(s) and the joint(s)
10. **chondritis** (kon-DRĪ-tis)	inflammation of cartilage	20. **osteochondritis** (os-tē-ō-kon-DRĪ-tis)	inflammation of the bone and cartilage

MEDICAL TERMS BUILT FROM WORD PARTS—cont'd

TERM	DEFINITION	TERM	DEFINITION
21. **osteomalacia** (os-tē-ō-ma-LĀ-sha)	softening of the bone	27. **sternocostal** (ster-nō-KOS-tal)	pertaining to the sternum and the rib(s) (Figure 10.16)
22. **osteonecrosis** (os-tē-ō-ne-KRŌ-sis)	abnormal condition of death of bone (tissue)	28. **subcostal** (sub-KOS-tal)	pertaining to below the ribs
23. **osteopathy** (os-tē-OP-a-thē)	disease of the bone	29. **tendinitis** (ten-di-NĪ-tis)	inflammation of the tendon(s)
24. **osteopenia** (os-tē-ō-PĒ-ne-a)	abnormal reduction of bone mass	30. **tenodesis** (ten-ō-DĒ-sis)	surgical fixation (fusion) of a tendon
25. **osteosarcoma** (os-tē-ō-sar-KŌ-ma)	tumor of the bone and the connective tissue (Figure 10.17)	31. **tenoplasty** (TEN-ō-plas-tē)	surgical repair of a tendon
26. **sternal** (STER-nal)	pertaining to the sternum (Figure 10.14)		

EXERCISE D   Pronounce and Spell MORE Terms Built from Word Parts

Practice pronunciation and spelling on paper and online.

1. **Practice on Paper**

    a. **Pronounce**: Read the phonetic spelling and say aloud the terms listed in the previous table, Review of MORE Terms Built from Word Parts.

    b. **Spell**: Have a study partner read the terms aloud. Write the spelling of the terms on a separate sheet of paper.

2. **Practice Online** 🌐

    a. **Access** online learning resources. Go to evolve.elsevier.com > Evolve Resources > Practice Student Resources.

    b. **Pronounce**: Select Audio Glossary > Lesson 10 > Exercise D. Select a term to hear its pronunciation and repeat aloud.

    c. **Spell**: Select Activities > Lesson 10 > Spell Terms > Exercise D. Select the audio icon and type the correct spelling of the term.

❑   Check the box when complete.

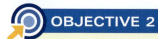

OBJECTIVE 2

Define, pronounce, and spell medical terms NOT built from word parts

The terms listed below may contain word parts, but are difficult to translate literally.

MEDICAL TERMS NOT BUILT FROM WORD PARTS

TERM	DEFINITION
carpal tunnel syndrome (CTS) (KAR-pl)(TUN-el) (SIN-drōm)	common nerve entrapment disorder of the wrist caused by compression of the median nerve. Symptoms include pain, tingling, and numbness in portions of the hand and fingers.
chiropractic (kī-rō-PRAK-tik)	system of treatment that consists of manipulation of the vertebral column
fracture (Fx) (FRAK-chūr)	broken bone
gout (gowt)	disease in which an excessive amount of uric acid in the blood causes sodium urate crystals to be deposited in the joints, especially that of the great toe, producing arthritis
hernia (HUR-nē-ah)	protrusion of an organ or structure through an abnormal opening. Hernias often occur due to weakness of the mucsles or ligaments in the surrounding area.
herniated disk (HER-nē-āt-ed) (disk)	rupture of the intervertebral disk cartilage, which allows the contents to protrude through it, putting pressure on the spinal nerve roots
Lyme disease (līm) (di-ZĒZ)	immune response caused by a bite from a deer tick infected with *Borrelia burgdorferi*; causes symptoms including fever, headache, and joint pain, and mimics other musculoskeletal diseases. A rash (target lesion) may initially arise at the site of the tick bite.
magnetic resonance imaging (MRI) (mag-NET-ik) (REZ-ō-nans) (IM-a-jing)	diagnostic imaging test producing scans that give information about the body's anatomy by placing the patient in a strong magnetic field
muscular dystrophy (MD) (MUS-kū-lar) (DIS-tro-fē)	group of hereditary diseases characterized by degeneration of muscle and weakness
nuclear medicine (NM) (NŪ-klē-er) (MED-i-sin)	diagnostic imaging test producing scans that give information about the body's anatomy and function by using radioactive material. Nuclear medicine is also used to treat various medical conditions.
orthopedics (ortho) (or-thō-PĒ-diks)	study and treatment of diseases and abnormalities of the musculoskeletal system
orthopedist (or-thō-PĒ-dist)	physician who specializes in the study and treatment of diseases and abnormalities of the musculoskeletal system
osteoporosis (os-tē-ō-po-RŌ-sis)	disease caused by abnormal loss of bone density occurring predominantly in postmenopausal women, which can lead to an increase in fractures of the ribs, thoracic and lumbar vertebrae, hips, and wrists
plantar fasciitis (PLAN-tar) (fas-ē-Ī-tis)	inflammation of the connective tissue of the sole of the foot; common cause of heel pain
rheumatoid arthritis (RA) (RŪ-ma-toyd) (ar-THRĪ-tis)	chronic systemic disease characterized by autoimmune inflammatory changes in the connective tissue throughout the body
spinal stenosis (SPĪ-nal) (ste-NŌ-sis)	narrowing of the spinal canal with compression of nerve roots. Symptoms include pain, numbness, and tingling in the thigh which radiates to lower extremities.

EXERCISE E   **Label**

Write the medical terms pictured and defined using the previous table of Medical Terms NOT Built from Word Parts. Check your work with the Answer Key in Appendix C.

1. _____

immune response caused by a bite from an infected deer tick; a rash (target lesion) may initially arise at the site of the tick bite

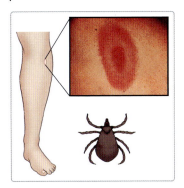

2. _____

common nerve entrapment disorder of the wrist caused by compression of the median nerve

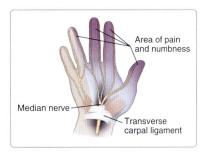

3. _____

broken bone

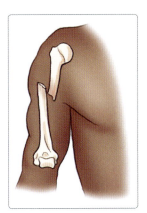

4. _____

disease in which an excessive amount of uric acid in the blood causes sodium urate crystals to be deposited in the joints

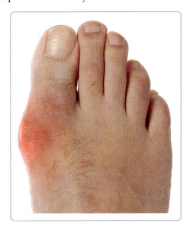

5. _____

disease caused by abnormal loss of bone density that may lead to an increase in fractures

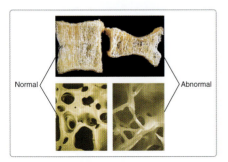

6. _____

rupture of the intervertebral disk cartilage, which allows the contents to protrude through it, putting pressure on the spinal nerve roots

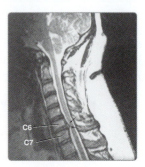

7. _____

narrowing of the spinal canal with compression of nerve roots.

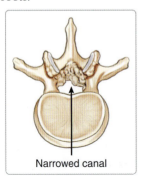

8. _____

inflammation of the connective tissue of the sole of the foot, common cause of heel pain

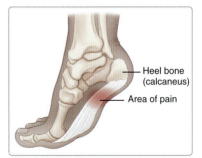

9. _____

diagnostic imaging test producing scans that give information about the body's anatomy and function by using radioactive material.

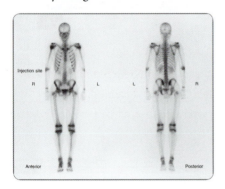

10. _____

diagnostic imaging test producing scans that give information about the body's anatomy by placing the patient in a strong magnetic field

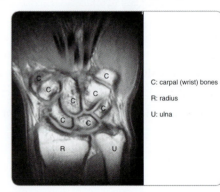

11. _____

chronic systemic disease characterized by autoimmune inflammatory changes in the connective tissue throughout the body

---

EXERCISE F   Learn Medical Terms NOT Built from Word Parts

Fill in the blanks with medical terms defined in bold using the Medical Terms NOT Built from Word Parts table. Answers are listed in Appendix C.

1. _____ is the branch of medicine dealing with the **study and treatment of diseases and abnormalities of the musculoskeletal system**. A **physician who specializes in the study and treatment of diseases and abnormalities of the musculoskeletal system** is called a(n) _____. This term was devised in 1740 and comes from *orthos* meaning straight, and *ped*, meaning children, and literally means to straighten children. At that time rickets, osteomyelitis, tuberculosis, and poliomyelitis were the main orthopedic problems, often resulting in deformities. Correcting these deformities by straightening or aligning bones was common. Today, an orthopedist may be required to repair a **broken bone,** or _____, fix a **rupture of the intervertebral disk cartilage,** or _____, or treat a patient with **narrowing of the spinal canal with compression of nerve roots**, or _____.

2. A rheumatologist may see a person with swelling, pain, and stiffness in a joint and request a blood test to diagnose a **chronic systemic disease characterized by autoimmune inflammatory changes in the connective tissue**, or _____.

3. _____, a **disease in which an excessive amount of uric acid in the blood causes sodium urate crystals to be deposited in the joints**, generally affects the great toe, but may also affect joints in the feet, ankles, wrists, and hands. The sharp sodium urate crystals cause inflammation and pain as they collect in the joints. Risk factors include diets high in red meat or seafood, excessive alcohol use, certain medications, and genetic predisposition.

4. Usually diagnosed in children by the age of 5 years, a **group of hereditary diseases characterized by degeneration of muscle and weakness,** or _____, is characterized by the replacement of muscle tissue with fat and scar tissue.

5. **Common nerve entrapment disorder of the wrist caused by compression of the median nerve,** or _____, can be caused by many factors, including repetitive work stress, traumatic injuries such as fractures or sprains, or arthritis in the wrist joint. Another condition that may be caused by repetitive stress, **inflammation of the connective tissue of the sole of the foot,** or _____, may occur in runners due to repeated stretching and small tears. Treatment may involve rest, ice packs, therapeutic exercises, massage, anti-inflammatory or steroidal medications, or surgery.

6. Utilized in the diagnosis of many musculoskeletal disorders, **diagnostic imaging test producing scans that give information about the body's anatomy by placing the patient in a strong magnetic field,** or _____, is an excellent radiographic tool aiding in the diagnosis of a multitude of conditions. Highly detailed, cross-sectional images of soft tissue are produced.

7. To generate images using **diagnostic imaging test producing scans that give information about the body's anatomy and function by using radioactive material,** or _____, the patient is first injected with intravenous low-dose radioactive tracer. As body tissues absorb the tracer, images are recorded with a special camera. This diagnostic procedure is especially helpful in evaluating musculoskeletal disorders such as bone tumors, fractures, and arthritis.

8. With increased prevalence in the aging population, this **disease caused by abnormal loss of bone density occurring predominantly in postmenopausal women,** or _____, can cause kyphosis of the spine and increased risk for fractures. Diets high in calcium and vitamin D and use of weight-bearing exercise over a lifetime can help prevent this debilitating chronic disease.

9. **A protrusion of an organ or structure through an abnormal opening,** or _____, often occurs within the abdominal cavity. Common types include inguinal, which occur near the groin, umbilical, which are around the umbilicus (belly button), and hiatal, in which a portion of the stomach pushes up through the diaphragm.

10. **System of treatment that consists of manipulation of the vertebral column,** or _____, is a health care profession that focuses on the relationship between the body's structure and its functioning. In North America, it is often considered a complementary health approach.

11. **Immune response caused by a bite from a deer tick infected with _Borrelia burgdorferi_,** or _____, may have symptoms similar to a number of other musculoskeletal diseases, including rheumatoid arthritis, gout, and ankylosing spondylitis. A two step process for diagnosing this disease is currently recommended to prevent misdiagnosis and improper treatment.

EXERCISE G | **Pronounce and Spell Terms NOT Built from Word Parts**

Practice pronunciation and spelling on paper and online.

1. **Practice on Paper**
   a. **Pronounce**: Read the phonetic spelling and say aloud the terms listed in the previous table of Terms NOT Built from Word Parts.
   b. **Spell**: Have a study partner read the terms aloud. Write the spelling of the terms on a separate sheet of paper.

2. **Practice Online** 🌐
   a. **Access** online learning resources. Go to evolve.elsevier.com > Evolve Resources > Practice Student Resources.
   b. **Pronounce**: Select Audio Glossary > Lesson 10 > Exercise G. Select a term to hear its pronunciation and repeat aloud.
   c. **Spell**: Select Activities > Lesson 10 > Spell Terms > Exercise G. Select the audio icon and type the correct spelling of the term.

❏ Check the box when complete.

OBJECTIVE 3

Write abbreviations.

ABBREVIATIONS RELATED TO THE MUSCULOSKELETAL SYSTEM

Use the online **flashcards** to familiarize yourself with the following abbreviations.

ABBREVIATION	TERM	ABBREVIATION	TERM
C1-C7	cervical vertebrae	NM	nuclear medicine
CTS	carpal tunnel syndrome	OA	osteoarthritis
DC	doctor of chiropractic	ortho	orthopedics
DO	doctor of osteopathy	OT	occupational therapy
EMG	electromyogram	PT	physical therapy
Fx	fracture	RA	rheumatoid arthritis
L1-L5	lumbar vertebrae	ROM	range of motion
MD	muscular dystrophy	T1-T12	thoracic vertebrae
MR	magnetic resonance	THA	total hip arthroplasty
MRI	magnetic resonance imaging	TKA	total knee arthroplasty

FYI The abbreviations **MR** and **MRI** are used interchangeably.

EXERCISE H Abbreviate Medical Terms

Write the correct abbreviation next to its medical term.

1. Diseases and Disorders:

 a. _____   carpal tunnel syndrome

 b. _____   fracture

 c. _____   muscular dystrophy

 d. _____   osteoarthritis

 e. _____   rheumatoid arthritis

2. Diagnostic Tests and Equipment:

 a. _____   electromyogram

 b. _____   magnetic resonance

 c. _____   magnetic resonance imaging

 d. _____   nuclear medicine

3. Surgical Procedures:

 a. _____   total knee arthroplasty

 b. _____   total hip arthroplasty

4. Specialties and Professions:

 a. _____   orthopedics

 b. _____   physical therapy

 c. _____   doctor of osteopathy

 d. _____   occupational therapy

 e. _____   doctor of chiropractic

5. Related Terms:

 a. _____   cervical vertebrae

 b. _____   lumbar vertebrae

 c. _____   thoracic vertebrae

 d. _____   range of motion

OBJECTIVE 4

Identify medical terms by clinical category.

Now that you have worked through the musculoskeletal system lesson, review and practice medical terms grouped by clinical category. Categories include signs and symptoms, diseases and disorders, diagnostic tests and equipment, surgical procedures, specialties and professions, and other terms related to the musculoskeletal system. Check your responses with the Answer Key in Appendix C.

EXERCISE I Signs and Symptoms

Write the medical terms for signs and symptoms next to their definitions.

1. _____   pain in the joint

2. _____   without development (process of wasting away)

3. _____   slow movement

4. _____   painful movement

5. _____   abnormal development

6. _____   excessive development

7. _____   muscle pain

8. _____   muscle weakness

9. _____   protrusion of an organ or structure through an abnormal
                                      opening

EXERCISE J   Diseases and Disorders

Write the medical terms for diseases and disorders next to their definitions.

1. _____   inflammation of the joint(s)

2. _____   inflammation of the connective tissue of the sole of the foot

3. _____   inflammation of the bursa

4. _____   common nerve entrapment disorder of the wrist caused by
                                      compression of the median nerve

5. _____   inflammation of cartilage

6. _____   softening of cartilage

7. _____   softening of the skull

8. _____   fissure of the skull

9. _____   broken bone

10. _____ disease in which an excessive amount of uric acid in the
                                      blood causes sodium urate crystals to be deposited in the
                                      joints, especially that of the great toe, producing arthritis

11. _____ rupture of the intervertebral disk cartilage, which allows the
                                      contents to protrude through it, putting pressure on the
                                      spinal nerve roots

12. _____ abnormal condition of a hump (thoracic spine)

13. _____ abnormal condition of bent forward (lumbar spine)

14. _____ group of hereditary diseases characterized by degeneration
                                      of muscle and weakness

15. _____ abnormal condition of death

16. _____ inflammation of the bone(s) and the joint(s)

17. _____ inflammation of the bone and cartilage

18. _____ softening of the bone

19. _____ abnormal condition of death of the bone (tissue)

20. _____ disease of the bone

21. _____ abnormal reduction of bone mass

22. _____   disease caused by abnormal loss of bone density occurring predominantly in postmenopausal women, which can lead to an increase in fractures of the ribs, thoracic and lumbar vertebrae, hips, and wrists

23. _____   tumor of the bone and the connective tissue

24. _____   fissure of the vertebral column

25. _____   chronic systemic disease characterized by autoimmune inflammatory changes in the connective tissue throughout the body

26. _____   abnormal condition of crooked, curved (spine)

27. _____   inflammation of the vertebral joints

28. _____   inflammation of the tendon(s)

29. _____   narrowing of the spinal canal with compression of nerve roots

30. _____   immune response caused by a bite from a deer tick infected with *Borrelia burgdorferi*; causes symptoms including fever, headache, and joint pain, and mimics other musculoskeletal diseases

EXERCISE K   Diagnostic Tests and Equipment

Write the medical terms for diagnostic tests and equipment next to their definitions.

1. _____   radiographic image of a joint

2. _____   pertaining to visual examination of a joint

3. _____   visual examination of a joint

4. _____   record of the electrical activity of a muscle

5. _____   diagnostic imaging test producing scans that give information about the body's anatomy by placing the patient in a strong magnetic field

6. _____   diagnostic imaging test producing scans that give information about the body's anatomy by using radioactive material

EXERCISE L   Surgical Procedures

Write the medical terms for surgical procedures next to their definitions.

1. _____   surgical puncture of a joint to remove fluid

2. _____   surgical fixation (fusion) of a joint

3. _____   surgical repair of a joint

4. _____   excision of a bursa

5. _____   incision into a bursa

6. _____   excision of a wrist (bone)

7. _____   excision of cartilage

8. _____   incision into the skull

9. _____   excision of a phalanx (any bone of the fingers or toes)

10. _____   incision into the vertebral column

11. _____   surgical fixation (fusion) of a tendon

12. _____   surgical repair of a tendon

13. _____   excision of a vertebra

14. _____   surgical repair of a vertebra

EXERCISE M   **Specialties and Professions**

Write the medical terms for specialties and professions next to their definitions.

1. _____   study and treatment of diseases and abnormalities of the musculoskeletal system

2. _____   physician who specializes in the study and treatment of diseases and abnormalities of the musculoskeletal system

3. _____   system of treatment that consists of manipulation of the vertebral column

---

EXERCISE N   **Medical Terms Related to the Musculoskeletal System**

Write the medical terms related to the musculoskeletal system next to their definitions.

1. _____   pertaining to the wrist

2. _____   pertaining to the ribs and cartilage

3. _____   pertaining to the femur

4. _____   pertaining to excessive development

5. _____   pertaining to the ilium

6. _____   pertaining to the ilium and the femur

7. _____   pertaining to between the ribs

8. _____   pertaining to between the vertebra(e)

9. _____   pertaining to within the skull

10. _____   pertaining to the ischium

11. _____   pertaining to the ischium and the pubis

12. _____   pertaining to a phalanx (any bone of the fingers or toes)

13. _____   pertaining to the sternum

14. _____   pertaining to the sternum and the ribs

15. _____   pertaining to below the ribs

16. _____   pertaining to the vertebrae

OBJECTIVE 5

Use medical language in clinical statements, the case study, and a medical record.

EXERCISE O   Use Medical Terms in Clinical Statements

Circle the medical terms and abbreviations defined in the bolded phrases. Answers are listed in Appendix C. For pronunciation practice, read the answers aloud.

1. Carmen McCroskey is experiencing pain in her ankle caused by traumatic **inflammation of the joint(s)** (arthralgia, arthritis, osteoarthritis) resulting from a **broken bone** (herniated disk, gout, fracture) several years ago. Her orthopedic surgeon will perform a triple **surgical fixation (fusion) of a joint** (arthrodesis, arthrogram, arthrocentesis) in an attempt to reduce the pain in the area.

2. If **radiographic image of a joint** (arthroscopy, arthrocentesis, arthrogram) findings indicate that surgery is needed, a(n) **visual examination of a joint** (arthroscopy, arthrocentesis, arthrodesis), may be performed to repair ligaments, fix a torn meniscus, or address other minor injuries. Common types of **pertaining to visual examination of a joint** (arthroplasty, arthroscopic, arthralgia) surgery include rotator cuff repair of the shoulder and meniscus repair of the knee.

3. Total hip replacement and total knee **surgical repair of a joint** (arthroscopy, arthrodesis, arthroplasty) are common orthopedic procedures. Various prostheses are used to rebuild joints that have been damaged by trauma or, more commonly, **inflammation of the bone(s) and the joint(s)** (osteochondritis, osteoarthritis, osteopathy).

4. During her lifetime, Abigail Carpenter experienced multiple changes to the curvature of her vertebral column. During elementary school, she was diagnosed with mild **abnormal condition of crooked, curved spine** (scoliosis, spondylarthritis, muscular dystrophy). While pregnant with twins, as her spine adjusted to the extra weight, she had prominent **abnormal condition of bent forward (lumbar spine)** (lordosis, rachischisis, scoliosis). After menopause, she lost two inches of height as she developed **abnormal condition of a hump (thoracic spine)** (scoliosis, kyphosis, hernia) due to **disease caused by abnormal loss of bone density** (muscular dystrophy, osteosarcoma, osteoporosis).

5. To assist in determining the patient's diagnosis of **a group of hereditary diseases characterized by degeneration of muscle and weakness** (myasthenia, rheumatoid arthritis, muscular dystrophy), the physician ordered a(n) **record of the electrical activity of a muscle** (arthroscopy, electromyogram, rachiotomy).

6. While playing soccer, Eli Kleinman experienced pain above the posterior aspect of his heel and could not continue playing. The **physician who specializes in the study and treatment of diseases and abnormalities of the musculoskeletal system** (chiropractic orthopedist, pulmonologist) told Eli's mother that he strained his Achilles tendon, causing **inflammation of his tendon** (tendinitis, bursitis, chondritis). The orthopedist prescribed analgesics and cautioned against physical activity to avoid the risk of a tendon rupture, which might require **surgical repair of a tendon** (arthroplasty, vertebroplasty, tenoplasty).

7. **Inflammation of a bursa** (Osteoarthritis, Chondritis, Bursitis) may be precipitated by **inflammation of the joint(s)** (bursitis, tendonitis, arthritis). The chief symptom is severe pain. In chronic cases a(n) **incision into a bursa** (rachiotomy, bursotomy, vertebrectomy) to remove calcium deposits may be required.

8. **Softening of cartilage** (Craniomalacia, Osteomalacia, Chondromalacia) of the patella (knee cap) may occur after a knee injury. It is characterized by swelling, pain, and degenerative changes. **Softening of the bone** (Craniomalacia, Osteomalacia, Chondromalacia) results from many diseases. It is caused by an inadequate amount of phosphorus and calcium in the blood, resulting in impaired mineralization of the bone.

9. **Excessive development** (Atrophy, Dystrophy, Hypertrophy) occurs when muscles are overdeveloped, which may result from weightlifting. Loss of muscle mass, **without development,** (atrophy, dystrophy, hypertrophy) occurs when muscles are not used, which may result from disability or a sedentary lifestyle.

10. George Robenowski was seen in the **system of treatment that consists of manipulation of the vertebral column** (chiropractic, orthopedic, physical therapy) clinic for chronic back pain; he was later referred to an orthopedist for his **narrowing of the spinal canal with compression of nerve roots** (plantar fasciitis, Lyme disease, spinal stenosis).

11. Medical terms are often used to indicate areas of the body when describing pain or observations. For example, the physician may write the following terms:
    - **pertaining to within the skull** (intracranial, intervertebral, intravascular) bleeding
    - **pertaining to between the ribs** (costochondral, sternocostal, intercostal) muscles
    - discomfort in the **pertaining to below the ribs** (subcostal, subdural, subxiphoid) region
    - **pertaining to the ischium and the pubis** (ischial, iliofemoral, ischiopubic) bruising
    - a lesion noted over the left **pertaining to the ilium** (iliac, ileal, ischial) region
    - pain in the left **pertaining to the sternum and the ribs** (costochondral, sternocostal, intercostal) region
    - stiffness in the **pertaining to the vertebra(e)** (vertebral, intervertebral, phalangeal) column
    - **pertaining to the femur** (femoral, carpal, ischial) artery occlusion
    - **pertaining to the sternum** (vertebral, sternal, intercostal) incision

---

EXERCISE P **Apply Medical Terms to the Case Study**

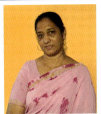

Think back to Shanti Mehra who was introduced in the case study at the beginning of the lesson. After working through Lesson 10 on the musculoskeletal system, consider the medical terms that might be used to describe her experience. List two terms relevant to the case study and their meanings. ▪

Medical Term	Definition
1.	
2.	

EXERCISE Q   Use Medical Terms in a Document

Mrs. Mehra went to the Emergency Department. After a nurse took her vital signs, an emergency physician examined her and ordered an x-ray [radiograph]. A radiologist reviewed the results. She was then given medication for pain and referred to an orthopedist. This visit is documented in the medical record below.

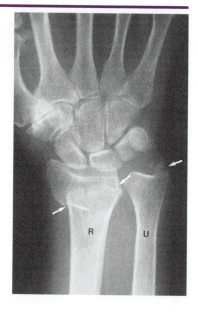

Use the definitions in numbers 1-9 to write medical terms within the document.

1. study and treatment of diseases and abnormalities of the musculoskeletal system

2. broken bone

3. muscle pain

4. abnormal condition of hump (thoracic spine)

5. pertaining to the vertebra(e)

6. pertaining to the ilium

7. pertaining to the wrist

8. pertaining to a phalanx

9. disease caused by abnormal loss of bone density occurring predominantly in postmenopausal women

Refer to the medical record to answer questions 10-13

10. In the physical examination section of the medical document, there are many anatomic terms that deal with parts of the body. For example, **iliac** means "pertaining to the ilium" and **carpal** means "pertaining to the wrist bones." Write the terms referring to the bones in the forearm that mean "pertaining to the radius" and "pertaining to the ulna." (Hint: the suffix "**ar**" is another word part meaning "pertaining to.")

   a. _____/_____
      wr   s

   b. _____/_____
      wr   s

11. The iliac crests are the curved superior portions of the ilium. When you put your hands on your hips, they are on the tops of the iliac crests. Try to find the iliac crests on yourself and on the diagram on Figure 10.10.

12. A contusion is an injury with no break in the skin, characterized by pain, swelling, and discoloration. Name a more common term for contusion: _____.

13. Identify two new medical terms in the medical record you would like to investigate. Use your medical dictionary or an online resource to look up the definition.

Medical Term	Definition
1. _____	_____
2. _____	_____

```
011107 MEHRA, Shanti                                                              _ □ X
File    Patient    Navigate    Custom Fields    Help

 <  >  👤  👥  🔲  🔲  📄  🏠  Rx  🕐  ⊘  ✂  📄  📇  ▦  ✓  🌐  🔍  ❓

Chart Review   Encounters   Notes   Labs   Imaging   Procedures   Rx   Documents   Referrals   Scheduling   Billing

Name: MEHRA, Shanti          MR#: 011107        Gender: F      │ Allergies: Codeine
                             DOB: 10/17/19XX     Age: 67       │ PCP: Kimbrell, Howard DO
```

Clinical Note
Encounter Date: 04/02/20XX

History: This 67-year-old woman is seen for a follow-up visit in (1.) _____.
She presented one week ago in the emergency department for treatment of a
(2.)_____ of the right wrist, with an accompanying right ulnar fracture.
She also experienced (3.) _____ and pain in her right hip. The patient
is postmenopausal with a history of cigarette smoking.

Physical Examination: The patient is 5'5" tall and weighs 117 lbs. She has prominent
dorsal (4.) _____ in the thoracic (5.) _____ column.
The examination of the right forearm and hand reveals normal color with minimal swelling.
She has contusions over the right (6.) _____ crest. AP and lateral
radiographs of the right wrist and hand reveal healing distal, radial and ulnar fractures.
There are no (7.) _____, metacarpal, or (8.) _____
abnormalities noted.

Diagnostic Studies: A DEXA scan assessing bone-mineral density shows evidence of
(9.) _____.

Impression: Healing right distal radial and ulnar fractures and osteoporosis.

Recommendation: The patient was advised to continue immobilization of the right forearm
for another three weeks. Calcium and vitamin D therapy were recommended. Smoking
cessation was strongly encouraged. Alendronate was prescribed as treatment for her
osteoporosis. A follow-up visit is scheduled in three weeks.

Electronically signed: Maxwell S. Kline, MD 04/02/20XX 16:30

```
 Start   Log On/Off   Print   Edit
```

EXERCISE R   **Use Medical Language in Electronic Health Records Online**

Select the correct medical terms to complete three medical records in one patient's electronic file.

🌐 Access online resources at evolve.elsevier.com > Evolve Resources > Practice Student Resources > Activities >
Lesson 10 > Electronic Health Records

Topic: Fracture Right Arm
Record 1: Admission Note
Record 2: Radiology Report
Record 3: Neurology Consultation

❏   Check the box when complete.

OBJECTIVE 6

Recall and assess knowledge of word parts, medical terms, and abbreviations.

EXERCISE S **Online Review of Lesson Content**

🌐 *Recall and assess your learning from working through the lesson by completing online learning activities. at evolveelsevier.com > Evolve Resources > Practice Student Resources. Keep track of your progress by placing a check mark next to completed activities.*

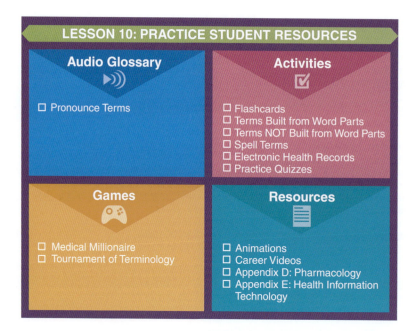

EXERCISE T **Lesson Content Quiz**

Test your knowledge of the terms and abbreviations introduced in this lesson. Circle the letter for the medical term or abbreviation related to the words in italics.

1. Sometimes, people with *immune response caused by a bite from a deer tick infected with Borrelia burgdorferi* do not have any memory of a tick bite or rash.
   a. rheumatoid arthritis
   b. Lyme disease
   c. chondritis

2. Orthopedists may perform *visual examination of a joint* to diagnose and sometimes treat problems in the knee, shoulder, or elbow.
   a. arthroscopy
   b. arthrogram
   c. arthrocentesis

3. A total hip *surgical repair of a joint* may be necessary in patients with severe osteoarthritis, if other measures are no longer effective.
   a. arthrodesis
   b. arthroplasty
   c. chondroplasty

4. The causes of *abnormal condition of bone death* are not always clear, but some known factors include steroid medications, alcohol use, previous injury, and increased pressure inside the bone.
   a. osteomalacia
   b. osteosarcoma
   c. osteonecrosis

5. Injuries from an automobile accident may result in *pertaining to the ribs and cartilage* pain.
   a. costochondral
   b. subcostal
   c. intercostal

6. Symptoms of Parkinson disease may include tremors, *slow movement* and dementia.
   a. dyskinesia
   b. bradykinesia
   c. hypertrophy

7. *Abnormal condition of crooked, curved (spine)* is more common in girls and is usually graded in terms of mild, moderate, or severe; braces or surgery may be recommended in some cases.
   a. lordosis
   b. kyphosis
   c. scoliosis

8. In patients with long standing diabetes mellitus, poor circulation may result in osteonecrosis of the toe, and may require *excision of any bone of the fingers or toes.*
   a. bursectomy
   b. phalangectomy
   c. condrectomy

9. If a herniated disk is suspected, a(n) *diagnostic imaging test producing scans that gives information about the body's anatomy by placing the patient in a strong magnetic field* may aid in the diagnosis.
   a. MRI
   b. NM
   c. EMG

10. In mild to moderate cases of *common nerve entrapment disorder of the wrist caused by compression of the median nerve*, the use of wrist splints at night can be very helpful.
    a. plantar fasciitis
    b. rheumatoid arthritis
    c. carpal tunnel syndrome

LESSON AT A GLANCE   **MUSCULOSKELETAL SYSTEM WORD PARTS**

COMBINING FORMS

arthr/o	necr/o
burs/o	oste/o
carp/o	phalang/o
chondr/o	pub/o
cost/o	rachi/o
crani/o	scoli/o
femor/o	spondyl/o
ili/o	stern/o
ischi/o	ten/o, tendin/o
kinesi/o	troph/o
kyph/o	vertebr/o
lord/o	

SUFFIXES

-asthenia
-desis
-malacia
-schisis

PREFIX

inter-

SIGNS AND SYMPTOMS
arthralgia
atrophy
bradykinesia
dyskinesia
dystrophy
hernia
hypertrophy
myalgia
myasthenia

DISEASES AND DISORDERS
arthritis
bursitis
carpal tunnel syndrome (CTS)
chondritis
chondromalacia
craniomalacia
cranioschisis
fracture (Fx)
gout
herniated disk
kyphosis
lordosis
Lyme disease
muscular dystrophy (MD)
necrosis
osteoarthritis (OA)
osteochondritis
osteomalacia
osteonecrosis
osteopathy
osteopenia
osteoporosis

osteosarcoma
plantar fasciitis
rachischisis
rheumatoid arthritis (RA)
scoliosis
spinal stenosis
spondylarthritis
tendinitis

DIAGNOSTIC TESTS AND EQUIPMENT
arthrogram
arthroscopic
arthroscopy
electromyogram (EMG)
magnetic resonance imaging (MRI)
nuclear medicine (NM)

SURGICAL PROCEDURES
arthrocentesis
arthrodesis
arthroplasty
bursectomy
bursotomy
carpectomy
chondrectomy
craniotomy
phalangectomy
rachiotomy
tenodesis
tenoplasty
vertebrectomy
vertebroplasty

RELATED TERMS
carpal
costochondral
femoral
hypertrophic
iliac
iliofemoral
intercostal
intervertebral
intracranial
ischial
ischiopubic
phalangeal
sternal
sternocostal
subcostal
vertebral

SPECIALTIES AND PROFESSIONS
chiropractic
orthopedics (ortho)
orthopedist

ABBREVIATIONS
C1–C7	MD	PT
CTS	MR	RA
DC	MRI	ROM
DO	NM	T1–T12
EMG	OA	THA
Fx	ortho	TKA
L1–L5	OT	

Koji Kaneshiro

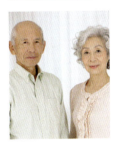

Kazuno Kaneshiro is worried about her husband, Koji. He was eating breakfast with her when he suddenly stopped speaking and dropped his spoon onto the table. "He never does that!" she thought. He wasn't making any sense, though he was definitely trying to say something. Also, his right arm was hanging limply by his side. She noticed that the left side of his face was also droopy. She had seen a billboard about strokes and was afraid he might be having one. She remembered the billboard saying that every minute counts so she called 911 immediately.

■ *Consider Koji's situation as you work through the lesson on the nervous system and behavioral health. At the end of the lesson, we will return to this case study and identify medical terms used to document Koji's experience and the care he receives.*

OBJECTIVES

1 ■ Build, translate, pronounce, and spell medical terms built from word parts (p. 332).

2 ■ Define, pronounce, and spell medical terms NOT built from word parts (p. 345).

3 ■ Write abbreviations (p. 352).

4 ■ Identify medical terms by clinical category (p. 353).

5 ■ Use medical language in clinical statements, the case study, and a medical record (p. 356).

6 ■ Recall and assess knowledge of word parts, medical terms, and abbreviations (p. 360).

INTRODUCTION TO THE NERVOUS SYSTEM

Anatomic Structures of the Nervous System

brain (brān)	central organ of the nervous system contained within the cranium that coordinates body activities and processes sensory information transmitted through nerves. Sections of the brain include the cerebellum, the cerebrum, and the brainstem.
brainstem (BRĀN-stem)	stemlike portion of the brain that connects with the spinal cord; contains centers that control respiration and heart rate. Three structures comprise the brainstem: midbrain, pons, and medulla oblongata.
central nervous system (CNS) (SEN-trel) (NUR-vus) (SIS-tum)	brain and spinal cord (Figures 11.1 and 11.3)
cerebellum (ser-a-BEL-um)	located under the posterior portion of the cerebrum; assists in the coordination of skeletal muscles to maintain balance
cerebrospinal fluid (CSF) (ser-ē-brō-SPĪ-nel) (FLOO-id)	clear, colorless fluid contained in ventricles; cushions brain and spinal cord from shock, transports nutrients, and clears metabolic waste

Anatomic Structures of the Nervous System—cont'd

cerebrum (se-RĒ-brum)	largest portion of the brain; divided into left and right hemispheres
meninges (me-NIN-jēz)	three layers of membranes that cover the brain and spinal cord. The dura mater is the tough outer layer, the arachnoid is the delicate, weblike, middle layer, and the pia mater is the thin, inner layer of the meninges.
nerve (nurv)	cordlike structure made up of fibers that carries impulses from one part of the body to another
peripheral nervous system (PNS) (puh-RIF-er-ul) (NUR-vus) (SIS-tum)	system of nerves extending from the brain and spinal cord (Figure 11.1)
spinal cord (SPĪ-nel) (kord)	tubelike bundle of nerve tissue extending from the brainstem to the lower portion of the spine; conducts nerve impulses to and from the brain
ventricles (VEN-tri-kuls)	spaces within the brain that contain cerebrospinal fluid

Functions of the Nervous System

- Control and integration of body functions
- Communication
- Mental activity, thought, and memory

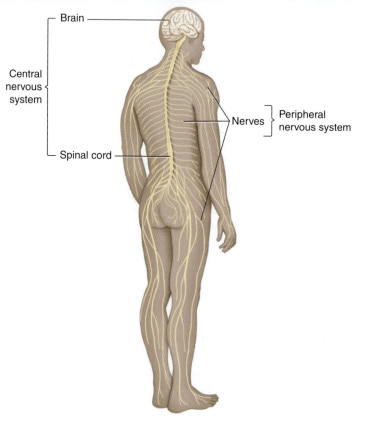

Figure 11.1 Nervous system.

How the Nervous System Works

The **brain, spinal cord,** and **nerves** form a complex communication system allowing for the coordination of body functions and activities. As a whole, the nervous system is designed to detect changes inside and outside the body, to evaluate this sensory information, and to send directions to muscles or glands in response. The nervous system may be divided into two parts: the **central nervous system** (CNS) and the **peripheral nervous system** (PNS) (Figure 11.1). The central nervous system, the **brain** and **spinal cord,** receives and processes sensory information and formulates outgoing responses. The largest portion of the brain, the **cerebrum,** controls skeletal muscles, contains centers for sight and hearing, and provides for mental activities such as thought, memory, and emotional reactions. The brain and spinal cord are covered by a three-layered membrane called the **meninges.** Further protection is provided by bone, the skull, and the spine. The peripheral nervous system forms a complex network of nerves extending from the brain and spinal cord. It carries sensory messages to the central nervous system and delivers responding messages to muscles and glands.

> **FYI**   The **meninges** are made up of three layers called the **dura mater,** the **arachnoid,** and the **pia mater.** Dura mater and pia mater were first named by a Persian physician in the tenth century. Dura mater, the outer tough layer, means tough mother. Pia mater, the delicate inner layer, means soft mother. The arachnoid resembles a spider web. Arachnida is the scientific name for spiders and is derived from Greek mythology.

Aspects of Behavioral Health

The terms "behavioral health" and "mental health" are closely related. Generally, these terms refer to our emotional, psychological, and social well-being. It reflects how we think, feel, and act. It has an impact on how we handle stress, make choices, and relate to the world around us. Behavioral health is part of an integrated approach to care of the patient as a whole. This lesson will serve as an introduction to a few common behavioral health terms.

CAREER FOCUS   **Professionals Who Work with the Nervous System and in Behavioral Health**

- **Speech-Language Pathology Aides** assist with screening exams and implementation of treatment plans addressing communication and swallowing disorders. They work closely with patients and are supervised by Speech-Language Pathologists.

- **Neurodiagnostic Technicians** use special equipment to monitor how well a patient's nervous system is working (Figure 11.2). These include electroencephalograms (EEGs), polysomnograms (sleep studies), and nerve conduction studies.

- **Psychiatric Aides** work under the direction of nurses and doctors to help mentally impaired or emotionally disturbed patients. They may assist with daily living activities, lead patients in educational and recreational activities, or accompany them to and from examinations and treatments.

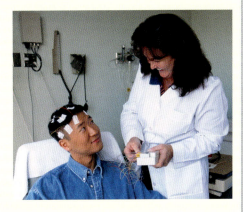

Figure 11.2 A neurodiagnostic technician performs an EEG on a patient.

 FOR MORE INFORMATION

- Access online resources at evolve.elsevier.com > Practice Student Resources > Other Resources > Career Videos to watch interviews with a **Neurodiagnostic Technologist** and a **Psychiatric Technician**.

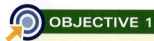

OBJECTIVE 1

Build, translate, pronounce, and spell medical terms built from word parts.

WORD PARTS Use the paper or online **flashcards** to familiarize yourself with the following word parts.

COMBINING FORM (WR + CV)	DEFINITION	COMBINING FORM (WR + CV)	DEFINITION
cerebr/o	cerebrum, brain	pleg/o	paralysis
encephal/o	brain	poli/o	gray matter
mening/o, meningi/o	meninges	psych/o	mind
myel/o	spinal cord	quadr/i	four (*Note: the combining form is an **i**.*)
phas/o	speech		

SUFFIX	DEFINITION
-us	no meaning

PREFIX	DEFINITION	PREFIX (P)	DEFINITION
hemi-	half	micro-	small

WORD PARTS PRESENTED IN PREVIOUS LESSONS   Used to Build Nervous System and Behavioral Health Terms

COMBINING FORM (WR + CV)	DEFINITION	COMBINING FORM (WR + CV)	DEFINITION
angi/o	blood vessel(s)	my/o	muscle(s), muscle tissue
arthr/o	joint(s)	neur/o	nerve(s), nerve tissue
cephal/o	head (upward)	path/o	disease
electr/o	electrical activity	thromb/o	blood clot
hydr/o	water		

SUFFIX	DEFINITION	SUFFIX (S)	DEFINITION
-al, -ic	pertaining to	-ia	diseased state, condition of
-algia	pain	-itis	inflammation
-cele	hernia, protrusion	-logist	one who studies and treats (specialist, physician)
-genic	producing, originating, causing	-logy	study of
-gram	record, radiographic image	-oma	tumor
-graph	instrument used to record	-osis	abnormal condition
-graphy	process of recording, radiographic imaging	-y	no meaning

PREFIX (P)	DEFINITION	PREFIX (P)	DEFINITION
a-	absence of, without	poly-	many, much
dys-	difficult, painful, abnormal		

Refer to Appendix A, Word Parts Used in *Basic Medical Language*, for alphabetical lists of word parts and their meanings.

EXERCISE A   Build and Translate Medical Terms Built from Word Parts

*Use the **Word Parts Tables** to complete the following questions. Check your responses with the Answer Key in Appendix C.*

1. **LABEL:** *Write the combining forms for anatomical structures of the nervous system on Figure 11.3. These anatomical combining forms will be used to build and translate medical terms in Exercise A.*

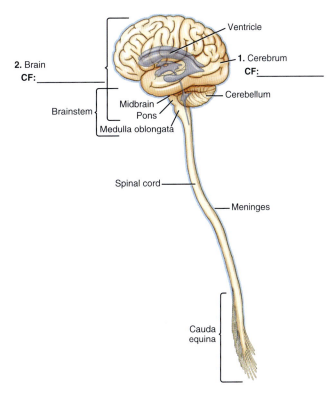

2. Brain
CF:_____

1. Cerebrum
CF:_____

Ventricle

Cerebellum

Brainstem

Midbrain
Pons
Medulla oblongata

Spinal cord

Meninges

Cauda equina

> **FYI** **Cauda equina**, horse's tail in Latin, refers to the bundle of nerves extending from the spinal cord near the end of the vertebral column.

Figure 11.3 The brain and spinal cord.

2. **MATCH:** *Draw a line to match the word part with its definition.*

   a. -al   blood clot
   b. angi/o   pertaining to
   c. -graphy   blood vessel(s)
   d. thromb/o   abnormal condition
   e. -osis   process of recording, radiographic imaging

3. **BUILD:** *Using the combining form **cerebr/o** and the word parts reviewed in the previous exercise, build the following terms related to the cerebrum. Remember, the definition usually starts with the meaning of the suffix.*

a. pertaining to the cerebrum

           _____/_____
                  wr   s

b. radiographic imaging of the blood vessels of the cerebrum

    cerebral _____/_o_/_____
                   wr   cv   s

c. abnormal condition of a blood clot in the cerebrum

    cerebral _____/_____
                   wr   s

4. **READ: Cerebral thrombosis** (se-RĒ-bral) (throm-BŌ-sis) is frequently caused by plaque formation or by an embolus (a blood clot or foreign material that enters the bloodstream and moves until it lodges at another point in the circulation). **Cerebral angiography** (se-RĒ-bral) (an-jē-OG-ra-fē) is an excellent test for diagnosing thrombosis and may also be used as therapy to break down the clot.

5. **LABEL:** *Write word parts to complete Figure 11.4.*

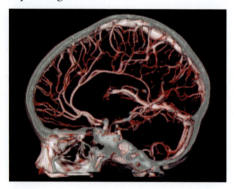

Figure 11.4 _____/_____   _____/o/_____ uses CT
            cerebrum   pertaining to   blood vessel   radiographic imaging
imaging to obtain images of the arterial and venous circulation.

6. **MATCH:** *Draw a line to match the word part with its definition.*

a. -itis   disease
b. -y   inflammation
c. path/o   no meaning

7. **BUILD:** *Using the combining form **encephal/o**, meaning brain, and the word parts reviewed in the matching exercise, build the following terms:*

a. disease of the brain

           _____/_o_/_____/y
                  wr   cv   wr   s

b. inflammation of the brain

           _____/_____
                  wr   s

8. **READ:** Viral infections are the most common causes of **encephalitis** (en-sef-a-LĪ-tis), which can sometimes be life-threatening. Fever, severe headache, or loss of consciousness are reasons to seek immediate medical care. The major symptom of **encephalopathy** (en-sef-a-LOP-a-thē) is an altered mental state. Frequent causes include infections, alcohol-related liver disease, kidney disease, trauma, and toxins.

9. **MATCH:** *Draw a line to match the word part with its definition.*

   a. electr/o   instrument used to record
   b. -graphy   electrical activity
   c. -graph   record, radiographic image
   d. -gram   process of recording, radiographic imaging

10. **TRANSLATE:** *Continue using the combining form **encephal/o** to complete the definitions of the following terms.*

   a. electr/o/encephal/o/gram   _____ of _____ activity of the brain
   b. electr/o/encephal/o/graph   _____used to record _____ _____of the brain
   c. electr/o/encephal/o/graphy   process of _____ the electrical activity of the _____

11. **READ:** An **electroencephalogram** (ē-lek-trō-en-SEF-a-lō-gram), abbreviated EEG, is a test that detects electrical activity in the brain using flat metal discs attached to the scalp (see Figure 11.2). The **electroencephalograph** (ē-lek-trō-en-SEF-a-lō-graf) detects electrical impulses that provide information about the activity of the brain cells. **Electroencephalography** (ē-lek-trō-en-sef-a-LOG-ra-fē) is very useful in diagnosing epilepsy (seizure disorder) and is also helpful in diagnosing sleep disorders.

> **FYI**   Compare **electroencephalogram** with **electromyogram** and **electrocardiogram**. Note that the combining form for the body part is the only difference between the words and therefore the meanings of each medical term.

12. **LABEL:** *Write word parts to complete Figure 11.5.*

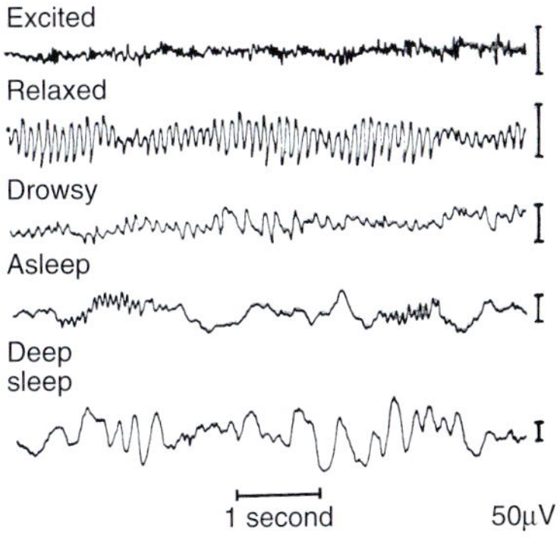

Excited

Relaxed

Drowsy

Asleep

Deep
sleep

1 second   50μV

Figure 11.5 Sample of recordings of different mental states obtained by

_____/o/_____/o/_____.

electrical activity   brain   process of recording

13. **MATCH:** *Draw a line to match the word part with its definition.*

    a. -al   pain
    b. -algia   pertaining to

14. **BUILD:** *Using the combining form* **neur/o**, *meaning nerve(s), and the word parts reviewed in the previous exercise, build the following terms.*

    a. pertaining to the nerve(s)   _____/_____
                                           wr   **s**

    b. pain in the nerve(s)   _____/_____
                                         wr   **s**

15. **READ:** The **neural** (NŪ-ral) foramen is an opening between the vertebrae; nerves leave the spine through these openings and extend to other parts of the body. Postherpetic **neuralgia** (nū-RAL-ja) can occur after shingles. This burning, stabbing, and sometimes very severe pain can occur anywhere on the body.

16. **LABEL:** *Write word parts to complete Figure 11.6.*

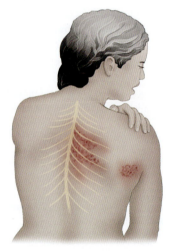

Figure 11.6 Postherpetic _____/_____
                         nerve(s)   pain
occurring on the right side of a patient's back.

17. **MATCH:** *Draw a line to match the word part with its definition.*

    a. -logist   no meaning
    b. -logy   one who studies and treats (specialist, physician)
    c. path/o   study of
    d. -y   disease

18. TRANSLATE: *complete the definitions of the following terms using the combining form **neur/o**.*

a. neur/o/logist   _____ who studies and treats diseases of the nervous system

b. neur/o/logy   study of the _____ (nervous system)

c. neur/o/path/y   _____ of the _____(nervous system)

19. READ: Diabetic peripheral **neuropathy** (nū-ROP-a-thē) usually occurs in patients who have had diabetes for at least two years. It causes decreased sensation in the feet and hands, and is often accompanied by pain. A **neurologist** (nū-ROL-o-jist) may perform special tests to determine the extent of the nerve damage. A **neurology** (nū-ROL-o-jē) consultation is especially important if the patient has developed sores or ulcers due to lack of sensation in the feet.

20. MATCH: *Draw a line to match the word part with its definition.*

a. -itis   joint(s)

b. -algia   nerve(s)

c. arthr/o   inflammation

d. my/o   muscle(s)

e. neur/o   pain

21. BUILD: *Use the prefix **poly-**, meaning many or much, and the word parts reviewed in the previous exercise to build the following terms.*

a. pain in many muscles   _____/_____/_____

                                              p   wr   s

b. inflammation of many joints   _____/_____/_____

                                              p   wr   s

c. inflammation of many nerves   _____/_____/_____

                                              p   wr   s

22. READ: **Polymyalgia** (pol-ē-mī-AL-ja) rheumatica, abbreviated PMR, is an inflammatory disorder that mainly affects adults over the age of 65. Patients complain of muscle pain and stiffness in the shoulders, neck, upper arms, and hips. Many types of **polyarthritis** (pol-ē-ar-THRĪ-tis) exist, including rheumatoid arthritis, lupus, viral arthritis, and gout. Guillain-Barré syndrome is a type of **polyneuritis** (pol-ē-nū-RĪ-tis), which causes rapid onset of numbness, weakness, and sometimes even paralysis of the legs, arms, breathing muscles, and face.

23. REVIEW OF NERVOUS SYSTEM AND BEHAVIORAL HEALTH TERMS BUILT FROM WORD PARTS: *The following is an alphabetical list of terms built and translated in the previous exercises.*

MEDICAL TERMS BUILT FROM WORD PARTS

TERM	DEFINITION	TERM	DEFINITION
1. **cerebral** (se-RĔ-bral)	pertaining to the cerebrum	9. **neural** (NŪ-ral)	pertaining to the nerve(s)
2. **cerebral angiography** (se-RĔ-bral) (an-jē-OG-ra-fē)	radiographic imaging of the blood vessels of the cerebrum (Figure 11.4)	10. **neuralgia** (nū-RAL-ja)	pain in the nerve(s) (Figure 11.6)
3. **cerebral thrombosis** (se-RĔ-bral) (throm-BŌ-sis)	abnormal condition of a blood clot in the cerebrum (Figure 11.11, *B*)	11. **neurologist** (nū-ROL-o-jist)	physician who studies and treats diseases of the nervous system
4. **electroencephalogram (EEG)** (ē-lek-trō-en-SEF-a-lō-gram)	record of electrical activity of the brain	12. **neurology** (nū-ROL-o-jē)	study of the nerves
5. **electroencephalograph** (ē-lek-trō-en-SEF-a-lō-graf)	instrument used to record electrical activity of the brain	13. **neuropathy** (nū-ROP-a-thē)	disease of the nerves
6. **electroencephalography** (ē-lek-trō-en-sef-a-LOG-ra-fē)	process of recording the electrical activity of the brain	14. **polyarthritis** (pol-ē-ar-THRĪ-tis)	inflammation of many joints
7. **encephalitis** (en-sef-a-LĪ-tis)	inflammation of the brain	15. **polymyalgia** (pol-ē-mī-AL-ja)	pain in many muscles
8. **encephalopathy** (en-sef-a-LOP-a-thē)	disease of the brain	16. **polyneuritis** (pol-ē-nū-RĪ-tis)	inflammation of many nerves

---

EXERCISE B   Pronounce and Spell Terms Built from Word Parts

Practice pronunciation and spelling on paper and online.

1. **Practice on Paper**
   a. **Pronounce:** Read the phonetic spelling and say aloud the terms listed in the previous table, Review Terms Built from Word Parts.
   b. **Spell:** Have a study partner read the terms aloud. Write the spelling of the terms on a separate sheet of paper.

2. **Practice Online** 🌐
   a. **Access** online learning resources. Go to evolve.elsevier.com > Evolve Resources > Practice Student Resources.
   b. **Pronounce:** Select Audio Glossary > Lesson 11 > Exercise B. Select a term to hear its pronunciation and repeat aloud.
   c. **Spell:** Select Activities > Lesson 11 > Spell Terms > Exercise B. Select the audio icon and type the correct spelling of the term.

❏ Check the box when complete.

EXERCISE C   **Build and Translate MORE Medical Terms Built from Word Parts**

*Use the **Word Parts Tables** to complete the following questions. Check your responses with the Answer Key in Appendix C.*

1. LABEL: *Write the combining forms for anatomical structures of the nervous system on Figure 11.7. These anatomical combining forms will be used to build and translate medical terms in Exercise C.*

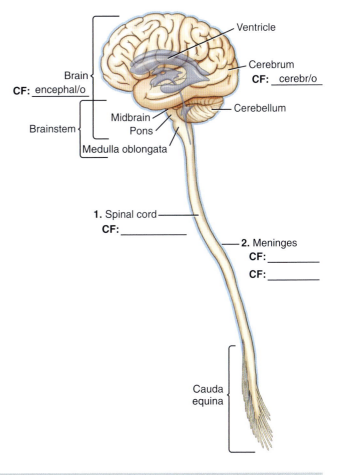

Ventricle

Cerebrum
CF: cerebr/o

Brain
CF: encephal/o

Cerebellum

Midbrain
Pons

Brainstem

Medulla oblongata

1. Spinal cord
CF: _____

2. Meninges
CF: _____
CF: _____

Cauda equina

Figure 11.7 The brain and spinal cord.

2. MATCH: *Draw a line to match the word part with its definition.*

a. -oma   hernia, protrusion
b. -itis   tumor
c. -cele   inflammation

3. BUILD: *Use the combining forms for meninges and the word parts reviewed in the previous exercise to build the following terms. Remember, the definition usually starts with the meaning of the suffix. Hint: use **mening/o** for a and b and **meningi/o** for c.*

a. hernia of the meninges   _____/ o /_____
                                          wr   cv   s

b. inflammation of the meninges _____/_____
                                          wr   s

c. tumor of the meninges   _____/_____
                                          wr   s

4. **READ:** Spina bifida occurs when the vertebral column doesn't close completely during development; this may result in a **meningocele** (me-NING-gō-sēl). A **meningioma** (me-nin-je-Ō-ma) is usually benign and slow growing, and occurs most often in the brains of older women. **Meningitis** (men-in-JĪ-tis) is usually caused by a bacterial or viral infection of the fluid surrounding the brain and spinal cord.

5. **LABEL:** Write word parts to complete Figure 11.8.

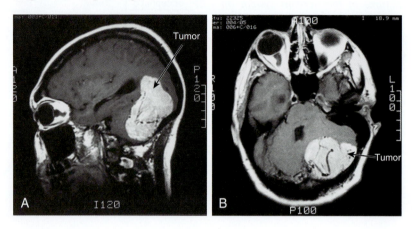

Figure 11.8 A large _____/_____ in a female patient.

meninges   tumor

6. **MATCH:** Draw a line to match the word part with its definition.

    a. -itis   gray matter
    b. poli/o   inflammation

7. **TRANSLATE:** Complete the definitions of the following terms using the combining form **myel/o**, meaning spinal cord. Use the meaning of the word parts to fill in the blanks. Remember, the definition usually starts with the meaning of the suffix.

    a. mening/o/myel/itis   _____ of the meninges and spinal cord
    b. poli/o/myel/itis   inflammation of the _____ matter of the _____ cord

8. **READ: Meningomyelitis** (me-ning-gō-mī-e-LĪ-tis) is a rare condition which is usually caused by a virus. **Poliomyelitis** (pō-lē-ō-mī-e-LĪ-tis) is often referred to as polio or infantile paralysis. It is a viral disease that has been eradicated from most countries in the world, thanks to the development of vaccines in 1952 and 1962 and mass vaccination campaigns.

9. **MATCH:** Draw a line to match the word part with its definition.

    a. -graphy   record, radiographic image
    b. -gram   process of recording, radiographic imaging

10. BUILD: *Continue using **myel/o**, along with the word parts reviewed in the previous exercise, to build the following terms related to the spinal cord.*

a. radiographic image of the spinal cord

                     _____ / o / _____
                             wr   cv   s

b. radiographic imaging of the spinal cord

                     _____ / o / _____
                             wr   cv   s

11. READ: **Myelography** (mī-e-LOG-ra-fē) is an invasive procedure that has been largely replaced by magnetic resonance imaging (MRI). For those who cannot have an MRI, such as a patient with a pacemaker, a CT **myelogram** (MĪ-e-lō-gram) is performed by injecting a contrast medium into the cerebrospinal fluid (CSF) that surrounds the spinal cord and obtaining images of the area in question.

12. LABEL: *Write word parts to complete Figure 11.9.*

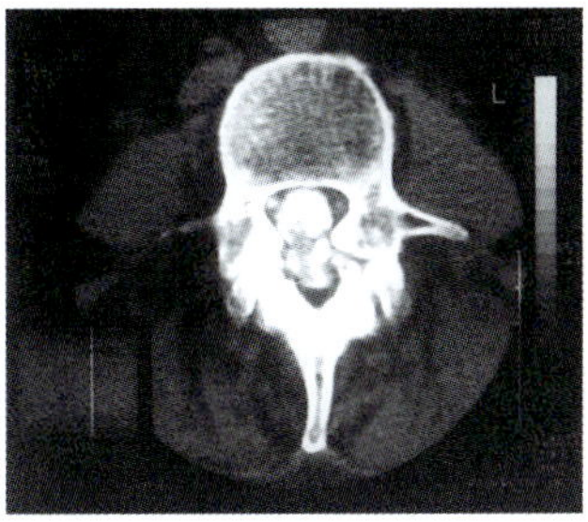

Figure 11.9 Image obtained by CT _____ /o/ _____.
                        spinal cord   radiographic imaging

13. MATCH: *Draw a line to match the word part with its definition.*

a. -algia   small
b. -us   pain
c. hydr/o   no meaning
d. micro-   water

14. TRANSLATE: *Complete the definitions of the following terms built from the combining form **cephal/o**, meaning head. Use the meaning of word parts to fill in the blanks.*

a. micro/cephal/us   small _____
b. hydr/o/cephal/us   _____(cerebrospinal fluid) in the _____ (brain)
c. ceph/algia   _____ in the head (headache)
*NOTE: the **al** is dropped from the combining form cephal/o in the term cephalgia.*

15. READ: **Cephalgia** (sef-AL-ja) refers to a headache and is used to describe cluster headaches associated with migraines and headaches accompanied by facial pain. **Microcephalus** (mī-krō-SEF-a-lus), also called microcephaly (mī-krō-SEF-a-lē), refers to an abnormally small circumference of a baby's head. It may be present at birth (congenital) or occur in the first few years of life (acquired). **Hydrocephalus** (hī-drō-SEF-a-lus) may be congenital or acquired and is caused by increased amounts of cerebrospinal fluid in the brain. Congenital hydrocephalus may result in an enlargement of the infant's cranium.

16. MATCH: *Draw a line to match the word part with its definition.*

a. a-   diseased state, condition of
b. dys-   half
c. hemi-   four
d. quadr/i   difficult, painful, abnormal
e. -ia   absence of, without

17. BUILD: *Use the combining form* **phas/o**, *meaning speech, along with the word parts reviewed in the previous exercise to build the following terms.*

a. condition of without speech   _____/_____/_____
                                           p   wr   s

b. condition of difficulty with speech _____/_____/_____
                                           p   wr   s

18. READ: Aphasia (a-FĀ-zha) describes a condition in which a person cannot communicate; it affects the ability to express oneself through both spoken and written language. **Dysphasia** (dis-FĀ-zha) is a less severe condition in which some speech and language abilities are preserved. Either may be the result of a stroke or head injury.

19. TRANSLATE: *Complete the definitions of the following terms built from the combining form* **pleg/o**, *meaning paralysis.*

a. hemi/pleg/ia   condition of _____ of half (right or left side of the body)
b. quadr/i/pleg/ia   condition of paralysis of _____ (limbs)

20. READ: Hemiplegia (hem-ē-PLĒ-ja) can affect either the left or right side of the body and is most commonly caused by a stroke. **Quadriplegia** (kwod-ri-PLĒ-ja) is usually a result of vertebral fractures that cause injury to the spinal cord.

21. LABEL: *Write word parts to complete Figure 11.10.*

FYI The term **paraplegia** is composed of the Greek words **para**, meaning beside, and **pleg**, meaning paralysis. Paraplegia has been used since Hippocrates' time and originally meant paralysis of any limb or side of the body. It has been used to mean paralysis from the waist down since the nineteenth century.

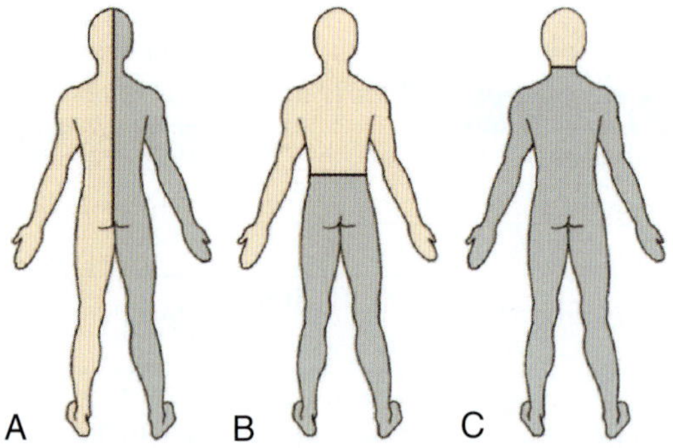

Figure 11.10 A. _____/_____/_____.
                         half   paralysis   condition of

B. Paraplegia. C. _____/i/_____/_____.
                          four   paralysis   condition of

22. MATCH: *Draw a line to match the word part with its definition.*

    a. -genic   no meaning
    b. path/o   producing, originating, causing
    c. -y   abnormal condition
    d. -osis   disease

23. BUILD: *Use the combining form **psych/o**, meaning mind, along with the word parts reviewed in the previous exercise, to build terms related to the mind.*

    a. originating in the mind   _____ / o / _____
                                                            wr   cv   s

    b. (any) disease of the mind   _____ / o / _____ / y
                                                            wr   cv   wr   s

    c. abnormal condition of the mind   _____ / _____
                                                             wr   s

24. READ: Psychogenic (sī-kō-JEN-ik) disorders arise from mental or emotional sources. While **psychopathy** (sī-KOP-a-thē) refers to any disease of the mind and may be mild or severe, **psychosis** (si-KŌ-sis) implies a severe impairment in perception of reality with hallucinations, incoherent speech or behavior, and a lack of awareness of this behavior on the part of the patient.

25. MATCH: *Draw a line to match the word part with its definition.*

    a. -logist   study of
    b. -logy   one who studies and treats (specialist, physician)

26. TRANSLATE: *Complete the definitions of the following terms. Use the meaning of word parts to fill in the blanks.*

    a. psych/o/logist   specialist who studies and treats the _____
    b. psych/o/logy   _____ of the mind

27. READ: The American Psychological Association describes **psychology** (sī-KOL-o-jē) as the study of the mind and behavior, which ranges from the functions of the brain to the actions of nations. A **psychologist** (sī-KOL-o-jist) may work in a private or group practice, or may work in schools, hospitals, nursing homes, mental health clinics, prisons, businesses, or places of worship.

28. REVIEW OF MORE NERVOUS SYSTEM AND BEHAVIORAL HEALTH TERMS BUILT FROM WORD PARTS: *the following is an alphabetical list of terms built and translated in the previous exercises.*

MEDICAL TERMS BUILT FROM WORD PARTS

TERM	DEFINITION	TERM	DEFINITION
1. aphasia (a-FĀ-zha)	condition of without speech (or loss of the ability to speak)	11. myelogram (MĪ-e-lō-gram)	radiographic image of the spinal cord
2. cephalgia (sef-AL-ja)	pain in the head (also called **headache**)	12. myelography (mī-e-LOG-ra-fē)	radiographic imaging of the spinal cord (Figure 11.9)
3. dysphasia (dis-FĀ-zha)	condition of difficulty with speech	13. poliomyelitis (pō-lē-ō-mī-e-LĪ-tis)	inflammation of the gray matter of the spinal cord
4. hemiplegia (hem-ē-PLĒ-ja)	condition of paralysis of half (of the body) (Figure 11.10, A)	14. psychogenic (sī-kō-JEN-ik)	originating in the mind
5. hydrocephalus (hī-drō-SEF-a-lus)	water in the head (increased amount of cerebrospinal fluid in the brain)	15. psychologist (sī-KOL-o-jist)	specialist who studies and treats the mind
6. meningioma (me-nin-je-Ō-ma)	tumor of the meninges (Figure 11.8)	16. psychology (sī-KOL-o-jē)	study of the mind
7. meningitis (men-in-JĪ-tis)	inflammation of the meninges	17. psychopathy (sī-KOP-a-thē)	(any) disease of the mind
8. meningocele (me-NING-gō-sēl)	hernia of the meninges	18. psychosis (si-KŌ-sis)	abnormal condition of the mind (major mental disorder characterized by extreme derangement, often with delusions and hallucinations)
9. meningomyelitis (me-ning-gō-mī-e-LĪ-tis)	inflammation of the meninges and the spinal cord		
10. microcephalus (mī-krō-SEF-a-lus)	small head (also called **microcephaly**)	19. quadriplegia (kwod-ri-PLĒ-ja)	condition of paralysis of four (limbs) (Figure 11.10, C)

EXERCISE D   Pronounce and Spell MORE Terms Built from Word Parts

Practice pronunciation and spelling on paper and online.

1. **Practice on Paper**
    a. **Pronounce:** Read the phonetic spelling and say aloud the terms listed in the previous table, Review of MORE Terms Built from Word Parts.
    b. **Spell:** Have a study partner read the terms aloud. Write the spelling of the terms on a separate sheet of paper.

2. **Practice Online**
   a. **Access** online learning resources. Go to evolve.elsevier.com > Evolve Resources > Practice Student Resources.
   b. **Pronounce**: Select Audio Glossary > Lesson 11 > Exercise D. Select a term to hear its pronunciation and repeat aloud.
   c. **Spell**: Select Activities > Lesson 11 > Spell Terms > Exercise D. Select the audio icon and type the correct spelling of the term.

❑   Check the box when complete.

OBJECTIVE 2

Define, pronounce, and spell medical terms NOT built from word parts.

The terms listed below may contain word parts, but are difficult to translate literally.

MEDICAL TERMS NOT BUILT FROM WORD PARTS

TERM	DEFINITION
Alzheimer disease (AD) (AWLTZ-hī-mer) (di-ZĒZ)	type of dementia caused by degeneration of brain tissue and occurring more frequently after age 65. The brain shrinks dramatically as nerve cells die and tissues atrophy. The disease is slowly progressive and usually results in profound dementia in 5 to 10 years. A prominent feature of AD is the inability to remember the recent past, while memories of the distant past remain intact.
anxiety disorder (ang-ZĪ-e-tē) (dis-OR-der)	disorder characterized by feelings of apprehension, tension, or uneasiness arising typically from the anticipation of unreal or imagined danger
bipolar disorder (bī-PŌ-lar) (dis-OR-der)	major psychological disorder typified by a disturbance in mood. The disorder is manifested by manic (elevated or irritated mood, excessive energy, impulsiveness) and depressive episodes that may alternate or elements of both may occur simultaneously.
concussion (kon-KUSH-un)	injury to the brain caused by major or minor head trauma; symptoms include vertigo, headache, and possible loss of consciousness
dementia (de-MEN-sha)	cognitive impairment characterized by loss of intellectual brain function. Patients have difficulty in various ways, including difficulty in performing complex tasks, reasoning, learning and retaining new information, orientation, word finding, and behavior. Dementia has several causes and is not considered part of normal aging.
depression (dē-PRESH-un)	mood disturbance characterized by feelings of sadness, despair, discouragement, hopelessness, lack of joy, altered sleep patterns, and difficulty with decision making and daily function. Depression ranges from normal feelings of sadness through dysthymia (mild depression), to major depression.
epidural nerve block (ep-i-DŪ-ral) (nurv) (blok)	procedure performed for spine-related pain, or for pain from other causes such as childbirth and labor, by injection of anesthetic agent into the epidural space. Injection may be between the vertebral spines, in the cervical, thoracic, or lumbar region.
lumbar puncture (LP) (LUM-bar) (PUNK-chur)	diagnostic procedure performed by insertion of a needle into the subarachnoid space, usually between the third and fourth lumbar vertebrae; performed for many reasons, including the removal of cerebrospinal fluid (also called **spinal tap**)

MEDICAL TERMS NOT BUILT FROM WORD PARTS—cont'd

TERM	DEFINITION
migraine (MĪ-grān)	an intense, throbbing headache, usually one-sided, and often associated with irritability, nausea, vomiting, and extreme sensitivity to light or sound. Migraines may occur with or without aura (sensory warning symptoms such as flashes of light, blind spots, or tingling in the arms or legs).
multiple sclerosis (MS) (MUL-ti-pul) (skle-RŌ-sis)	chronic degenerative disease characterized by sclerotic patches along the brain and spinal cord; signs and symptoms fluctuate over the course of the disease; more common symptoms include fatigue, balance and coordination impairments, numbness, and vision problems
paraplegia (par-a-PLĒ-ja)	paralysis from the waist down caused by damage to the lower level of the spinal cord
Parkinson disease (PD) (PAR-kin-sun) (di-ZĒZ)	chronic degenerative disease of the central nervous system; symptoms include resting tremors of the hands and feet, rigidity, expressionless face, shuffling gait, and eventually dementia. It usually occurs after the age of 50 years.
psychiatrist (sī-KĪ-a-trist)	physician with additional training and experience in the diagnosis, prevention, and treatment of mental disorders; can prescribe medications and direct therapy
sciatica (sī-AT-i-ka)	inflammation of the sciatic nerve, causing pain that travels from the buttock through the leg to the foot and toes; can be caused by injury, infection, arthritis, herniated disk, or from prolonged pressure on the nerve from sitting for long periods
seizure (SĒ-zher)	sudden, abnormal surge of electrical activity in the brain, resulting in involuntary body movements or behaviors
stroke (strōk)	interruption of blood supply to a region of the brain, depriving nerve cells in the affected area of oxygen and nutrients (also called **cerebrovascular accident [CVA]**) (Figure 11.11)
subarachnoid hemorrhage (SAH) (sub-e-RAK-noyd) (HEM-o-rij)	bleeding between the pia mater and arachnoid layers of the meninges (subarachnoid space) caused by a ruptured blood vessel (usually a ruptured cerebral aneurysm). The patient may experience an intense, sudden headache accompanied by nausea, vomiting, and neck pain. SAH is a critical condition which must be recognized and treated immediately to prevent permanent brain damage or death. (Figure 11.11, *A*)
syncope (SINK-o-pē)	fainting or sudden loss of consciousness caused by lack of blood supply to the cerebrum
transient ischemic attack (TIA) (TRAN-sē-ent) (is-KĒ-mik) (a-TAK)	sudden deficient supply of blood to the brain lasting a short time. The symptoms may be similar to those of stroke, but are temporary and the usual outcome is complete recovery. TIAs are often warning signs for eventual occurrence of a stroke

> **FYI** **Parkinson disease** is also called **parkinsonism**, **paralysis agitans**, and **shaking palsy**. It was described by James Parkinson, an English professor, in 1817 in his **Essay on the Shaking Palsy**.

> **FYI** **Epilepsy** (EP-i-lep-sē) is a general term given to a group of neurologic disorders, all characterized by abnormal electrical activity in the brain.

EXERCISE E   Label

Write the medical terms pictured and defined using the previous table of Medical Terms NOT Built from Word Parts. Check your work with the Answer Key in Appendix C.

1. _____
sudden deficient supply of blood to the brain lasting a short time

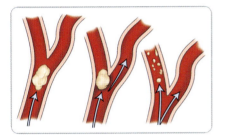

2. _____
interruption of blood supply to a region of the brain depriving nerve cells in the affected area of oxygen and nutrients

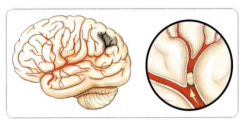

3. _____
bleeding between the pia mater and arachnoid layers of the meninges caused by a ruptured blood vessel

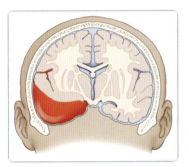

4. _____
cognitive impairment characterized by loss of intellectual brain function, including difficulty in performing complex tasks, reasoning, learning and retaining new information, orientation, word finding, and behavior.

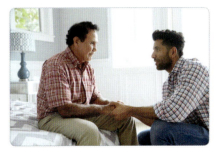

5. _____

type of dementia caused by degeneration of brain tissue and occurring more frequently after age 65

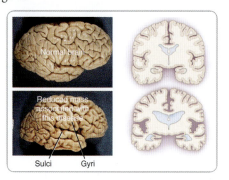

Normal brain

Reduced mass associated with this disease

Sulci   Gyri

6. _____

diagnostic procedure performed for the removal of cerebrospinal fluid (for testing)

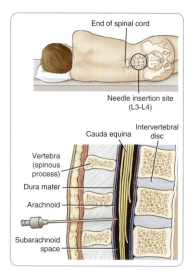

End of spinal cord

Needle insertion site (L3-L4)

Intervertebral disc

Cauda equina

Vertebra (spinous process)

Dura mater

Arachnoid

Subarachnoid space

7. _____

paralysis from the waist down

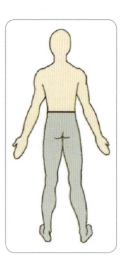

8. _____

inflammation of the sciatic nerve, causing pain that travels from the thigh through the leg to the foot and toes

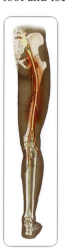

FYI The **sciatic nerve**, the longest in the body, travels through the hip from the spine to the thigh and continues with branches throughout the lower leg and foot. Sciatica is inflammation of the nerve along its course.

9. _____

an intense, throbbing headache, usually one-sided, and often associated with irritability, nausea, vomiting, and extreme sensitivity to light or sound

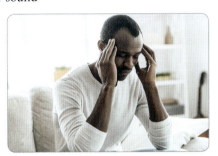

10. _____

physician with additional training and experience in the diagnosis, prevention, and treatment of mental disorders; can prescribe medications and direct therapy

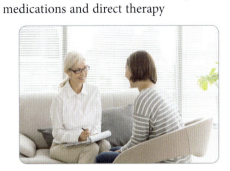

EXERCISE F   Learn Medical Terms NOT Built from Word Parts

Fill in the blanks with medical terms defined in bold using the Medical Terms NOT Built from Word Parts table. Answers are listed in Appendix C.

1. More than twice as likely to affect women than men, **chronic degenerative disease characterized by sclerotic patches along the brain and spinal cord**, or _____, abbreviated as _____, is likely to be diagnosed between the ages of 20 and 40 years. Symptoms of MS vary widely and may include fatigue, pain, numbness, or problems with vision or coordination.

2. Another **chronic degenerative disease of the central nervous system**, or _____ _____, abbreviated as _____, is usually diagnosed after the age of 50 years. A hallmark symptom of PD is a resting tremor, or uncontrolled movement of a limb when at rest, that stops during purposeful, voluntary movement. Other symptoms include rigidity, expressionless face, shuffling gait, and eventually dementia.

3. **Cognitive impairment characterized by loss of intellectual brain function**, or _____, has several causes and is not considered a part of normal aging. The **type of dementia caused by degeneration of brain tissue and occurring more frequently after age 65**, or _____ (AD), is the most common type of dementia, making up 60-80% of all cases. It causes death of nerve cells throughout the brain, leading to tissue loss and shrinkage.

4. Vertigo and loss of consciousness can be symptoms of **injury to the brain caused by major or minor head trauma**, or _____. Major head trauma can result in **sudden, abnormal surge of electrical activity in the brain, resulting in involuntary body movements or behaviors**, or _____. In some cases, patients may develop epilepsy years after a severe concussion.

5. **Inflammation of the sciatic nerve, causing pain that travels from the buttock through the leg to the foot and toes**, or _____, may be caused by arthritis in the vertebrae or by a herniated disk.

Procedure performed for spine-related pain by injection of anesthetic agent into the epidural space, or _____ may be needed in severe cases and usually incorporates a steroid like cortisone for long-term relief.

6. **An intense, throbbing headache, usually one sided, and often associated with irritability, nausea, vomiting, and extreme sensitivity to light or sound**, or _____, may be triggered by hormonal changes in women, or by certain foods, food additives (like aspartame or MSG), alcohol, stress, or changes in sleep patterns.

7. A **diagnostic procedure performed by insertion of a needle into the subarachnoid space usually between the third and fourth lumbar vertebrae, or** _____, abbreviated _____, is also called a spinal tap. It may be used to diagnose normal pressure hydrocephalus, which is a form of hydrocephalus with a gradual onset, usually affecting those 60 years of age and older.

8. **Interruption of blood supply to a region of the brain, depriving nerve cells in the affected area of oxygen and nutrients**, or _____, (also called **cerebrovascular accident** and abbreviated as _____), can be best understood by categorizing the underlying cause of the interruption of blood flow (Figure 11.11). One type of stroke is caused by bleeding within the brain or cranial space, known as hemorrhagic stroke. Another type is an ischemic stroke, which is due to a blocked vessel caused by a cerebral thrombosis or a cerebral embolus.

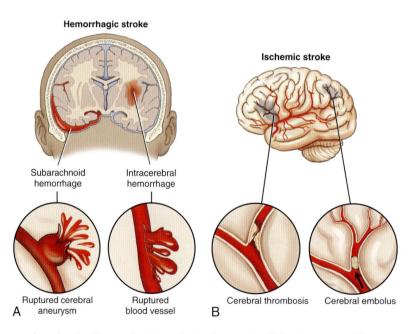

Figure 11.11 Causes of stroke. **A.** Hemorrhagic stroke is the result of bleeding caused by an intracerebral hemorrhage or a subarachnoid hemorrhage, usually a result of a ruptured cerebral aneurysm. **B.** Ischemic stroke is the result of a blocked blood vessel caused by a cerebral thrombosis or cerebral embolus.

9. **Bleeding between the pia mater and arachnoid layers of the meninges (subarachnoid space) caused by a ruptured blood vessel**, or _____, is usually the result of a ruptured brain aneurysm, and can result in a hemorrhagic stroke.

10. **A sudden deficient supply of blood to the brain lasting a short time**, or _____ _____, abbreviated _____, usually lasts only a few minutes and causes no permanent damage. It is considered a warning sign for an ischemic stroke. Symptoms may include hemiplegia, dysphasia, loss of vision, and **fainting or sudden loss of consciousness caused by lack of blood supply to the cerebrum**, or _____.

11. **Paralysis from the waist down caused by damage to the lower level of the spinal cord**, or _____ _____, may be caused by vertebral fracture or dislocation (Figure 11.10, *B*).

12. **Disorder characterized by feelings of apprehension, tension, or uneasiness**, or _____ _____, may be treated with psychotherapy (talk therapy) and/or medications. Making lifestyle changes, learning coping mechanisms, and relaxation therapy can also help.

13. **Mood disturbance characterized by feelings of sadness, despair, and discouragement**, or _____ _____, may range from normal feelings of sadness (resulting from personal loss or tragedy), through dysthymia (mild depressive symptoms that come and go), to major depressive disorder (persistent depressed feelings that impact everyday life). Both dysthymia and major depression can be treated with psychotherapy and/or medications.

14. **Major psychological disorder typified by a disturbance in mood, manifested by manic or depressive episodes**, or _____ has symptoms that range from feelings of hopelessness and despair (depression) to elevated or irritated mood, excessive energy, and impulsiveness (mania). Mood shifts may occur only a few times a year, or as often as several times a day. Sometimes bipolar disorder causes symptoms of depression and mania at the same time. Medication is the main treatment for bipolar disorder, although psychotherapy is also very important.

15. **A physician with additional training and experience in the diagnosis, prevention, and treatment of mental disorders**, or a _____, is trained to assess mental and physical aspects of psychological problems. They can order and perform a variety of laboratory and psychological tests to make diagnoses and formulate treatment plans.

EXERCISE G   Pronounce and Spell Terms NOT Built from Word Parts

Practice pronunciation and spelling on paper and online.

1. **Practice on Paper**
   a. **Pronounce**: Read the phonetic spelling and say aloud the terms listed in the previous Terms NOT Built from Word Parts table.
   b. **Spell**: Have a study partner read the terms aloud. Write the spelling of the terms on a separate sheet of paper.

2. **Practice Online** 🌐

    a. **Access** online learning resources. Go to evolve.elsevier.com > Evolve Resources > Practice Student Resources.

    b. **Pronounce:** Select Audio Glossary > Lesson 11 > Exercise G. Select a term to hear its pronunciation and repeat aloud.

    c. **Spell:** Select Activities > Lesson 11 > Spell Terms > Exercise G. Select the audio icon and type the correct spelling of the term.

❏   Check the box when complete.

OBJECTIVE 3

Write abbreviations.

ABBREVIATIONS RELATED TO THE NERVOUS SYSTEM AND BEHAVIORAL HEALTH

Use the online **flashcards** to familiarize yourself with the following abbreviations.

ABBREVIATION	TERM	ABBREVIATION	TERM
AD	Alzheimer disease	**LP**	lumbar puncture
ADL, ADLs	activities of daily living (such as personal hygiene, dressing, eating, ability to use the restroom, and transferring to and from a standing position)	**MS**	multiple sclerosis
CNS	central nervous system	**PD**	Parkinson disease
CSF	cerebrospinal fluid	**PNS**	peripheral nervous system
CVA	cerebrovascular accident	**SAH**	subarachnoid hemorrhage
EEG	electroencephalogram	**TIA**	transient ischemic attack

EXERCISE H   Abbreviate Medical Terms

Write the correct abbreviation next to its medical term.

1. Diseases and Disorders:

    a. _____ Alzheimer disease

    b. _____ cerebrovascular accident

    c. _____ multiple sclerosis

    d. _____ Parkinson disease

    e. _____ subarachnoid hemorrhage

    f. _____ transient ischemic attack

2. Diagnostic Tests and Equipment:

    a. _____ electroencephalogram

    b. _____ lumbar puncture

3. Related Terms:

    a. _____ central nervous system

    b. _____ cerebrospinal fluid

    c. _____ peripheral nervous system

    d. _____, _____ activities of daily living

⊙ OBJECTIVE 4

Identify medical terms by clinical category.

Now that you have worked through the nervous system and behavioral health lesson, review and practice medical terms grouped by clinical category. Categories include signs and symptoms, diseases and disorders, diagnostic tests and equipment, surgical procedures, specialties and professions, and other terms related to the nervous system and behavioral health. Check your responses with the Answer Key in Appendix C.

EXERCISE I **Signs and Symptoms**

Write the medical terms for signs and symptoms next to their definitions.

1. _____ condition of without speech (or loss of the ability to speak)

2. _____ pain in the head (also called headache)

3. _____ condition of difficulty with speech

4. _____ pain in the nerve(s)

5. _____ inflammation of many joints

6. _____ pain in many muscles

7. _____ inflammation of many nerves

8. _____ sudden, abnormal surge of electrical activity in the brain, resulting in involuntary body movements or behaviors

9. _____ fainting or sudden loss of consciousness caused by lack of blood supply to the cerebrum

EXERCISE J   Diseases and Disorders

Write the medical terms for diseases and disorders next to their definitions.

1. _____ type of dementia caused by degeneration of brain tissue and occurring more frequently after age 65

2. _____ disorder characterized by feelings of apprehension, tension or uneasiness arising typically from the anticipation of unreal or imagined danger

3. _____ major psychological disorder typified by a disturbance in mood

4. _____ abnormal condition of a blood clot in the cerebrum

5. _____ injury to the brain caused by major or minor head trauma

6. _____ cognitive impairment characterized by loss of intellectual brain function

7. _____ mood disturbance characterized by feelings of sadness, despair, discouragement, hopelessness, lack of joy, altered sleep patterns, and difficulty with decision making and daily function.

8. _____ inflammation of the brain

9. _____ disease of the brain

10. _____ condition of paralysis of half (of the body)

11. _____ water in the head (increased amount of cerebrospinal fluid in the brain)

12. _____ tumor of the meninges

13. _____ inflammation of the meninges

14. _____ hernia of the meninges

15. _____ inflammation of the meninges and the spinal cord

16. _____ an intense, throbbing headache, usually one-sided, and often associated with irritability, nausea, vomiting, and extreme sensitivity to light or sound

17. _____ chronic degenerative disease characterized by sclerotic patches along the brain and spinal cord

18. _____ disease of the nerves

19. _____ paralysis from the waist down caused by damage to the lower level of the spinal cord

20. _____ chronic degenerative disease of the central nervous system; symptoms include resting tremors of the hands and feet, rigidity, expressionless face, shuffling gait, and eventually dementia

21. _____ inflammation of the gray matter of the spinal cord

22. _____ (any) disease of the mind

23. _____ abnormal condition of the mind (major mental disorder characterized by extreme derangement, often with delusions and hallucinations)

24. _____ condition of paralysis of four (limbs)

25. _____ inflammation of the sciatic nerve, causing pain that travels from the buttock through the leg to the foot and toes

26. _____ interruption of blood supply to a region of the brain, depriving nerve cells in the affected area of oxygen and nutrients

27. _____ bleeding between the pia mater and arachnoid layers of the meninges caused by a ruptured blood vessel

28. _____ sudden deficient supply of blood to the brain lasting a short time

29. _____ small head

EXERCISE K   Diagnostic Tests and Equipment

Write the medical terms for diagnostic tests and equipment next to their definitions.

1. _____ radiographic imaging of the blood vessels of the cerebrum

2. _____ record of electrical activity of the brain

3. _____ instrument used to record electrical activity of the brain

4. _____ process of recording the electrical activity of the brain

5. _____ diagnostic procedure performed by insertion of a needle into the subarachnoid space, usually between the third and fourth lumbar vertebrae (also called a spinal tap)

6. _____ radiographic image of the spinal cord

7. _____ radiographic imaging of the spinal cord

EXERCISE L   Surgical Procedure

Write the medical term for the surgical procedure next to its definition.

_____ procedure performed for spine-related pain by injection of anesthetic agent into the epidural space

EXERCISE M   Specialties and Professions

Write the medical terms for specialties and professions next to their definitions.

1. _____   physician who studies and treats diseases of the nervous system

2. _____   study of the nerves (nervous system)

3. _____   specialist who studies and treats the mind

4. _____   study of the mind

5. _____   physician with additional training and experience in the diagnosis, prevention, and treatment of mental disorders; can prescribe medications and direct therapy

EXERCISE N   Medical Terms Related to the Nervous System and Behavioral Health

Write the medical terms related to the nervous system and behavioral health next to their definitions.

1. _____   pertaining to the cerebrum

2. _____   pertaining to a nerve

3. _____   originating in the mind

OBJECTIVE 5

Use medical language in clinical statements, the case study, and a medical record.

Check responses for the following exercises in Appendix C.

EXERCISE O   Use Medical Terms in Clinical Statements

Circle the medical terms and abbreviations defined in the bolded phrases. Answers are listed in Appendix C. For pronunciation practice, read the answers aloud.

1. **Mood disturbance characterized by feelings of sadness, despair, and hopelessness** (Anxiety Disorder, Depression, Psychosis) is a diagnosis frequently encountered in the field of **study of the mind** (psychology, neurology, endocrinology). It may be accompanied by **disorder characterized by feelings of apprehension, tension, or uneasiness** (bipolar disorder, dementia, anxiety disorder). Fortunately, there are medications, which may be prescribed by a **physician with additional training and experience in the diagnosis, prevention, and treatment of mental disorders who can prescribe medications and direct therapy** (psychiatrist, psychologist, psych tech), that are helpful in treating both conditions. Psychotherapy performed by a **specialist who studies and treats the mind** (psychologist, physiologist, neurologist) can also be very helpful.

2. The manic phase of **major psychological disorder typified by a disturbance in mood** (anxiety disorder, somatoform disorder, bipolar disorder) can be very dangerous to the patient. In addition to euphoria and recklessness, some patients experience **major mental disorder characterized by extreme derangement**

(psychosis, neurosis, thrombosis) in which they may hear voices or see things that aren't there. Lithium was previously the most commonly used medication for bipolar disease, but newer options also exist.

3. **Pain in the head or headache** (Neuralgia, Arthralgia, Cephalgia) is generally classified by type. **An intense, throbbing headache, usually one-sided** (Sciatica, Migraine, TIA), tension headache, and cluster headaches account for nearly 90% of all headaches. Other types of headaches include posttraumatic headaches, giant cell (temporal) arteritis, sinus headaches, brain tumor, and chronic daily headache. **Bleeding between the pia mater and arachnoid layers of the meninges caused by a ruptured blood vessel** (Cerebral thrombosis, Meningitis, Subarachnoid hemorrhage) may cause a headache that the patient describes as "the worst in my entire life."

4. In **process of recording the electrical activity of the brain** (electroencephalography, electrocardiography, myelography), electrodes are attached to areas of the patient's scalp. The electrical impulses are transmitted by an **instrument used for recording the electrical activity of the brain** (echocardiograph, electrocardiograph, electroencephalograph) that amplifies them and records them as brain waves on a moving strip of paper known as a(n) **record of electrical activity of the brain** (arteriogram, esophagram, electroencephalogram). The process of recording the electrical activity of the brain is used to diagnose intracranial lesions and to evaluate the brain's electrical activity in **sudden, abnormal surge of electrical activity in the brain** (multiple sclerosis, Parkinson disease, seizures), **injury to the brain caused by major or minor head trauma** (concussions, seizures, psychoses), **inflammation of the meninges** (meningioma, meningitis, meningocele), and **inflammation of the brain** (encephalitis, meningomyelitis, polyneuritis).

5. Common symptoms of a(n) **interruption of blood supply to a region of the brain**, (stroke, syncope, concussion) include **condition of without speech** (aphagia, dysphasia, aphasia), **condition of paralysis of half (of the body)** (quadriplegia, hemiplegia, myalgia), and facial drooping. Prompt diagnosis and treatment are critical. While the majority of strokes are ischemic, resulting from blockage in a **pertaining to the cerebrum** (cerebellar, celiac, cerebral) artery, some are hemorrhagic, caused by intracranial bleeding. A CT or MRI can usually help tell the difference. Early treatment with thrombolytic agents (which break up clots) can help save lives but can be very dangerous if given to a patient with a brain bleed. A **sudden deficient supply of blood to the brain lasting a short time** (SAH, CVA, TIA) usually does not require treatment.

6. The most common type of **cognitive impairment characterized by loss of intellectual brain function** (dementia, dysphasia, psychopathy) is caused by **degeneration of brain tissue and occurring more frequently after age 65** (Parkinson disease, multiple sclerosis, Alzheimer disease), accounting for 60-80% of all cases. Other types include vascular dementia, **chronic degenerative disease of the central nervous system** (Parkinson disease, encephalopathy, meningitis), normal pressure **water in the head (increased amount of cerebrospinal fluid in the brain)** (encephalitis, meningomyelitis, hydrocephalus), and Huntington disease.

EXERCISE P   **Apply Medical Terms to the Case Study**

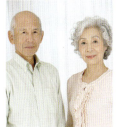

Think back to Koji Kaneshiro who was introduced in the case study at the beginning of the lesson. After working through Lesson 11 on the nervous system and behavioral health, consider the medical terms that might be used to describe his experience. List two terms relevant to the case study and their meanings. ■

Medical Term	Definition
1. _____	_____
2. _____	_____

EXERCISE Q Use Medical Terms in a Document

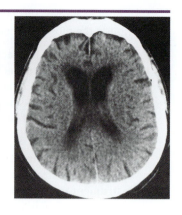

The ambulance came and took Mr. Kaneshiro to the local emergency department. A neurology consultation was obtained. The neurologist's report is provided below.

Use the definitions in numbers 1-11 to write medical terms within the document on the next page.

1. condition of without speech (or loss of the ability to speak)

2. condition of paralysis of half (of the body)

3. cognitive impairment characterized by loss of intellectual brain function

4. condition of difficulty with speech

5. bleeding between the pia mater and arachnoid layers of the meninges caused by a ruptured blood vessel

6. CVA

7. abnormal condition of a blood clot in the cerebrum

8. radiographic imaging of the blood vessels of the cerebrum

9. pertaining to the cerebrum

10. study of the nerves (nervous system)

11. physician who studies and treats diseases of the nervous system

Refer to the medical document to answer questions 12-13.

12. In the history section, Mrs. Kaneshiro describes an event that occurred about one year ago, in which her husband had a brief episode of partial paralysis. The medical term for this event is: _____ _____ _____.

13. Identify two new medical terms in the medical record you would like to investigate. Use your medical dictionary or an online reference to look up the definition.

   Medical Term   **Definition**

   1. _____   _____

   2. _____   _____

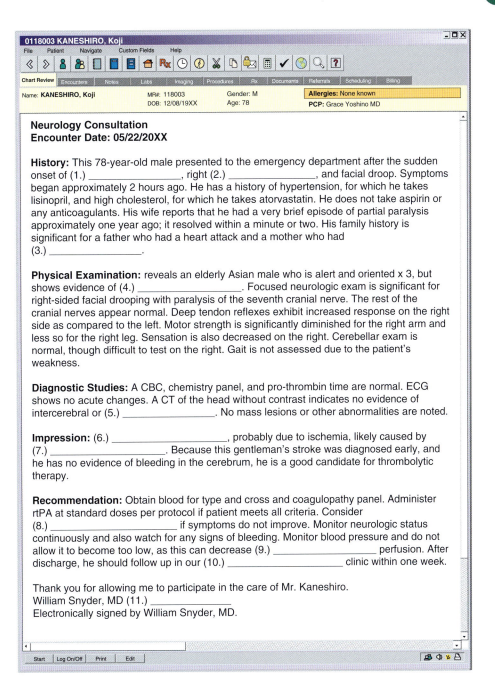

File   Patient   Navigate   Custom Fields   Help

Chart Review   Encounters   Notes   Labs   Imaging   Procedures   Rx   Documents   Referrals   Scheduling   Billing

Name: **KANESHIRO, Koji**   MR#: 118003   Gender: M   **Allergies:** None known
                                    DOB: 12/08/19XX   Age: 78   **PCP:** Grace Yoshino MD

Neurology Consultation
Encounter Date: 05/22/20XX

History: This 78-year-old male presented to the emergency department after the sudden onset of (1.) _____, right (2.) _____, and facial droop. Symptoms began approximately 2 hours ago. He has a history of hypertension, for which he takes lisinopril, and high cholesterol, for which he takes atorvastatin. He does not take aspirin or any anticoagulants. His wife reports that he had a very brief episode of partial paralysis approximately one year ago; it resolved within a minute or two. His family history is significant for a father who had a heart attack and a mother who had (3.) _____.

Physical Examination: reveals an elderly Asian male who is alert and oriented x 3, but shows evidence of (4.) _____. Focused neurologic exam is significant for right-sided facial drooping with paralysis of the seventh cranial nerve. The rest of the cranial nerves appear normal. Deep tendon reflexes exhibit increased response on the right side as compared to the left. Motor strength is significantly diminished for the right arm and less so for the right leg. Sensation is also decreased on the right. Cerebellar exam is normal, though difficult to test on the right. Gait is not assessed due to the patient's weakness.

Diagnostic Studies: A CBC, chemistry panel, and pro-thrombin time are normal. ECG shows no acute changes. A CT of the head without contrast indicates no evidence of intercerebral or (5.) _____. No mass lesions or other abnormalities are noted.

Impression: (6.) _____, probably due to ischemia, likely caused by (7.) _____. Because this gentleman's stroke was diagnosed early, and he has no evidence of bleeding in the cerebrum, he is a good candidate for thrombolytic therapy.

Recommendation: Obtain blood for type and cross and coagulopathy panel. Administer rtPA at standard doses per protocol if patient meets all criteria. Consider (8.) _____ if symptoms do not improve. Monitor neurologic status continuously and also watch for any signs of bleeding. Monitor blood pressure and do not allow it to become too low, as this can decrease (9.) _____ perfusion. After discharge, he should follow up in our (10.) _____ clinic within one week.

Thank you for allowing me to participate in the care of Mr. Kaneshiro.
William Snyder, MD (11.) _____
Electronically signed by William Snyder, MD.

Start   Log On/Off   Print   Edit

EXERCISE R   Use Medical Language in Electronic Health Records Online

Select the correct medical terms to complete three medical records in one patient's electronic file.

 Access online resources at evolve.elsevier.com > Evolve Resources > Practice Student Resources > Activities > Lesson 11 > Electronic Health Records

Topic: Multiple Sclerosis
Record 1: Ophthalmology Report
Record 2: Cytology Report
Record 3: Neurology Office Visit

❏   Check the box when complete.

OBJECTIVE 6

Recall and assess knowledge of word parts, medical terms, and abbreviations.

EXERCISE S   Online Review of Lesson Content

Recall and assess your learning from working through the lesson by completing online learning activities at evolve. elsevier.com > Evolve Resources > Practice Student Resources. Keep track of your progress by placing a check mark next to completed activities.

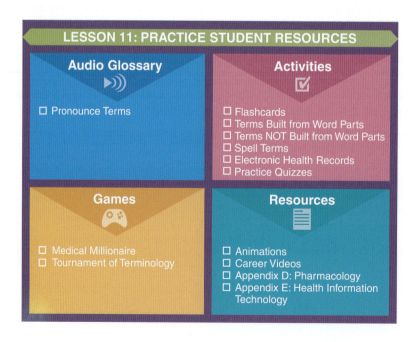

LESSON 11: PRACTICE STUDENT RESOURCES

Audio Glossary
☐ Pronounce Terms

Activities
☐ Flashcards
☐ Terms Built from Word Parts
☐ Terms NOT Built from Word Parts
☐ Spell Terms
☐ Electronic Health Records
☐ Practice Quizzes

Games
☐ Medical Millionaire
☐ Tournament of Terminology

Resources
☐ Animations
☐ Career Videos
☐ Appendix D: Pharmacology
☐ Appendix E: Health Information Technology

EXERCISE T Lesson Content Quiz

Test your knowledge of the terms and abbreviations introduced in this lesson. Circle the letter for the medical term or abbreviation related to the words in italics.

1. The 71-year-old man with right leg pain was told he had *pain in the nerve(s)*.
   a. neuropathy
   b. neuralgia
   c. polyneuritis

2. An elderly gentleman was brought to the emergency department following an episode of *syncope*.
   a. confusion
   b. throbbing headache
   c. fainting

3. The linebacker on the high school football team sustained *an injury to the brain caused by head trauma* during yesterday's game.
   a. concussion
   b. seizure
   c. migraine

4. A 60-year-old man with Type 2 diabetes was found to have peripheral *disease of the nerves* after undergoing a nerve conduction study.
   a. neuralgia
   b. neuropathy
   c. sciatica

5. A 55-year-old woman who complained of upper back and arm pain was diagnosed with *polymyalgia*.
   a. pain in one muscle
   b. disease of many muscles
   c. pain in many muscles

6. A diagnosis of *a chronic degenerative disease characterized by sclerotic patches along the brain and spinal cord* was made on a 32-year-old woman who presented with a history of leg weakness and muscle cramps.
   a. transient ischemic attack
   b. multiple sclerosis
   c. Parkinson disease

7. *Cerebral angiography* was performed on a 58-year-old man who presented with an acute onset of right arm and leg weakness. Cerebral angiography produced images of the
   a. veins of the cerebrum only
   b. arteries of the cerebrum only
   c. blood vessels of the cerebrum

8. The 25-year-old man was diagnosed with a *major psychological disorder typified by a disturbance in mood*.
   a. depression
   b. bipolar disorder
   c. anxiety disorder

9. An 18-year-old female who presented with an acute onset of headache and fever of 102F underwent a *diagnostic procedure performed by insertion of a needle into the subarachnoid space between vertebrae* to exclude acute meningitis.
   a. lumbar puncture
   b. epidural nerve block
   c. electroencephalography

10. An *ADL* scale is used to assess the ability to perform basic self-care tasks.
    a. activities of daily life
    b. acts of daily living
    c. activities of daily living

LESSON AT A GLANCE | NERVOUS SYSTEM AND BEHAVIORAL HEALTH WORD PARTS

COMBINING FORMS

cerebr/o
encephal/o
mening/o, meningi/o
myel/o
phas/o

pleg/o
poli/o
psych/o
quadr/i

PREFIXES

hemi-
micro-

SUFFIX

-us

LESSON AT A GLANCE | NERVOUS SYSTEM AND BEHAVIORAL HEALTH MEDICAL TERMS AND ABBREVIATIONS

SIGNS AND SYMPTOMS

aphasia
cephalgia
dysphasia
neuralgia
polyarthritis
polymyalgia
polyneuritis
seizure
syncope

DISEASES AND DISORDERS

Alzheimer disease (AD)
anxiety disorder
bipolar disorder
cerebral thrombosis
concussion
dementia
depression
encephalitis
encephalopathy
hemiplegia
hydrocephalus
meningioma

meningitis
meningocele
meningomyelitis
microcephalus
migraine
multiple sclerosis (MS)
neuropathy
paraplegia
Parkinson disease (PD)
poliomyelitis
psychopathy
psychosis
quadriplegia
sciatica
stroke
subarachnoid hemorrhage (SAH)
transient ischemic attack (TIA)

DIAGNOSTIC TESTS AND EQUIPMENT

cerebral angiography
electroencephalogram (EEG)
electroencephalograph
electroencephalography

lumbar puncture (LP)
myelogram
myelography

SURGICAL PROCEDURES

epidural nerve block

SPECIALTIES AND PROFESSIONS

neurologist
neurology
psychiatrist
psychologist
psychology

RELATED TERMS

cerebral
neural
psychogenic

ABBREVIATIONS

AD	CVA	PD
ADL, ADLs	EEG	PNS
CNS	LP	SAH
CSF	MS	TIA

Nascha Tohe

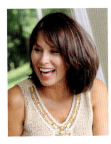

Nascha generally thinks of herself as being healthy. Lately, though, she's been really tired. She's also thirsty all the time and drinks 3-4 quarts of water every day. Now Nascha has to get up 2 or 3 times at night to go to the bathroom, and she goes more during the day, too. Her father has diabetes. He has to see a special doctor and have his sugar level tested all the time. She is worried that she might have the same problem. Her sister convinced her to come to the clinic to get checked out.

■ *Consider Nascha's situation as you work through the lesson on the endocrine system. We will return to this case study and identify medical terms used to describe and document her experiences.*

OBJECTIVES

1 ■ Build, translate, pronounce, and spell medical terms built from word parts (p. 365).

2 ■ Define, pronounce, and spell medical terms NOT built from word parts (p. 371).

3 ■ Write abbreviations (p. 375).

4 ■ Identify medical terms by clinical category (p. 376).

5 ■ Use medical language in clinical statements, the case study, and a medical record (p. 378).

6 ■ Recall and assess knowledge of word parts, medical terms, and abbreviations (p. 381).

INTRODUCTION TO THE ENDOCRINE SYSTEM

Anatomic Structures of the Endocrine System

adrenal glands (a-DRĒ-nal) (glans)	glands located above the kidneys that secrete various hormones, including cortisone and adrenaline
hormone (HŌR-mōn)	chemical substance secreted by an endocrine gland that is carried by the blood to a target tissue
islets of Langerhans (Ī-litz) (LAHNG-er-hahnz)	clusters of endocrine tissue found throughout the pancreas, made up of different cell types that secrete various hormones, including insulin (Figure 12.4)
metabolism (ma-TAB-a-liz-am)	sum total of all the chemical processes that take place in a living organism
pancreas (PAN-krē-as)	long organ that lies transversely across the upper abdomen that has a role in digestion as well as hormone secretion; contains the islets of Langerhans, which perform endocrine functions
pituitary gland (pi-TOO-i-tār-ē) (gland)	pea-sized gland located at the base of the brain; produces hormones that stimulate the function of other endocrine glands

Anatomic Structures of the Endocrine System—cont'd

thymus (THĪ-mas)	lymphatic organ located behind the sternum; plays an important role in the development of the body's immune system, particularly from infancy to puberty
thyroid gland (THĪ-roid) (gland)	butterfly-shaped gland located anteriorly in the neck and inferior to the larynx; secretes hormones that regulate the metabolism of carbohydrates, proteins, and fats needed for growth, development, and basal metabolic rate

Functions of the Endocrine System

- Regulates body activities
- Secretes hormones
- Influences growth, development, and metabolism

How the Endocrine System Works

The endocrine system is made up of glands that secrete hormones to assist in the regulation of body activities (see Figure 12.2). The nervous system also regulates body activities but does so through nerve impulses. Nervous system regulation takes place quickly, and the effects only last a short while. The endocrine system communicates through **hormones,** or chemical messengers, which take longer to produce results; however, the effects of endocrine system regulation usually last longer.

Hormones produced by endocrine glands are released directly into the bloodstream and are transported throughout the body. Target tissues are designed to respond to the specific hormone that influences their activities. Each endocrine gland secretes specialized hormones that affect various body systems. The **pituitary gland** is referred to as the master gland because it secretes several hormones that influence the activities of other endocrine glands. Testes and ovaries, presented in Lesson 6, are also considered endocrine glands because they secrete hormones.

CAREER FOCUS   **Professionals Who Work with the Endocrine System**

- **Medical Assistants** are a critical part of the healthcare team. They work in physicians' offices, hospitals, nursing homes, or clinics. Responsibilities may include answering phones and scheduling appointments, greeting patients, taking vital signs, explaining procedures to patients, performing tests and labs, and maintaining electronic health records (EHRs).

- **Certified Diabetes Educators (CDEs)** are licensed healthcare professionals, such as nurses, dietitians, pharmacists, podiatrists, and exercise physiologists, who have received special training in teaching diabetes self-management skills.

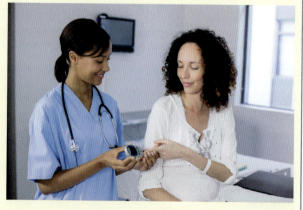

Figure 12.1 Medical assistant checking a patient's blood sugar with a glucometer.

CAREER FOCUS Professionals Who Work with the Endocrine System—cont'd

FOR MORE INFORMATION

- For more information about **Certified Diabetes Educators** visit the webpages of the National Certification Board of Diabetes Educators and the American Association of Diabetic Educators.

OBJECTIVE 1

Build, translate, pronounce, and spell medical terms built from word parts.

WORD PARTS Use the paper or online **flashcards** to familiarize yourself with the following word parts.

COMBINING FORM (WR + CV)	DEFINITION	COMBINING FORM (WR + CV)	DEFINITION
adrenal/o	adrenal gland	glyc/o	sugar
crin/o	to secrete	thym/o	thymus gland
dips/o	thirst	thyroid/o	thyroid gland
SUFFIX (S)	**DEFINITION**		
-ism	state of		

WORD PARTS PRESENTED IN PREVIOUS LESSONS Used to Build Terms for the Endocrine System

COMBINING FORM (WR+CV)	DEFINITION	COMBINING FORM (WR + CV)	DEFINITION
acr/o	extremities	path/o	disease
aden/o	gland	ur/o	urine, urination, urinary tract
SUFFIX (S)	**DEFINITION**	**SUFFIX (S)**	**DEFINITION**
-e, -y	no meaning	-itis	inflammation
-ectomy	surgical removal, excision	-logist	one who studies and treats (specialist, physician)
-emia	blood condition	-logy	study of
-ia	diseased state, condition of	-megaly	enlargement
-ic	pertaining to	-oma	tumor
PREFIX (P)	**DEFINITION**	**PREFIX (P)**	**DEFINITION**
endo-	within	hypo-	below, deficient, under
hyper-	above, excessive	poly-	many, much

Refer to Appendix A, Word Parts Used in *Basic Medical Language*, for alphabetical lists of word parts and their meanings.

EXERCISE A   **Build and Translate Terms Built from Word Parts**

*Use the **Word Parts Tables** to complete the following questions. Check your responses with the Answer Key in Appendix C.*

1. **LABEL:** *Write the combining forms for anatomical structures of the endocrine system on Figure 12.2. These anatomical combining forms will be used to build and translate medical terms in Exercise A.*

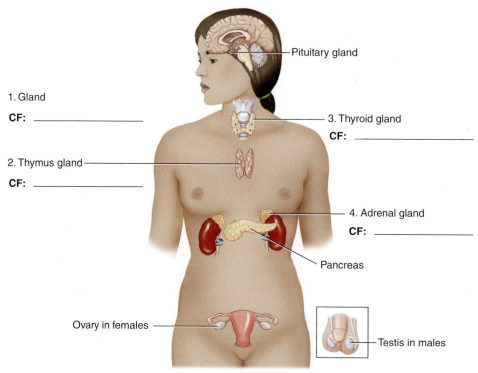

1. Gland
   CF: _____

2. Thymus gland
   CF: _____

Pituitary gland

3. Thyroid gland
   CF: _____

4. Adrenal gland
   CF: _____

Pancreas

Ovary in females

Testis in males

Figure 12.2 The endocrine system with combining forms.

2. **MATCH:** *Draw a line to match the word part with its definition.*

   a. acr/o   pertaining to
   b. -ic   tumor
   c. -itis   inflammation
   d. -ectomy   extremities
   e. -oma   enlargement
   f. -megaly   excision

3. **BUILD:** *Using the combining forms **aden/o** and **adrenal/o**, build the following terms. Remember, the definition usually starts with the meaning of the suffix.*

   a. inflammation of the adrenal gland   _____ / _____
                                                         wr   s

   b. excision of the adrenal gland   _____ / _____
                                                         wr   s

c. tumor composed of a gland (glandular tissue)

_____/_____
wr   s

d. enlargement of the extremities (and facial features)

_____/_o_/_____
wr   cv   s

e. enlargement (of one or both) of the adrenal glands

_____/_o_/_____
wr   cv   s

---

4. READ: Adrenalitis (a-drē-nal-Ī-tis) of an autoimmune origin may lead to primary adrenal insufficiency called Addison disease. An **adrenalectomy** (ad-rē-nal-EK-to-mē) may be performed to treat adrenal cancer or adrenal **adenoma** (ad-e-NŌ-ma). Adenomas are usually benign tumors and may occur in several locations in the body, including the pituitary gland, thyroid gland, and adrenal gland. They may also occur in organs such as the colon, breast, and kidney. A pituitary adenoma may excrete human growth hormone causing **acromegaly** (ak-rō-MEG-a-lē) in adults, which is evidenced by enlarged hands, feet, and facial features. Causes of **adrenomegaly** (a-drē-nō-MEG-a-lē) include infections like tuberculosis, diseases like sarcoidosis, genetic abnormalities, malignancies, and hemorrhage.

---

5. LABEL: *Write word parts to complete Figure 12.3.*

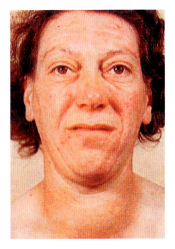

Figure 12.3 _____/o/_____ is a metabolic disorder
wr   s
characterized by marked enlargement of the bones of the face, jaw, and extremities.

---

6. TRANSLATE: *Complete the definitions of the following terms describing the thymus gland and thyroid gland. Remember, the definition usually starts with the meaning of the suffix.*

a. thym/ic   _____ to the _____ gland
b. thym/oma   _____ of the thymus _____
c. thym/ectomy   _____ of the thymus gland
d. thyroid/ectomy   _____ of the thyroid _____
e. thyroid/itis   _____ of the _____ gland

7. **READ:** Thymectomy (thī-MEK-to-mē) is a surgical procedure, which may be performed to treat **thymoma** (thī-MŌ-ma) and **thymic** (THĪ-mik) carcinoma. A **thyroidectomy** (thī-royd-EK-to-mē) may be performed to treat thyroid adenoma (nodules), thyroid cancer, goiter, and severe hyperthyroidism. **Thyroiditis** (thī-royd-Ī-tis) has many causes, including autoimmune diseases, viral and bacterial infections, drug reactions, and radiation therapy.

8. **MATCH:** *Draw a line to match the word part with its definition.*

   a. hyper-   blood condition
   b. hypo-   above, excessive
   c. -emia   sugar
   d. -ism   below, deficient, under
   e. glyc/o   state of

9. **BUILD:** *Build the following terms using the combining form **thyroid/o**.*

   a. state of excessive thyroid gland (activity)

   _____/_____/_____
      p   wr   s

   b. state of deficient thyroid gland (activity)

   _____/_____/_____
      p   wr   s

10. **READ:** In **hyperthyroidism** (hī-per-THĪ-royd-izm), an excessive amount of thyroid hormone is released into the bloodstream, potentially leading to nervousness, sleep disruption, weight loss, goiter, and other symptoms. In **hypothyroidism** (hī-pō-THĪ-royd-izm), deficient amounts of thyroid hormone are produced, potentially leading to fatigue, depression, weight gain, increased sensitivity to cold, and other symptoms.

11. **TRANSLATE:** *Complete the definitions by using the meaning of word parts to fill in the blanks.*

   a. glyc/emia   condition of _____ in the blood
   b. hyper/glyc/emia   _____ of excessive _____ in the _____
   c. hypo/glyc/emia   condition of _____ sugar in the _____

12. **READ:** **Glycemia** (glī-SĒ-mē-a) refers to the sugar level in the blood and is measured by several lab tests, including glycosylated hemoglobin (HbA1c). **Hyperglycemia** (hī-per-glī-SĒ-mē-a) is most often associated with diabetes and occurs when insulin is not available to process sugar or when it is not used effectively. **Hypoglycemia** (hī-pō-glī-SĒ-mē-a) can be a result of an overproduction of insulin, alcohol consumption, systemic infection, and hormonal imbalances. It can also be an unwanted side effect of medications used to treat diabetes.

13. **MATCH:** *Draw a line to match the word part with its definition.*

   a. poly-   thirst
   b. ur/o   many, much
   c. dips/o   diseased state, condition of
   d. -ia   urination, urine, urinary tract

14. BUILD: *Write word parts to build the following terms.*

    a. condition of much thirst   _____/_____/_____

                                              p   wr   s

    b. condition of much urine   _____/_____/_____

                                              p   wr   s

15. READ: **Polydipsia** (pol-ē-DIP-sē-a), or excessive thirst, may be a symptom of hyperglycemia. **Polyuria** (pol-ē-Ū-rē-a) refers to increased amount of urine. Polydipsia and polyuria are common symptoms of diabetes mellitus.

16. MATCH: *Draw a line to match the word part with its definition.*

    a. endo-   to secrete

    b. crin/o   disease

    c. path/o   within

    d. -logist   one who studies and treats (specialist, physician)

    e. -logy   no meaning

    f. -e, -y   study of

17. TRANSLATE: *Complete the definitions by using the meaning of word parts to fill in the blanks.*

    a. endo/crin/e   to _____ within

    b. endo/crin/o/logy   _____ of the endocrine system

    c. endo/crin/o/logist   physician who _____and treats diseases of the _____ system

    d. endo/crin/o/path/y   (any) _____ of the endocrine _____

> **FYI**   The combination of the prefix **endo-** and the combining form **crin/o** will be translated as **endocrine system** in terms with suffixes or combining forms that add meaning. Examples include: endocrinology, endocrinologist, and endocrinopathy.

18. READ: The **endocrine** (EN-dō-krin) system is made up of glands that "secrete within" the body by releasing hormones directly into the bloodstream. **Endocrinopathy** (en-dō-kri-NOP-a-thē) refers to disease processes of the endocrine system, which usually manifest as hormonal imbalances. **Endocrinology** (en-dō-kri-NOL-o-jē) is the subspecialty of internal medicine focused on diagnosing and treating endocrinopathies. An **endocrinologist** (en-dō-kri-NOL-o-jist) is a physician who cares for patients affected by disease and disorders of the endocrine system.

19. REVIEW OF ENDOCRINE SYSTEM TERMS BUILT FROM WORD PARTS: *the following is an alphabetical list of terms built and translated in the previous exercises.*

MEDICAL TERMS BUILT FROM WORD PARTS

TERM	DEFINITION	TERM	DEFINITION
1. acromegaly (ak-rō-MEG-a-lē)	enlargement of the extremities (and facial features) (Figure 12.3)	**12. hyperthyroidism** (hī-per-THĪ-royd-izm)	state of excessive thyroid activity
2. adenoma (ad-e-NŌ-ma)	tumor composed of a gland (glandular tissue)	**13. hypoglycemia** (hī-pō-glī-SĒ-mē-a)	condition of deficient sugar in the blood
3. adrenalectomy (ad-rē-nal-EK-to-mē)	excision of the adrenal gland	**14. hypothyroidism** (hī-pō-THĪ-royd-izm)	state of deficient thyroid activity
4. adrenalitis (a-drē-nal-Ī-tis)	inflammation of the adrenal gland	**15. polydipsia** (pol-ē-DIP-sē-a)	condition of much thirst
5. adrenomegaly (a-drē-nō-MEG-a-lē)	enlargement (of one or both) of the adrenal glands	**16. polyuria** (pol-ē-Ū-rē-a)	condition of much urine
6. endocrine (EN-dō-krin)	to secrete within	**17. thymectomy** (thī-MEK-to-mē)	excision of the thymus gland
7. endocrinologist (en-dō-kri-NOL-o-jist)	physician who studies and treats disease of the endocrine system	**18. thymic** (THĪ-mik)	pertaining to the thymus gland
8. endocrinology (en-dō-kri-NOL-o-jē)	study of the endocrine system	**19. thymoma** (thī-MŌ-ma)	tumor of the thymus gland
9. endocrinopathy (en-dō-kri-NOP-a-thē)	(any) disease of the endocrine system	**20. thyroidectomy** (thī-royd-EK-to-mē)	excision of the thyroid gland
10. glycemia (glī-SĒ-mē-a)	condition of sugar in the blood	**21. thyroiditis** (thī-royd-Ī-tis)	inflammation of the thyroid gland
11. hyperglycemia (hī-per-glī-SĒ-mē-a)	condition of excessive sugar in the blood		

EXERCISE B   Pronounce and Spell Terms Built from Word Parts

Practice pronunciation and spelling on paper and online.

1. Practice on Paper

    a. Pronounce: Read the phonetic spelling and say aloud the terms listed in the previous table, Review of Terms Built from Word Parts.

    b. Spell: Have a study partner read the terms aloud. Write the spelling of the terms on a separate sheet of paper.

2. **Practice Online**

   a. **Access** online learning resources. Go to evolve.elsevier.com > Evolve Resources > Practice Student Resources.

   b. **Pronounce**: Select Audio Glossary > Lesson 12 > Exercise B. Select a term to hear its pronunciation and repeat aloud.

   c. **Spell**: Select Activities > Lesson 12 > Spell Terms > Exercise B. Select the audio icon and type the correct spelling of the term.

❏   Check the box when complete.

OBJECTIVE 2

Define, pronounce, and spell medical terms NOT built from word parts.

The terms listed below may contain word parts, but are difficult to translate literally.

MEDICAL TERMS NOT BUILT FROM WORD PARTS

TERM	DEFINITION
Addison disease (AD-i-sun) (di-ZĒZ)	chronic syndrome resulting from a deficiency in the hormonal secretion of the adrenal gland with symptoms of weight loss, hypotension, and skin darkening (also called **primary adrenal insufficiency**)
diabetes mellitus (DM) (dī-a-BĒ-tēz) (MEL-li-tus)	chronic disease involving a disorder of carbohydrate metabolism caused by underactivity of the insulin-producing islets of Langerhans (Figure 12.4) in the pancreas and characterized by elevated blood sugar; it can also be caused by resistance of the tissues to insulin.
fasting blood sugar (FBS) (FAST-ing) (blud) (SHOO-ger)	blood test to determine the amount of glucose (sugar) in the blood after fasting for 8 to 10 hours. Elevation may indicate diabetes mellitus.
fine needle aspiration (FNA) (FĪN) (NĒ-del) (as-pi-RĀ-shen)	biopsy technique that uses a narrow hollow needle to obtain tiny amounts of tissue for pathologic examination. Thyroid nodules are frequently biopsied using FNA.
glycosylated hemoglobin (HbA1c) (glī-KŌ-sa-lāt-ad) (HĒ-mō-glō-bin)	blood test used to diagnose diabetes and monitor its treatment by measuring the amount of glucose (sugar) bound to hemoglobin in the blood; provides an indication of blood sugar level over the past three months, covering the 120-day lifespan of the red blood cell (also called **glycated hemoglobin**, **hemoglobin A1c**)
goiter (GOY-ter)	enlargement of the thyroid gland
Graves disease (grāvz) (di-ZĒZ)	disorder of the thyroid gland characterized by the presence of hyperthyroidism, goiter, and exophthalmos (protrusion of the eyes)
metabolic syndrome (met-a-BOL-ik) (SIN-drōm)	group of signs and symptoms including insulin resistance, obesity characterized by excessive fat around the area of the waist and abdomen, hypertension, hyperglycemia, elevated triglycerides, and low levels of the "good" cholesterol HDL (also called **syndrome X** and **insulin resistance syndrome**)

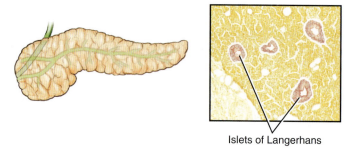

Islets of Langerhans

Figure 12.4 Pancreas, with islets of Langerhans.

FYI   Diabetes Mellitus

Two major forms of diabetes mellitus are **type 1**, previously called insulin-dependent diabetes mellitus (IDDM) or juvenile-onset diabetes, and **type 2**, previously called noninsulin-dependent diabetes mellitus (NIDDM) or adult-onset diabetes mellitus (AODM). Type 2 diabetes mellitus has reached epidemic proportions and is a major cause of cardiovascular disease.

Type 1 Diabetes Mellitus

Cause	beta cells of the pancreas that produce insulin are destroyed and eventually no insulin is produced
Characteristics	abrupt onset, occurs primarily in childhood or adolescence; patients often are thin
Symptoms	polyuria, polydipsia, weight loss, hyperglycemia, acidosis, and ketosis
Treatment	insulin injections and diet

Type 2 Diabetes Mellitus

Cause	resistance of body cells to the action of insulin, which may eventually lead to a decrease in insulin secretion
Characteristics	slow onset, usually occurs in adults; many patients are obese
Symptoms	fatigue, blurred vision, polydipsia, and hyperglycemia; may have neural or vascular complications
Treatment	diet, exercise, oral or injected medication, and perhaps insulin

Long-Term Complications of Diabetes Mellitus
Macrovascular Complications
• coronary artery disease → myocardial infarction
• cerebrovascular disease → stroke
• peripheral artery disease → leg pain when walking (intermittent vascular claudication)

Microvascular Complications
• diabetic retinopathy → loss of vision
• diabetic nephropathy → chronic kidney disease, renal failure
• neuropathy → loss of feeling in extremities, amputation

EXERCISE C   Label

Write the medical terms pictured and defined using the previous table of Medical Terms NOT Built from Word Parts. Check your work with the Answer Key in Appendix C.

1. _____

disorder of the thyroid gland characterized by the presence of hyperthyroidism, goiter, and exophthalmos (protrusion of the eyes)

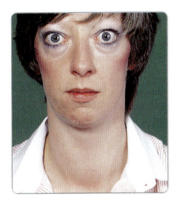

2. _____

group of signs and symptoms including insulin resistance, obesity characterized by excessive fat around the area of the waist and abdomen, hypertension, hyperglycemia, elevated triglycerides, and low levels of the "good" cholesterol HDL

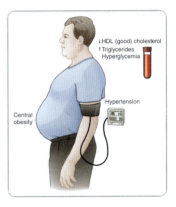

3. _____

enlargement of the thyroid gland

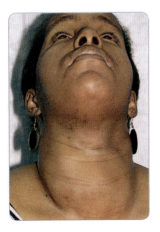

4. _____

chronic syndrome resulting from a deficiency in a hormonal section of the adrenal gland with symptoms of weight loss, hypotension, and skin darkening

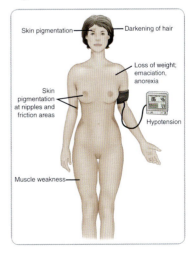

EXERCISE D   Learn Medical Terms NOT Built from Word Parts

Fill in the blanks with medical terms defined in bold using the Medical Terms NOT Built from Word Parts table. Answers are listed in Appendix C.

1. The **chronic disease involving a disorder of carbohydrate metabolism caused by underactivity of the insulin-producing islets of Langerhans in the pancreas and characterized by elevated blood sugar**, or _____ may be diagnosed based on the results of the glucose tolerance test, the **blood test to determine the amount of glucose (sugar) in the blood after fasting for 8 to 10 hours**, or _____, and the **blood test used to diagnose diabetes and monitor its treatment by measuring the amount of glucose (sugar) bound to hemoglobin in the blood**, or _____. After a diabetes diagnosis, the HbA1c will likely be ordered by a provider two to four times a year to monitor effectiveness of treatment over time.

2. **Enlargement of the thyroid gland**, or _____, may occur when the thyroid gland cannot produce enough hormones to meet the body's needs. If symptoms become significant, such as breathing difficulties, a thyroidectomy may be performed.

3. Goiter may be a symptom of a **disorder of the thyroid gland characterized by the presence of hyperthyroidism, goiter, and exophthalmos**, or _____. Goiter may also be caused by thyroiditis or a thyroid nodule, which is a mass on the thyroid gland that can sometimes be palpated.

4. A patient with a diagnosis of **chronic syndrome resulting from a deficiency in the hormonal secretion of the adrenal gland**, or _____, may have weakness, darkening of skin, loss of appetite, and/or depression.

5. **Biopsy technique that uses a narrow hollow needle to obtain tiny amounts of tissue for pathologic examination**, or _____, is frequently performed on thyroid nodules. Small biopsy needles are used to obtain multiple tissue samples, which are sent to the pathologist to evaluate for the possibility of malignant cells.

6. **Group of signs and symptoms including insulin resistance, obesity characterized by excessive fat around the area of the waist and abdomen, hypertension, hyperglycemia, elevated triglycerides, and low levels of the "good" cholesterol HDL**, or _____, increases the risks of developing type 2 diabetes mellitus, coronary artery disease, or stroke.

EXERCISE E   Pronounce and Spell Terms NOT Built from Word Parts

Practice pronunciation and spelling on paper and online.

1. Practice on Paper
    a. **Pronounce**: Read the phonetic spelling and say aloud the terms listed in the previous table, Medical Terms NOT Built from Word Parts.
    b. **Spell**: Have a study partner read the terms aloud. Write the spelling of the terms on a separate sheet of paper.

2. **Practice Online**

    a. **Access** online learning resources. Go to evolve.elsevier.com > Evolve Resources > Practice Student Resources.

    b. **Pronounce**: Select Audio Glossary > Lesson 12 > Exercise E. Select a term to hear its pronunciation and repeat aloud.

    c. **Spell**: Select Activities > Lesson 12 > Spell Terms > Exercise E . Select the audio icon and type the correct spelling of the term.

❏ Check the box when complete.

OBJECTIVE 3

Write abbreviations.

ABBREVIATIONS RELATED TO THE ENDOCRINE SYSTEM

Use the online **flashcards** to familiarize yourself with the following abbreviations.

ABBREVIATION	TERM	ABBREVIATION	TERM
DM	diabetes mellitus	**HbA1c**	glycosylated hemoglobin
FBS	fasting blood sugar	**T1DM**	type 1 diabetes mellitus
FNA	fine needle aspiration	**T2DM**	type 2 diabetes mellitus

EXERCISE F   Abbreviate Medical Terms

Write the correct abbreviation next to its medical term.

1. Diseases and Disorders:

    a. _____   diabetes mellitus

    b. _____   type 1 diabetes mellitus

    c. _____   type 2 diabetes mellitus

2. Diagnostic Tests:

    a. _____   fasting blood sugar

    b. _____   glycosylated hemoglobin

    c. _____   fine needle aspiration

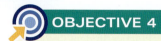

OBJECTIVE 4

Identify medical terms by clinical category.

Now that you have worked through the lesson on the endocrine system, review and practice medical terms grouped by clinical category. Categories include signs and symptoms, diseases and disorders, diagnostic tests, surgical procedures, specialties and professions, and other terms related to the endocrine system. Check your responses with the Answer Key in Appendix C.

EXERCISE G   Signs and Symptoms

Write the medical terms for signs and symptoms next to their definitions.

1. _____   condition of excessive sugar in the blood

2. _____   condition of deficient sugar in the blood

3. _____   condition of much thirst

4. _____   condition of much urine

5. _____   enlargement (of one or both) of the adrenal glands

EXERCISE H   Diseases and Disorders

Write the medical terms for diseases and disorders next to their definitions.

1. _____   (any) disease of the endocrine system

2. _____   chronic syndrome resulting from a deficiency in the hormonal secretion of the adrenal gland

3. _____   inflammation of the adrenal gland

4. _____   disorder of the thyroid gland characterized by the presence of hyperthyroidism, goiter, and exophthalmos (protrusion of the eyes)

5. _____   enlargement of the thyroid gland

6. _____   state of excessive thyroid activity

7. _____   state of deficient thyroid activity

8. _____   tumor composed of a gland (glandular tissue)

9. _____   enlargement of the extremities (and facial features)

10. _____   tumor of the thymus gland

11. _____   inflammation of the thyroid gland

12. _____ chronic disease involving a disorder of carbohydrate
metabolism caused by underactivity of the insulin-producing
islets of Langerhans in the pancreas and characterized by
elevated blood sugar

13. _____ group of signs and symptoms including insulin resistance,
obesity characterized by excessive fat around the area of the
waist and abdomen, hypertension, hyperglycemia, elevated
triglycerides, and low levels of the "good" cholesterol HDL

EXERCISE I   Diagnostic Tests

Write the medical terms for diagnostic tests and equipment next to their definitions.

1. _____ blood test used to diagnose diabetes and monitor its treatment
by measuring the amount of glucose (sugar) bound to
hemoglobin in the blood

2. _____ blood test to determine the amount of glucose (sugar) in the
blood after fasting for 8 to 10 hours

3. _____ biopsy technique that uses a narrow hollow needle to obtain
tiny amounts of tissue for pathologic examination

EXERCISE J   Surgical Procedures

Write the medical terms for surgical procedures next to their definitions.

1. _____ excision of the adrenal gland

2. _____ excision of the thymus gland

3. _____ excision of the thyroid gland

EXERCISE K   Specialties and Professions

Write the medical terms for specialties and professions next to their definitions.

1. _____ physician who studies and treats diseases of the endocrine
system

2. _____ study of the endocrine system

EXERCISE L   Medical Terms Related to the Endocrine System

Write the medical terms related to the endocrine system next to their definitions.

1. _____ to secrete within

2. _____ condition of sugar in the blood

3. _____ pertaining to the thymus gland

OBJECTIVE 5

Use medical language in clinical statements, the case study, and a medical record.

Check responses for the following exercises in Appendix C.

EXERCISE M   Use Medical Terms in Clinical Statements

Circle the medical terms and abbreviations defined in the bolded phrases. For pronunciation practice read the answers aloud.

1. A **biopsy technique that uses a narrow hollow needle to obtain tiny amounts of tissue for pathologic examination** (glycosylated hemoglobin, fine needle aspiration, fasting blood sugar) is frequently performed on thyroid nodules. Sonography is often used to localize the lesion. The procedure may be performed by a(n) **physician who studies and treats diseases of the endocrine system** (endocrinologist, pathologist, hematologist), or by a radiologist.

2. Unlike the results of **fasting blood sugar** (HbA1c, FNA, FBS), **glycosylated hemoglobin** (HbA1c, FNA, FBS) test results are not altered by what was eaten prior to the test.

3. **Condition of much thirst** (Polyuria, Polydipsia, Polyneuritis) and **condition of much urine** (polyuria, polydipsia, polyneuritis) may be caused by uncontrolled diabetes mellitus.

4. Graves disease is characterized by **state of excessive thyroid activity** (hypoglycemia, hyperthyroidism, hypothyroidism), **enlargement of the thyroid gland** (adenoma, goiter, acromegaly), and exophthalmos.

5. **Pertaining to the thymus gland** (Glycemia, Thymic, Endocrine) hypoplasia is a congenital condition caused by the absence or underdevelopment of the thymus gland.

6. A pituitary **tumor composed of a glandular tissue** (adrenalitis, thymoma, adenoma) can lead to an overproduction of growth hormone, which may cause **enlargement of the extremities** (thyroiditis, goiter, acromegaly) in adults, which primarily affects the bones of the hands, feet, and jaw.

7. Autoimmune **inflammation of the adrenal gland** (adenoma, thyroiditis, adrenalitis) is a common cause of **chronic syndrome resulting from a deficiency in the hormonal secretion of the adrenal gland** (diabetes mellitus, Addison disease, Graves disease).

EXERCISE N   Apply Medical Terms to the Case Study

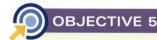

Think back to Nascha introduced in the case study at the beginning of the lesson. After working through Lesson 12 on the endocrine system, consider the medical terms that might be used to describe her experiences. List two terms relevant to the case study and their meanings. ■

Medical Term	Definition
1. _____	_____
2. _____	_____

EXERCISE O   **Use Medical Terms in a Document**

Nascha was able to see a healthcare provider. The following medical record documents her experiences.

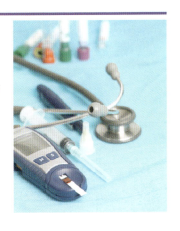

Use the definitions in numbers 1-9 to write medical terms within the history and physical report on the next page.

1. condition of much urine

2. condition of much thirst

3. disorder of the thyroid gland characterized by the presence of hyperthyroidism, goiter, and exophthalmos

4. chronic disease involving a disorder of carbohydrate metabolism and characterized by elevated blood sugar

5. blood test to determine the amount of glucose (sugar) in the blood after fasting for 8 to 10 hours

6. blood test used to diagnose diabetes and monitor its treatment by measuring the amount of glucose (sugar) bound to hemoglobin in the blood

7. condition of excessive sugar in the blood

8. condition of deficient sugar in the blood

9. study of the endocrine system

Refer to the History and Physical on the next page to answer questions 10 and 11.

10. Several terms used in the medical record were presented in previous lessons. Can you identify them and recall their meanings? Identify two.

Medical Term   **Definition**

1. _____   _____

2. _____   _____

11. Identify two new medical terms in the medical record you would like to investigate. Use your medical dictionary or an online reference to look up the definitions.

Medical Term   **Definition**

1. _____   _____

2. _____   _____

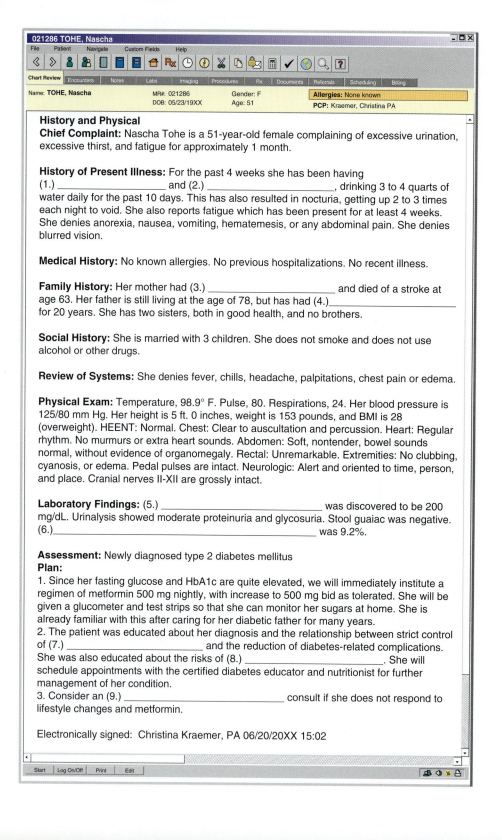

021286 TOHE, Nascha

File   Patient   Navigate   Custom Fields   Help

Chart Review | Encounters | Notes | Labs | Imaging | Procedures | Rx | Documents | Referrals | Scheduling | Billing

Name: **TOHE, Nascha**   MR#: 021286   Gender: F   **Allergies:** None known
                                DOB: 05/23/19XX   Age: 51   PCP: Kraemer, Christina PA

History and Physical

Chief Complaint: Nascha Tohe is a 51-year-old female complaining of excessive urination, excessive thirst, and fatigue for approximately 1 month.

History of Present Illness: For the past 4 weeks she has been having (1.) _____ and (2.) _____, drinking 3 to 4 quarts of water daily for the past 10 days. This has also resulted in nocturia, getting up 2 to 3 times each night to void. She also reports fatigue which has been present for at least 4 weeks. She denies anorexia, nausea, vomiting, hematemesis, or any abdominal pain. She denies blurred vision.

Medical History: No known allergies. No previous hospitalizations. No recent illness.

Family History: Her mother had (3.) _____ and died of a stroke at age 63. Her father is still living at the age of 78, but has had (4.)_____ for 20 years. She has two sisters, both in good health, and no brothers.

Social History: She is married with 3 children. She does not smoke and does not use alcohol or other drugs.

Review of Systems: She denies fever, chills, headache, palpitations, chest pain or edema.

Physical Exam: Temperature, 98.9° F. Pulse, 80. Respirations, 24. Her blood pressure is 125/80 mm Hg. Her height is 5 ft. 0 inches, weight is 153 pounds, and BMI is 28 (overweight). HEENT: Normal. Chest: Clear to auscultation and percussion. Heart: Regular rhythm. No murmurs or extra heart sounds. Abdomen: Soft, nontender, bowel sounds normal, without evidence of organomegaly. Rectal: Unremarkable. Extremities: No clubbing, cyanosis, or edema. Pedal pulses are intact. Neurologic: Alert and oriented to time, person, and place. Cranial nerves II-XII are grossly intact.

Laboratory Findings: (5.) _____ was discovered to be 200 mg/dL. Urinalysis showed moderate proteinuria and glycosuria. Stool guaiac was negative. (6.)_____ was 9.2%.

Assessment: Newly diagnosed type 2 diabetes mellitus
Plan:
1. Since her fasting glucose and HbA1c are quite elevated, we will immediately institute a regimen of metformin 500 mg nightly, with increase to 500 mg bid as tolerated. She will be given a glucometer and test strips so that she can monitor her sugars at home. She is already familiar with this after caring for her diabetic father for many years.
2. The patient was educated about her diagnosis and the relationship between strict control of (7.) _____ and the reduction of diabetes-related complications. She was also educated about the risks of (8.) _____. She will schedule appointments with the certified diabetes educator and nutritionist for further management of her condition.
3. Consider an (9.) _____ consult if she does not respond to lifestyle changes and metformin.

Electronically signed: Christina Kraemer, PA 06/20/20XX 15:02

Start | Log On/Off | Print | Edit

EXERCISE P   **Use Medical Language in Electronic Health Records Online**

Select the correct medical terms to complete three medical records in one patient's electronic file

 Access online resources at evolve.elsevier.com > Evolve Resources > Practice Student Resources > Activities > Lesson 12 > Electronic Health Records .

Topic: Thymoma
Record 1: Pre-operative Note
Record 2: Radiology Report
Record 3: Pathology Report

❏   Check the box when complete.

OBJECTIVE 6

Recall and assess knowledge of word parts, medical terms, and abbreviations.

EXERCISE Q   **Online Review of Lesson Content**

 Recall and assess your learning from working through the lesson by completing learning activities at evolve.elsevier. com > Evolve Resources > Practice Student Resources. Keep track of your progress by placing a check mark next to completed activities.

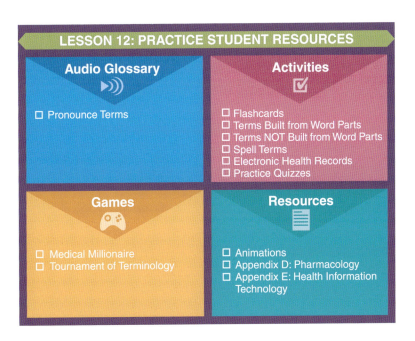

LESSON 12: PRACTICE STUDENT RESOURCES

Audio Glossary
▶))

❏ Pronounce Terms

Activities
☑

❏ Flashcards
❏ Terms Built from Word Parts
❏ Terms NOT Built from Word Parts
❏ Spell Terms
❏ Electronic Health Records
❏ Practice Quizzes

Games
🎮

❏ Medical Millionaire
❏ Tournament of Terminology

Resources
📄

❏ Animations
❏ Appendix D: Pharmacology
❏ Appendix E: Health Information
   Technology

EXERCISE R Lesson Content Quiz

Test your knowledge of the terms and abbreviations introduced in this lesson. Circle the letter for the medical term or abbreviation related to the words in italics.

1. *Enlargement of the extremities (and facial features) is usually a result of excess human growth hormone in adults,* while gigantism is due to excess growth hormone before puberty.
   a. adrenomegaly
   b. acromegaly
   c. adrenalitis

2. Myasthenia gravis, an autoimmune disorder affecting the connection between nerves and muscles, is associated with thymus abnormalities. *Excision of the thymus gland* is frequently required in these patients.
   a. thymectomy
   b. thyroidectomy
   c. adrenalectomy

3. *Condition of much urine* and *condition of much thirst* are two common initial symptoms of diabetes mellitus.
   a. polydipsia; polyuria
   b. polyuria; polydipsia
   c. polysomnia; polydipsia

4. *A blood test to determine the amount of glucose (sugar) in the blood after fasting for 8-10 hours* is very important in helping patients manage their diabetes treatment.
   a. HbA1c
   b. FNA
   c. FBS

5. An increase in the risk of type 2 diabetes mellitus, coronary heart disease, and stroke is associated with *group of signs and symptoms including insulin resistance, obesity characterized by excessive fat around the area of the waist and abdomen, hypertension, hyperglycemia, elevated triglycerides, and low levels of the "good" cholesterol HDL.*
   a. metabolic syndrome
   b. Addison disease
   c. Graves disease

6. *Disorder of the thyroid gland characterized by the presence of hyperthyroidism, goiter, and exophthalmos* and Hashimoto thyroiditis are both autoimmune diseases affecting the thyroid.
   a. hyperglycemia
   b. Graves disease
   c. hypothyroidism

7. A(n) *physician who studies and treats diseases of the endocrine system* may treat thyroid disease, diabetes mellitus, or any other *disease of the endocrine system* such as Addison disease or Cushing syndrome.
   a. dermatologist; dermatopathy
   b. endocrinology; endocrinologist
   c. endocrinologist; endocrinopathy

8. A fine needle aspiration of the thyroid may be performed to help distinguish between a(n) *tumor composed of a gland* and thyroid carcinoma.
   a. adenoma
   b. thymoma
   c. hematoma

LESSON AT A GLANCE ENDOCRINE SYSTEM WORD PARTS

COMBINING FORMS

adrenal/o	glyc/o
crin/o	thym/o
dips/o	thyroid/o

SUFFIX

-ism

LESSON AT A GLANCE ENDOCRINE SYSTEM MEDICAL TERMS AND ABBREVIATIONS

SIGNS AND SYMPTOMS

adrenomegaly
hyperglycemia
hypoglycemia
polydipsia
polyuria

DISEASES AND DISORDERS

acromegaly
Addison disease
adenoma
adrenalitis
diabetes mellitus (DM)
endocrinopathy
goiter
Graves disease

hyperthyroidism
hypothyroidism
metabolic syndrome
thymoma
thyroiditis

DIAGNOSTIC TESTS AND EQUIPMENT

fasting blood sugar (FBS)
fine needle aspiration (FNA)
glycosylated hemoglobin (HbA1c)

SURGICAL PROCEDURES

adrenalectomy
thymectomy
thyroidectomy

SPECIALTIES AND PROFESSIONS

endocrinologist
endocrinology

RELATED TERMS

endocrine
glycemia
thymic

ABBREVIATIONS

DM	HbA1c
FBS	T1DM
FNA	T2DM

WORD PART	TYPE	DEFINITION	LESSON
a-	prefix	absence of, without	4
-a	suffix	no meaning	3
abdomin/o	combining form	abdomen, abdominal cavity	8
-ac	suffix	pertaining to	7
acr/o	combining form	extremities	3
-ad	suffix	toward	2
aden/o	combining form	gland(s); (node(s) when combined with lymph/o)	7
adrenal/o	combining form	adrenal gland	12
-al	suffix	pertaining to	1,2
-algia	suffix	pain	8
an-	prefix	absence of, without	4
an/o	combining form	anus	8
angi/o	combining form	blood vessel(s)	7
anter/o	combining form	front	2
append/o	combining form	appendix	8
appendic/o	combining form	appendix	8
arteri/o	combining form	artery (*s.*), arteries (*pl.*)	7
arthr/o	combining form	joint(s)	10
-ary	suffix	pertaining to	4
-asthenia	suffix	weakness	10
audi/o	combining form	hearing	9
blephar/o	combining form	eyelid	9
brady-	prefix	slow	7
bronch/o	combining form	bronchus (s), bronchi (pl)	4

WORD PART	TYPE	DEFINITION	LESSON
burs/o	combining form	bursa	10
capn/o	combining form	carbon dioxide	4
carcin/o	combining form	cancer	1
cardi/o	combining form	heart	7
carp/o	combining form	carpals, wrist (bone)	10
caud/o	combining form	tail (downward)	2
-cele	suffix	hernia, protrusion	6
-centesis	suffix	surgical puncture to remove fluid (with a sterile needle)	4
cephal/o	combining form	head (upward)	2
cerebr/o	combining form	cerebrum, brain	11
cervic/o	combining form	cervix (or neck)	6
chol/e	combining form	gall, bile	8
chondr/o	combining form	cartilage	10
col/o	combining form	colon	8
colon/o	combining form	colon	8
colp/o	combining form	vagina	6
cost/o	combining form	rib(s)	10
crani/o	combining form	skull (cranium)	10
crin/o	combining form	to secrete	12
cutane/o	combining form	skin	3

WORD PART	TYPE	DEFINITION	LESSON
cyan/o	combining form	blue	3
cyst/o	combining form	bladder, sac	5
cyt/o	combining form	cell(s)	1
derm/o	combining form	skin	3
dermat/o	combining form	skin	3
-desis	suffix	surgical fixation, fusion	10
dips/o	combining form	thirst	12
dist/o	combining form	away (from the point of attachment)	2
dors/o	combining form	back	2
duoden/o	combining form	duodenum	8
dys-	prefix	difficult, painful, abnormal	4
-e	suffix	no meaning	3
-eal	suffix	pertaining to	4
ech/o	combining form	sound	7
-ectomy	suffix	surgical removal, excision	4
electr/o	combining form	electrical activity	7
-emia	suffix	blood condition	5
encephal/o	combining form	brain	11
endo-	prefix	within	4
endometri/o	combining form	endometrium	6
enter/o	combining form	intestines (the small intestine)	8
epi-	prefix	on, upon, over	3
epitheli/o	combining form	epithelium, epithelial tissue	1
erythr/o	combining form	red	3
esophag/o	combining form	esophagus	8
femor/o	combining form	femur (upper leg bone)	10
gastr/o	combining form	stomach	8

WORD PART	TYPE	DEFINITION	LESSON
-genic	suffix	producing, originating, causing	1
gingiv/o	combining form	gums	8
gloss/o	combining form	tongue	8
glyc/o	combining form	sugar	12
-gram	suffix	record, radiographic image	4
-graph	suffix	instrument used to record	7
-graphy	suffix	process of recording, radiographic imaging	4
gynec/o	combining form	woman	6
hem/o	combining form	blood	5
hemat/o	combining form	blood	5
hemi-	prefix	half	11
hepat/o	combining form	liver	8
hist/o	combining form	tissue(s)	1
hydr/o	combining form	water	5
hyper-	prefix	above, excessive	4
hypo-	prefix	below, deficient, under	3
hyster/o	combining form	uterus	6
-ia	suffix	diseased state, condition of	4
-iasis	suffix	condition	5
-ic	suffix	pertaining to	2
ile/o	combining form	ileum	8
ili/o	combining form	ilium (upper, wing-shaped part on each side of the pelvis)	10
infer/o	combining form	below	2
inter-	prefix	between	10
intra-	prefix	within	3
-ior	suffix	pertaining to	2

WORD PART	TYPE	DEFINITION	LESSON
ir/o	combining form	iris	9
irid/o	combining form	iris	9
ischi/o	combining form	ischium (lower, posterior portion of the pelvis on which one sits)	10
-ism	suffix	state of	12
-itis	suffix	inflammation	3
jejun/o	combining form	jejunum	8
kerat/o	combining form	cornea (also means hard, horny tissue)	9
kinesi/o	combining form	movement, motion	10
kyph/o	combining form	hump (thoracic spine)	10
lapar/o	combining form	abdomen, abdominal cavity	8
laryng/o	combining form	larynx (voice box)	4
later/o	combining form	side	2
leuk/o	combining form	white	3
lingu/o	combining form	tongue	8
lip/o	combining form	fat, fat tissue	1
lith/o	combining form	stone(s), calculus (pl. calculi)	5
-logist	suffix	one who studies and treats (specialist, physician)	1
-logy	suffix	study of	1
lord/o	combining form	bent forward (lumbar spine)	10
lymph/o	combining form	lymph, lymphatic tissue	7
-lysis	suffix	dissolution, separating	3
-malacia	suffix	softening	10
mamm/o	combining form	breast	6
mast/o	combining form	breast	6
meat/o	combining form	meatus (opening)	5

WORD PART	TYPE	DEFINITION	LESSON
medi/o	combining form	middle	2
-megaly	suffix	enlargement	7
melan/o	combining form	black	3
men/o	combining form	menstruation, menstrual	6
mening/o	combining form	meninges	11
meningi/o	combining form	meninges	11
meta-	prefix	beyond	1
-meter	suffix	instrument used to measure	4
-metry	suffix	measurement	9
micro-	prefix	small	11
muc/o	combining form	mucus	4
my/o	combining form	muscle(s), muscle tissue	1
myc/o	combining form	fungus	3
myel/o	combining form	spinal cord	11
myring/o	combining form	eardrum (tympanic membrane)	9
nas/o	combining form	nose	4
necr/o	combining form	death	10
neo-	prefix	new	1
nephr/o	combining form	kidney	5
neur/o	combining form	nerve(s), nerve tissue	1
noct/i	combining form	night	5
-oid	suffix	resembling	1
olig/o	combining form	scanty, few	5
-oma	suffix	tumor	1
onc/o	combining form	tumor(s)	1
onych/o	combining form	nail	3
oophor/o	combining form	ovary	6

WORD PART	TYPE	DEFINITION	LESSON
ophthalm/o	combining form	eye	9
opt/o	combining form	vision	9
or/o	combining form	mouth	8
orchi/o	combining form	testis (testicle)	6
-osis	suffix	abnormal condition	3
oste/o	combining form	bone(s)	10
ot/o	combining form	ear	9
-ous	suffix	pertaining to	3
ox/i	combining form	oxygen	4
pancreat/o	combining form	pancreas	8
path/o	combining form	disease	1
-penia	suffix	abnormal reduction (in number)	7
peps/o	combining form	digestion	8
per-	prefix	through	3
-pexy	suffix	surgical fixation, suspension	6
phag/o	combining form	swallowing, eating	8
phalang/o	combining form	phalanx (*pl.* phalanges) (any bone of the fingers or toes)	10
pharyng/o	combining form	pharynx (throat)	4
phas/o	combining form	speech	11
phleb/o	combining form	vein(s)	7
-plasm	suffix	growth (substance or formation)	1
-plasty	suffix	surgical repair	5
pleg/o	combining form	paralysis	11
-plegia	suffix	paralysis	9
-pnea	suffix	breathing	4

WORD PART	TYPE	DEFINITION	LESSON
pneum/o	combining form	lung, air	4
pneumon/o	combining form	lung, air	4
poli/o	combining form	gray matter	11
poly-	prefix	many, much	4
poster/o	combining form	back, behind	2
proct/o	combining form	rectum	8
prostat/o	combining form	prostate gland	6
proxim/o	combining form	near (the point of attachment	2
psych/o	combining form	mind	11
-ptosis	suffix	drooping, sagging, prolapse	9
pub/o	combining form	pubis (anterior portion of the pelvis)	10
pulmon/o	combining form	lung	4
py/o	combining form	pus	5
pyel/o	combining form	renal pelvis	5
quadr/i	combining form	four	11
rachi/o	combining form	vertebra, spine, vertebral column	10
radi/o	combining form	x-rays (ionizing radiation)	1
rect/o	combining form	rectum	8
ren/o	combining form	kidney	5
retin/o	combining form	retina	9
rhin/o	combining form	nose	4
-rrhagia	suffix	rapid flow of blood, excessive bleeding	4
-rrhaphy	suffix	suturing, repairing	6
-rrhea	suffix	flow, discharge	4
-rrhexis	suffix	rupture	6

WORD PART	TYPE	DEFINITION	LESSON
salping/o	combining form	uterine tube (fallopian tube)	6
sarc/o	combining form	flesh, connective tissue	1
-schisis	suffix	split, fissure	10
scler/o	combining form	sclera	9
-sclerosis	suffix	hardening	7
scoli/o	combining form	crooked, curved (spine)	10
-scope	suffix	instrument used for visual examination	4
-scopic	suffix	pertaining to visual examination	4
-scopy	suffix	visual examination	4
scrot/o	combining form	scrotum	6
sigmoid/o	combining form	sigmoid colon	8
sinus/o	combining form	sinus (s), sinuses (pl)	4
somn/o	combining form	sleep	4
son/o	combining form	sound	6
spir/o	combining form	breathe, breathing	4
splen/o	combining form	spleen	7
spondyl/o	combining form	vertebra, spine, vertebral column	10
-stasis	suffix	control, stop	1
stern/o	combining form	sternum (breast bone)	10
-stomy	suffix	creation of an artifical opening	4
sub-	prefix	below, under	3
super/o	combining form	above	2
tachy-	prefix	rapid, fast	7
ten/o	combining form	tendon(s)	10
tendin/o	combining form	tendon(s)	10

WORD PART	TYPE	DEFINITION	LESSON
thorac/o	combining form	chest, chest cavity	4
-thorax	suffix	chest, chest cavity	4
thromb/o	combining form	blood clot	7
thym/o	combining form	thymus gland	12
thyroid/o	combining form	thyroid gland	12
-tomy	suffix	cut into, incision	4
trache/o	combining form	trachea (windpipe)	4
-trans	suffix	through, across, beyond	3
-tripsy	suffix	surgical crushing	5
troph/o	combining form	development	10
tympan/o	combining form	middle ear	9
ur/o	combining form	urination, urine, urinary tract	5
ureter/o	combining form	ureter	5
urethr/o	combining form	urethra	5
urin/o	combining form	urination, urine, urinary tract	5
-us	suffix	no meaning	11
vagin/o	combining form	vagina	6
vas/o	combining form	vessel, duct (in male reproductive system, refers to vas deferens)	6
ven/o	combining form	vein(s)	7
ventr/o	combining form	belly (front)	2
vertebr/o	combining form	vertebra, spine, vertebral column	10
viscer/o	combining form	internal organs	1
xanth/o	combining form	yellow	3
-y	suffix	no meaning	3

Abbreviations

Topics include:

Common Medical Abbreviations, pp. 389-394

Institute for Safe Medical Practices' (ISMP) List of Error-Prone Abbreviations, Symbols, and Dose Designations, includes The Joint Commission's "Do Not Use" list, pp. 395-398

Abbreviations are written as they appear most commonly in the medical and healthcare environment. Some may also appear in both capital and lowercase letters and with or without periods. A plural is formed by adding a lower case s. Consult with the healthcare facility for an approved list of abbreviations.

COMMON MEDICAL ABBREVIATIONS	DEFINITION
A&P	auscultation and percussion; anatomy and physiology
A1c	glycosylated hemoglobin (see also HgbA1c)
a.c.	before meals
ABE	acute bacterial endocarditis
ABGs	arterial blood gases
ACS	acute coronary syndrome
AD	Alzheimer disease
ADL, ADLs	activities of daily living
AFib	atrial fibrillation
AICD	automatic implantable cardioverter-defibrillator
AIDS	acquired immune deficiency syndrome
AKA	above-knee amputation
ALL	acute lymphocytic leukemia
ALS	amyotrophic lateral sclerosis
AM	between midnight and noon
AMA	against medical advice; American Medical Association
AMB	ambulate, ambulatory
AMI	acute myocardial infarction
AML	acute myelocytic leukemia
amp	ampule
amt	amount
ant	anterior
AOM	acute otitis media

COMMON MEDICAL ABBREVIATIONS	DEFINITION
AP	anteroposterior
APR	abdominoperineal resection
ARDS	acute respiratory distress syndrome; adult respiratory distress syndrome
ARF	acute renal failure
ARMD	age-related macular degeneration
AROM	artificial rupture of membranes
ASA	aspirin
as tol	as tolerated
AST	astigmatism
ASCVD	arteriosclerotic cardiovascular disease
ASD	atrial septal defect
ASHD	arteriosclerotic heart disease
AV	arteriovenous; atrioventricular
AVR	aortic valve replacement
ax	axillary
BA	bronchial asthma
BBB	bundle branch block
BCC	basal cell carcinoma
BE	barium enema
b.i.d.	twice a day
BKA	below-knee amputation
BM	bowel movement
BMI	body mass index
BOM	bilateral otitis media
BP	blood pressure
BPH	benign prostatic hyperplasia

COMMON MEDICAL ABBREVIATIONS	DEFINITION
BR	bedrest
BRP	bathroom privileges
BS	blood sugar; bowel sounds; breath sounds
BSO	bilateral salpingo-oophorectomy
BUN	blood urea nitrogen
Bx	biopsy
C	Celsius
C1-C7	cervical vertebrae
c̄	with
C&S	culture and sensitivity
c/o	complains of
Ca (or Ca++)	calcium
CA	cancer, carcinoma
CA-MRSA	community-associated methicillin-resistant *Staphylococcus aureus*
CABG	coronary artery bypass graft
CAD	coronary artery disease
cal	calorie
cap	capsule
CAPD	continuous ambulatory peritoneal dialysis
cath	catheterization, catheter
CBC	complete blood count
CBC with diff	complete blood count and differential
CBR	complete bedrest
CC	chief complaint, cubic centimeter*
CCU	coronary care unit
CDE	certified diabetes educator
CDH	congenital dislocation of the hip
C. diff	*Clostridium difficile* (bacteria)
CEA	carcinoembryonic antigen
CF	cystic fibrosis
CHB	complete heart block
CHD	coronary heart disease
chemo	chemotherapy
CHF	congestive heart failure
CHO	carbohydrate
chol	cholesterol
circ	circumcision
CKD	chronic kidney disease
Cl (or Cl−)	chloride
cl liq	clear liquid

COMMON MEDICAL ABBREVIATIONS	DEFINITION
CLD	chronic liver disease
CLL	chronic lymphocytic leukemia
cm	centimeter
CMA	certified medical assistant
CML	chronic myelogenous leukemia
CMP	comprehensive metabolic panel
CMV	cytomegalovirus
CNA	certified nursing assistant
CNM	certified nurse midwife
CNS	central nervous system
CO	carbon monoxide
CO_2	carbon dioxide
comp	compound
COPD	chronic obstructive pulmonary disease
CP	cerebral palsy
CPAP	continuous positive airway pressure
CPK	creatine phosphokinase
CPR	cardiopulmonary resuscitation
creat	creatinine
CRF	chronic renal failure
CRP	C-reactive protein
CS, C-sect, C-section	cesarean section
CSF	cerebrospinal fluid
CT	computed tomography
CTS	carpal tunnel syndrome
Cu	copper
CVA	cerebrovascular accident (stroke)
CVD	cardiovascular disease
CVP	central venous pressure
Cx	cervix
CXR	chest radiograph
D&C	dilation and curettage
D/S	dextrose in saline
D/W	dextrose in water
DAT	diet as tolerated
DC	doctor of chiropractic
DCIS	ductal carcinoma in situ
DERM	dermatology
DEXA	dual-energy x-ray absorptiometry (scan)

*CC, mistaken in pharmacology for "units," is used in laboratory, pathology, and prostate measurements.

COMMON MEDICAL ABBREVIATIONS	DEFINITION
DI	diabetes insipidus
diff	differential (part of complete blood count)
disch	discharge
DM	diabetes mellitus
DO	doctor of osteopathy
DOA	dead on arrival
DOB	date of birth
DRE	digital rectal examination
DSA	digital subtraction angiography
DVT	deep vein thrombosis
DW	distilled water
Dx	diagnosis
EBL	estimated blood loss
ECG	electrocardiogram
ECHO	echocardiogram
ECT	electroconvulsive therapy
ED	erectile dysfunction; emergency department
EEG	electroencephalogram
EENT	eyes, ears, nose, and throat
EGD	esophagogastroduodenoscopy
EHR	electronic health record
EKG	electrocardiogram
elix	elixir
EMG	electromyogram
EMR	electronic medical record
ENG	electronystagmography
ENT	ears, nose, and throat; otolaryngologist
ERCP	endoscopic retrograde cholangiopancreatography
ESR	erythrocyte sedimentation rate
ESRD	end-stage renal disease
ESWL	extracorporeal shock wave lithotripsy
ET	endotracheal
exam	examination
F	Fahrenheit
FBS	fasting blood sugar
Fe	iron
FHT	fetal heart tones
flu	influenza
FNA	fine needle aspiration
Fr	French (catheter size)

COMMON MEDICAL ABBREVIATIONS	DEFINITION
FSH	follicle-stimulating hormone
FTT	failure to thrive
FUO	fever of undetermined origin
Fx	fracture
g	gram
GB	gall bladder
GERD	gastroesophageal reflux disease
GI	gastrointestinal
GSW	gunshot wound
gtt	drop
GTT	glucose tolerance test
GU	genitourinary
Gyn	gynecology
h	hour
H&H	hemoglobin and hematocrit
H&P	history and physical
H_2O	water
H_2O_2	hydrogen peroxide (hydrogen dioxide)
HA-MRSA	hospital-associated methicillin-resistant *Staphylococcus aureus*
HB	heart block
HbA1c	glycosylated hemoglobin
HBV	hepatitis B virus
HCl	hydrochloric acid
HCO_3	bicarbonate
Hct	hematocrit
HCVD	hypertensive cardiovascular disease
HD	hemodialysis
HgbA1c	glycosylated hemoglobin (see also HbA1c)
HF	heart failure
Hg	mercury
Hgb	hemoglobin
HHD	hypertensive heart disease
HIT	health information technology
HIV	human immunodeficiency virus
HMD	hyaline membrane disease
HNP	herniated nucleus pulposus
HOB	head of bed
HOH	hard of hearing
HPI	history of present illness
HPV	human papillomavirus
HRT	hormone replacement therapy

COMMON MEDICAL ABBREVIATIONS	DEFINITION
HSG	hysterosalpingogram
ht	height
HTN	hypertension
Hx	history
hypo	hypodermic
I&D	incision and drainage
I&O	intake and output
IBS	irritable bowel syndrome
ICU	intensive care unit
ID	intradermal
IDDM	insulin-dependent diabetes mellitus
IHD	ischemic heart disease
IM	intramuscular
inf	inferior
IOP	intraocular pressure
IPPB	intermittent positive pressure breathing
irrig	irrigation
isol	isolation
IUD	intrauterine device
IV	intravenous
IVC	inferior vena cava
IVP	intravenous pyelogram
K	potassium
KCl	potassium chloride
kg	kilogram
KUB	kidneys, ureters, bladder
KVO	keep vein open
L	liter
L1–L5	lumbar vertebrae
L&D	labor and delivery
lab	laboratory
lac	laceration
lat	lateral
LE	lupus erythematosus
LFT	liver function tests
lg	large
LLL	left lower lobe
LLQ	left lower quadrant
LMP	last menstrual period
LP	lumbar puncture
LPN	licensed practical nurse
LR	lactated Ringer (IV solution)

COMMON MEDICAL ABBREVIATIONS	DEFINITION
lt	left
LTB	laryngotracheobronchitis
LUL	left upper lobe
LUQ	left upper quadrant
MA	medical assistant
med	medial
MCH	mean corpuscular hemoglobin
MCV	mean corpuscular volume
MD	muscular dystrophy; medical doctor
mEq	milliequivalent
mets	metastasis, metastases
mg	milligram
MH	mental health
MI	myocardial infarction
mL	milliliter
mm	millimeter
MM	multiple myeloma
MOM	milk of magnesia
MR	magnetic resonance
MRI	magnetic resonance imaging
MRSA	methicillin-resistant *Staphylococcus aureus*
MS	multiple sclerosis
MVP	mitral valve prolapse
N&V	nausea and vomiting
NA	nursing assistant
Na	sodium
NaCl	sodium chloride (salt)
NAS	no added salt
NB	newborn
neg	negative
neuro	neurology
NG	nasogastric
NICU	neurologic intensive care unit; neonatal intensive care unit
NIDDM	noninsulin-dependent diabetes mellitus
NKDA	no known drug allergies
NM	nuclear medicine
noc, noct	night
NP	nurse practitioner
NPO	nothing by mouth
NS	normal saline

COMMON MEDICAL ABBREVIATIONS	DEFINITION
NSAID	nonsteroidal antiinflammatory drug
NSR	normal sinus rhythm
NVS	neurologic vital signs
O₂	oxygen
OA	osteoarthritis
OAB	overactive bladder
OB	obstetrics
OB/GYN	obstetrician-gynecologist
OBS	organic brain syndrome
OD	overdose
oint	ointment
OM	otitis media
OOB	out of bed
OP	outpatient
Ophth	ophthalmology
OR	operating room
Ortho, ortho	orthopedics
OSA	obstructive sleep apnea
OT	occupational therapy
oz	ounce
P	pulse
p̄	after
PA	posteroanterior; physician's assistant
PAC	premature atrial contraction
PAD	peripheral artery disease
PAT	paroxysmal atrial tachycardia
PATH	pathology
p.c.	after meals
PCI	percutaneous coronary intervention
PCP	primary care physician; *Pneumocystis carinii* pneumonia
PCT	patient care technician
PCU	progressive care unit
PCV	packed cell volume
PD	Parkinson disease
PDA	patent ductus arteriosus
PE	pulmonary edema; pulmonary embolism
Peds	pediatrics
PEEP	positive end expiratory pressure
PEG	percutaneous endoscopic gastrostomy
per	by

COMMON MEDICAL ABBREVIATIONS	DEFINITION
PERLA	pupils equal, reactive to light and accommodation
PET	positron emission tomography (scan)
PFTs	pulmonary function tests
PICU	pediatric intensive care unit
PID	pelvic inflammatory disease
PKD	polycystic kidney disease
PKU	phenylketonuria
PM	between noon and midnight
PMH	past medical history
PMR	polymyalgia rheumatica
PNS	peripheral nervous system
PO	orally; phone order
post	posterior
post-op	postoperatively
PP	postpartum; postprandial (after meals)
PPD	purified protein derivative
PRBC	packed red blood cells
PRN	whenever necessary
PSA	prostate-specific antigen
PSG	polysomnography
pt	patient; pint
PT	physical therapy; prothrombin time
PTA	physical therapist assistant
PTCA	percutaneous transluminal coronary angioplasty
PT/INR	prothrombin time/international normalized ratio
PTSD	posttraumatic stress disorder
PTT	partial thromboplastin time (pro time)
PUL	percutaneous ultrasound lithotripsy, pulmonary
PVC	premature ventricular contraction
PVD	peripheral vascular disease
Px	prognosis
q	every
q_h	every number of hours (e.g., q2h)
qt	quart
R	respirations
RA	rheumatoid arthritis
RBC	erythrocyte; red blood cell count; red blood cell
RCP	respiratory care practitioner
RD	registered dietitian

COMMON MEDICAL ABBREVIATIONS	DEFINITION
reg	regular
REM	rapid eye movement
resp	respirations
RHD	rheumatic heart disease
RLL	right lower lobe
RLQ	right lower quadrant
RN	registered nurse
R/O	rule out
ROM	range of motion
ROS	review of systems
RP	radical prostatectomy
RR	recovery room
rt	right; routine
RT	respiratory therapist; radiologic technologist; respiratory therapy
RUL	right upper lobe
RUQ	right upper quadrant
Rx	prescription
$\bar{s}$	without
SAH	subarachnoid hemorrhage
SBE	subacute bacterial endocarditis
SCC	squamous cell carcinoma
SH	social history
SIDS	sudden infant death syndrome
SLE	systemic lupus erythematosus
SMAC	sequential multiple analysis computer
SNF	skilled nursing facility
SO_2	oxygen saturation
SOB	shortness of breath
SSE	soapsuds enema
staph	staphylococcus, staphylococci
stat	immediately
STD	sexually transmitted disease
STI	sexually transmitted infection
strep	streptococcus, streptococci
subcut	subcutaneous
sup	superior
SVN	small volume nebulizer
T	temperature
T1–T12	thoracic vertebrae
T1DM	type 1 diabetes mellitus
T2DM	type 2 diabetes mellitus

COMMON MEDICAL ABBREVIATIONS	DEFINITION
T&A	tonsillectomy and adenoidectomy
tab	tablet
TAH	total abdominal hysterectomy
TAH/BSO	total abdominal hysterectomy [and] bilateral salpingo-oophorectomy
TB	tuberculosis
TBI	traumatic brain injury
TCDB	turn, cough, deep breathe
TD	transdermal
temp	temperature
THA	total hip arthroplasty
TIA	transient ischemic attack
tid	three times a day
TKA	total knee arthroplasty
TPN	total parenteral nutrition
trach	tracheostomy
TRUS	transrectal ultrasound
TURP	transurethral resection of the prostate gland
TVH	total vaginal hysterectomy
TWE	tap water enema
Tx	treatment; traction
UA	urinalysis
UC	ulcerative colitis
UGI series	upper GI (gastrointestinal) series
UPPP	uvulopalatopharyngoplasty
URI	upper respiratory infection
US	ultrasound
UTI	urinary tract infection
VA	visual acuity
vag	vaginal
VCUG	voiding cystourethrogram
VDRL	venereal disease research laboratory
v fib	ventricular fibrillation
V/Q scan	lung ventilation/perfusion scan
VRE	vancomycin-resistant *Enterococcus*
VS	vital signs
W/C	wheelchair
WA	while awake
WBC	leukocyte; white blood cell
wt	weight
XRT	radiation therapy

INSTITUTE FOR SAFE MEDICATION PRACTICES' LIST OF ERROR-PRONE ABBREVIATIONS, SYMBOLS, AND DOSE DESIGNATIONS

The abbreviations, symbols, and dose designations found in this table have been reported to ISMP through the ISMP National Medication Errors Reporting Program (ISMP MERP) as being frequently misinterpreted and involved in harmful medication errors. They should **NEVER** be used when communicating medical information. This includes internal communications, telephone/verbal prescriptions, computer-generated labels, labels for drug storage bins, medication administration records, as well as pharmacy and prescriber computer order entry screens.

The Joint Commission established a National Patient Safety Goal specifying certain abbreviations, acronyms, and symbols that must appear on an accredited organization's "do not use" list; these are called to your attention with a double asterisk (**). However, we hope that you consider others beyond the minimum Joint Commission requirements. By using and promoting safe practices, and by educating one another about hazards, we can better protect our patients.

ABBREVIATIONS	INTENDED MEANING	MISINTERPRETATION	CORRECTION
μg	Microgram	Mistaken as "mg"	Use "mcg"
AD, AS, AU	Right ear, left ear, each ear	Mistaken as OD, OS, OU (right eye, left eye, each eye)	Use "right ear," "left ear," or "each ear"
OD, OS, OU	Right eye, left eye, each eye	Mistaken as AD, AS, AU (right ear, left ear, each ear)	Use "right eye," "left eye," or "each eye"
BT	Bedtime	Mistaken as "BID" (twice daily)	Use "bedtime"
cc	Cubic centimeters	Mistaken as "u" (units)	Use "mL"
D/C	Discharge or discontinue	Premature discontinuation of medications if D/C (intended to mean "discharge") has been misinterpreted as "discontinued" when followed by a list of discharge medications	Use "discharge" and "discontinue"
IJ	Injection	Mistaken as "IV" or "intrajugular"	Use "injection"
IN	Intranasal	Mistaken as "IM" or "IV"	Use "intranasal" or "NAS"
HS	Half-strength	Mistaken as bedtime	Use "half-strength" or "bedtime"
hs	At bedtime, hours of sleep	Mistaken as half-strength	
IU**	International unit	Mistaken as IV (intravenous) or 10 (ten)	Use "units"
o.d. or OD	Once daily	Mistaken as "right eye" (OD-oculus dexter), leading to oral liquid medications administered in the eye	Use "daily"
OJ	Orange juice	Mistaken as OD or OS (right or left eye); drugs meant to be diluted in orange juice may be given in the eye	Use "orange juice"
Per os	By mouth, orally	The "os" can be mistaken as "left eye" (OS-oculus sinister)	Use "PO," "by mouth," or "orally"
q.d. or QD**	Every day	Mistaken as q.i.d., especially if the period after the "q" or the tail of the "q" is misunderstood as an "i"	Use "daily"
qhs	Nightly at bedtime	Mistaken as "qhr" or every hour	Use "nightly"
qn	Nightly or at bedtime	Mistaken as "qh" (every hour)	Use "nightly" or "at bedtime"
q.o.d. or QOD**	Every other day	Mistaken as "q.d." (daily) or "q.i.d." (four times daily) if the "o" is poorly written	Use "every other day"

ABBREVIATIONS	INTENDED MEANING	MISINTERPRETATION	CORRECTION
q1d	Daily	Mistaken as q.i.d. (four times daily)	Use "daily"
q6PM, etc.	Every evening at 6 PM	Mistaken as every 6 hours	Use "daily at 6 PM" or "6 PM daily"
SC, SQ, sub q	Subcutaneous	SC mistaken as SL (sublingual); SQ mistaken as "5 every;" the "q" in "sub q" has been mistaken as "every" (e.g., a heparin dose ordered "sub q 2 hours before surgery" misunderstood as every 2 hours before surgery)	Use "subcut" or "subcutaneously"
ss	Sliding scale (insulin) or $\frac{1}{2}$ (apothecary)	Mistaken as "55"	Spell out "sliding scale;" use "one-half" or "$\frac{1}{2}$"
SSRI	Sliding scale regular insulin	Mistaken as selective-serotonin reuptake inhibitor	Spell out "sliding scale (insulin)"
SSI	Sliding scale insulin	Mistaken as Strong Solution of Iodine (Lugol's)	
i/d	One daily	Mistaken as "tid"	Use "1 daily"
TIW or tiw	3 times a week	Mistaken as "3 times a day" or "twice in a week"	Use "3 times weekly"
U or u**	Unit	Mistaken as the number 0 or 4, causing a 10-fold overdose or greater (e.g., 4U seen as "40" or 4u seen as "44"); mistaken as "cc" so dose given in volume instead of units (e.g., 4u seen as 4cc)	Use "unit"
UD	As directed ("ut dictum")	Mistaken as unit dose (e.g., diltiazem 125 mg IV infusion "UD" misinterpreted as meaning to give the entire infusion as a unit [bolus] dose)	Use "as directed"

DOSE DESIGNATIONS AND OTHER INFORMATION	INTENDED MEANING	MISINTERPRETATION	CORRECTION
Trailing zero after decimal point (e.g., 1.0 mg)**	1 mg	Mistaken as 10 mg if the decimal point is not seen	Do not use trailing zeros for doses expressed in whole numbers
"Naked" decimal point (e.g., .5 mg)**	0.5 mg	Mistaken as 5 mg if the decimal point is not seen	Use zero before a decimal point when the dose is less than a whole unit
Abbreviations such as mg. or mL. with a period following the abbreviation	mg mL	The period is unnecessary and could be mistaken as the number 1 if written poorly	Use mg, mL, etc. without a terminal period
Dose Designations and Other Information	Intended Meaning	Misinterpretation	Correction
Drug name and dose run together (especially problematic for drug names that end in "l" such as Inderal 40 mg; Tegretol 300 mg)	Inderal 40 mg Tegretol 300 mg	Mistaken as Inderal 140 mg Mistaken as Tegretol 1300 mg	Place adequate space between the drug name, dose, and unit of measure

DOSE DESIGNATIONS AND OTHER INFORMATION	INTENDED MEANING	MISINTERPRETATION	CORRECTION
Numerical dose and unit of measure run together (e.g., 10mg, 100mL)	10 mg 100 mL	The "m" is sometimes mistaken as a zero or two zeros, risking a 10- to 100-fold overdose	Place adequate space between the dose and unit of measure
Large doses without properly placed commas (e.g., 100000 units; 1000000 units)	100,000 units 1,000,000 units	100000 has been mistaken as 10,000 or 1,000,000; 1000000 has been mistaken as 100,000	Use commas for dosing units at or above 1,000, or use words such as 100 "thousand" or 1 "million" to improve readability

DRUG NAME ABBREVIATIONS	INTENDED MEANING	MISINTERPRETATION	CORRECTION

To avoid confusion, do not abbreviate drug names when communicating medical information. Examples of drug name abbreviations involved in medication errors include:

APAP	acetaminophen	Not recognized as acetaminophen	Use complete drug name
ARA A	vidarabine	Mistaken as cytarabine (ARA C)	Use complete drug name
AZT	zidovudine (Retrovir)	Mistaken as azathioprine or aztreonam	Use complete drug name
CPZ	Compazine (prochlorperazine)	Mistaken as chlorpromazine	Use complete drug name
DPT	Demerol-Phenergan-Thorazine	Mistaken as diphtheria-pertussis-tetanus (vaccine)	Use complete drug name
DTO	Diluted tincture of opium, or deodorized tincture of opium (Paregoric)	Mistaken as tincture of opium	Use complete drug name
HCl	hydrochloric acid or hydrochloride	Mistaken as potassium chloride (The "H" is misinterpreted as "K")	Use complete drug name unless expressed as a salt of a drug
HCT	hydrocortisone	Mistaken as hydrochlorothiazide	Use complete drug name
HCTZ	hydrochlorothiazide	Mistaken as hydrocortisone (seen as HCT250 mg)	Use complete drug name
MgSO4**	magnesium sulfate	Mistaken as morphine sulfate	Use complete drug name
MS, MSO4**	morphine sulfate	Mistaken as magnesium sulfate	Use complete drug name
MTX	methotrexate	Mistaken as mitoxantrone	Use complete drug name
PCA	procainamide	Mistaken as patient controlled analgesia	Use complete drug name
PTU	propylthiouracil	Mistaken as mercaptopurine	Use complete drug name
T3	Tylenol with codeine No. 3	Mistaken as liothyronine	Use complete drug name
TAC	triamcinolone	Mistaken as tetracaine, Adrenalin, cocaine	Use complete drug name
TNK	TNKase	Mistaken as "TPA"	Use complete drug name
ZnSO4	zinc sulfate	Mistaken as morphine sulfate	Use complete drug name

STEMMED DRUG NAMES	INTENDED MEANING	MISINTERPRETATION	CORRECTION
"Nitro" drip	nitroglycerin infusion	Mistaken as sodium nitroprusside infusion	Use complete drug name
"Norflox"	norfloxacin	Mistaken as Norflex	Use complete drug name
"IV Vanc"	intravenous vancomycin	Mistaken as Invanz	Use complete drug name

SYMBOLS	INTENDED MEANING	MISINTERPRETATION	CORRECTION
℥	Dram	Symbol for dram mistaken as "3"	Use the metric system
ℳ	Minim	Symbol for minim mistaken as "mL"	
x3d	For three days	Mistaken as "3 doses"	Use "for three days"
> and <	Greater than and less than	Mistaken as opposite of intended; mistakenly use incorrect symbol; "< 10" mistaken as "40"	Use "greater than" or "less than"
/ (slash mark)	Separates two doses or indicates "per"	Mistaken as the number 1 (e.g., "25 units/10 units" misread as "25 units and 110" units)	Use "per" rather than a slash mark to separate doses
@	At	Mistaken as "2"	Use "at"
&	And	Mistaken as "2"	Use "and"
+	Plus or and	Mistaken as "4"	Use "and"
°	Hour	Mistaken as a zero (e.g., q2° seen as q 20)	Use "hr," "h," or "hour"
Φ or ⊘	zero, null sign	Mistaken as numerals 4, 6, 8, and 9	Use 0 or zero, or describe intent using whole words

Visit www.jointcommission.org for more information about this Joint Commission requirement.

LESSON 1

Exercise A

Identify Origins of Medical Language

1. a; 2. c; 3. d; 4. b
5. a. acronym; MRSA
   b. eponym; Parkinson disease
   c. modern language; posttraumatic stress disorder
   d. Greek and Latin; arthritis

Exercise B

Define Word Parts, Combining Form, and Categories of Medical Terms

A.
1. c; 2. e; 3. a; 4. g; 5. f; 6. b; 7. d
B.
1. word root; 2. end; beginning;
3. suffix; prefix; pertaining to within a vein; 4. combining vowel; inflammation of the bone and joint

Exercise C

Build and Translate Terms Built from Word Parts

1. **Match:** a. -al; pertaining to; b. -logy; study of; c. -oma; tumor
2. **Label:** Figure 1.3, (1) hist/o; (2) cyt/o
3. **Translate:** hist/o/logy; study of tissue(s)
4. **Reading Exercise**
5. **Label:** Figure 1.4, (1) neur/o, (2) epitheli/o; (3) sarc/o; (4) my/o
6. **Build:** a. my/oma; b. epitheli/oma; c. sarc/oma
7. **Reading Exercise**
8. **Match:** a. lip/o; fat, fat tissue; b. cyt/o; cell(s); c. -oma; tumor; d. -oid; resembling
9. **Translate:** a. lip/oma; tumor (composed of) fat tissue; b. lip/oid; resembling fat; c. cyt/oid; resembling a cell
10. **Reading Exercise**
11. **Label:** Figure 1.5, lip/oma
12. **Label:** Figure 1.6, 1. viscer/o
13. **Build:** a. viscer/al, b. epitheli/al
14. **Match:** a. path/o; disease b. -genic; producing, originating, causing;

c. -logy; study of; d. -logist; one who studies and treats (specialist, physician)
15. **Translate:** a. path/o/logist; physician who studies disease; b. path/o/genic; producing disease; c. path/o/logy; study of disease
16. **Reading Exercise**
17. a. radi/o/logy; b. radi/o/logist
18. **Reading Exercise**
19. **Match:** a. carcin/o; cancer; b. -oma; tumor; c. -genic; producing, originating, causing; d. meta-; beyond; e. neo-; new; f. -plasm; growth (substance or formation); g. -stasis; control, stop
20. **Build:** a. neo/plasm; b. meta/stasis; c. carcin/o/genic; d. carcin/oma
21. **Reading Exercise**
22. **Label:** Figure 1.7, carcin/oma
23. **Reading Exercise**
24. **Label:** Figure 1.8, meta/stasis
25. **Match:** a. onc/o; tumor(s); b. -logy; study of; c. -logist; one who studies and treats (specialist, physician)
26. **Translate:** a. onc/o/logy; study of tumors; b. onc/o/logist; physician who studies and treats tumors
27. **Reading Exercise**
28. **Term Table: Review of Body Structure and Oncology Terms Built from Word Parts**

Exercise D

Pronounce and Spell Medical Terms Built from Word Parts

1. Check responses with the Term Table in Exercise C, #28
2. Check answers with online resources

Exercise E

Label

1. staphylococcus (s.); staphylococci (pl.); 2. streptococcus (s.); streptococci (pl.); 3. infection; 4. biopsy;
5. chemotherapy; 6. radiation therapy;
7. malignant

Exercise F

Learn Medical Terms NOT Built from Word Parts

1. benign; malignant; biopsy;
2. diagnosis; prognosis;
3. chemotherapy; radiation therapy; remission; 4. inflammation;
5. infection; staphylococcus; streptococcus

Exercise G

Pronounce and Spell Medical Terms NOT Built from Word Parts

1. Check responses with the Table for Terms NOT Built from Word Parts
2. Check answers with online resources

Exercise H

Abbreviate Medical Terms

1. Disease and disorders: CA
2. Descriptive of the disease process: a. mets; b. Dx; c. Px
3. Surgical procedures: Bx
4. Treatments: a. XRT; b. chemo
5. Specialties: PATH
6. Related terms: a. lab; b. staph; c. strep

Exercise I

Body Structure Terms

1. cytoid; 2. lipoid; 3. epithelial; 4. visceral

Exercise J

Oncology Terms
Signs and Symptoms
1. inflammation
Disease and Disorders
2. neoplasm; 3. epithelioma;
4. neuroma; 5. sarcoma; 6. lipoma;
7. myoma; 8. carcinoma; 9. infection
Descriptive of Disease and Disease Processes
10. diagnosis; 11. prognosis;
12. malignant; 13. benign; 14. remission;
15. metastasis
Surgical Procedures:
16. biopsy

Treatments
17. radiation therapy; 18. chemotherapy
Specialties and Professions
19. pathologist; 20. oncologist;
21. oncology; 22. histology;
23. pathology; 24. cytology;
25. radiology; 26. radiologist
Related Terms
27. carcinogenic; 28. pathogenic;
29. streptococcus; 30. staphylococcus

Exercise K

Use Medical Terms in Clinical Statements

1. Pathogenic; carcinogenic;
2. diagnosis; CA; oncologist;
3. neoplasm; cytology; benign; malignant; 4. pathologist; lipoid;
5. pathology; sarcoma; metastasis; oncology; Px

Exercise L

Apply Medical Terms to Case Study
Answers will vary and may include: diagnosis, prognosis, and remission along with their respective definitions.

Exercise M

Use Medical Language in Documents

1. biopsy; 2. cytology; 3. pathologist;
4. diagnosis; 5. carcinoma;
6. inflammation; 7. metastasis;
8. malignant; 9. oncologist;
10. chemotherapy; 11. prognosis;
12. Radiation therapy
13. F; "no evidence of metastasis" (beyond control) means the cancer has not spread to surrounding organs.
14. F; prognosis means "prediction of a possible outcome of a disease"; diagnosis means "identification of a disease."
15. F; an oncologist treats patients with cancer; a pathologist studies body changes caused by disease, usually from a specimen.
16. Answers will vary and may include: Bx, biopsy; Dx, diagnosis; mets, metastasis; chemo, chemotherapy; Px, prognosis; XRT, radiation therapy; CA, and cancer along with the terms they abbreviate.
17. Research exercise; answers will vary

Exercise N

Online Review of Lesson Content
Completed with online resources

Exercise O

Lesson Content Quiz

1. b; 2. a; 3. c; 4. a; 5. c; 6. b; 7. b;
8. a; 9. c; 10. b

LESSON 2

Exercise A

Build and Translate Directional Terms Built from Word Parts

1. **Match:** a. -al, -ic, -ior; pertaining to; b. -ad; toward
2. **Label:** Figure 2.3, (1) dors/o; (2) poster/o; (3) anter/o; (4) ventr/o
3. **Translate:** a. ventr/al; pertaining to the belly; b. dors/al; pertaining to the back; c. anter/ior; pertaining to the front; d. poster/ior; pertaining to the back (behind)
4. **Reading Exercise**
5. **Label:** Figure 2.4, (1) dors/al, poster/ior; (2) anter/ior; (3) ventr/al
6. **Translate:** a. poster/o/anter/ior (PA); pertaining to the back and to the front; b. anter/o/poster/ior (AP); pertaining to the front and to the back
7. **Reading Exercise**
8. **Label:** Figure 2.5, a. poster/o/anter/ior; b. anter/o/poster/ior
9. **Label:** Figure 2.6, (1) super/o; (2) cephal/o; (3) caud/o; (4) infer/o
10. **Translate:** a. super/ior; pertaining to above; b. infer/ior; pertaining to below; c. anter/o/super/ior; pertaining to the front and above
11. **Reading Exercise**
12. **Translate:** a. cephal/ic; pertaining to the head; b. caud/al; pertaining to the tail; c. cephal/ad; toward the head; d. caud/ad; toward the tail
13. **Reading Exercise**
14. **Label:** Figure 2.7, (1) super/ior; (2) cephal/ic; (3) cephal/ad; (4) caud/ad; (5) infer/ior; (6) caud/al
15. **Label:** Figure 2.8, (1) later/o; (2) medi/o; (3) proxim/o; (4) dist/o
16. **Build:** a. proxim/al; b. dist/al
17. **Reading Exercise**
18. **Build:** a. medi/al; b. later/al
19. **Reading Exercise**
20. **Label:** Figure 2.11, later/al
21. **Build:** a. medi/o/later/al; b. anter/o/medi/al; c. poster/o/later/al; d. super/o/later/al; e. infer/o/later/al; f. anter/o/later/al
22. **Term Table: Review of Directional Terms Built from Word Parts**

Exercise B

Pronounce and Spell Medical Terms Built from Word Parts

1. Check responses with the Term Table in Exercise A, #22
2. Check answers with online resources

Exercise C

Learn Anatomic Planes, Abdominopelvic Regions, and Patient Positions

1. **Label:** Figure 2.14, (1) axial; (2) coronal; (3) sagittal
2. **Label:** Figure 2.16, (1) Right hypochondriac region; (2) Right lumbar region; (3) Right iliac region; (4) Hypogastric region; (5) Epigastric region; (6) Left hypochondriac region; (7) Umbilical region; (8) Left lumbar region; (9) Left iliac region
3. **Label:** Figure 2.17, (1) supine; (2) prone; (3) Fowler; (4) orthopnea; (5) Trendelenburg; (6) Sims

Exercise D

Pronounce and Spell Anatomic Planes, Abdominopelvic Regions, and Patient Positions

1. Check responses with the Term Tables for Anatomic Planes, Abdominopelvic Regions, and Patient Positions
2. Check answers with online resources

Exercise E

Abbreviate Medical Terms

1. Directional Terms
   a. sup; b. inf; c. med; d. lat; e. PA; f. AP; g. post; h. ant
2. Abdominopelvic Quadrants
   a. RUQ; b. RLQ; c. LUQ; d. LLQ

Exercise F

Directional Terms

1. cephalic; 2. superior;
3. superolateral; 4. posterolateral;
5. posteroanterior; 6. posterior;
7. dorsal; 8. mediolateral;
9. anteromedial; 10. medial; 11. lateral;
12. inferolateral; 13. inferior;
14. proximal; 15. distal; 16. caudad;
17. cephalad; 18. caudal; 19. ventral;
20. anterior; 21. anterosuperior;
22. anteroposterior; 23. anterolateral

Exercise G

Anatomic Planes

1. axial; 2. coronal; 3. sagittal

Exercise H

Abdominopelvic Regions

1. umbilical; 2. epigastric; 3. hypogastric;
4. hypochondriac; 5. lumbar; 6. iliac

Exercise I

Patient Positions

1. supine; 2. prone; 3. orthopnea;
4. Trendelenburg; 5. Sims; 6. Fowler

Exercise J

Use Medical Terms in Clinical Statements

1. Underlined Terms: distal, lateral, anterior, medial, inferior, anterolateral, proximal, inferior, medial, anterosuperior, posterior, inferior, medial, dorsal, lateral 2. b; 3. a; 4. a; 5. distal; 6. AP; 7. lateral; sagittal; 8. medial; 9. superior; 10. lumbar; 11. anterior; 12. coronal; axial; 13. anterior; 14. orthopnea; 15. Trendelenburg; 16. Dorsal; 17. cephalic; 18. caudal

Exercise K

Apply Medical Terms

Answers will vary and may include: distal, proximal, ventral, anterior, dorsal, posterior, umbilical region, iliac region(s), and lumbar region(s) along with their respective definitions.

Exercise L

Use Medical Language in Documents

1. iliac; 2. lumbar; 3. distal; 4. medial; 5. lateral; 6. proximal; 7. superolaterally; pertaining to above and to the side; 8. anteroposterior; pertaining to the front and to the back

Exercise M

Online Review of Lesson Content

Completed with online resources

Exercise N

Lesson Content Quiz

1. c; 2. a; 3. b; 4. c; 5. b; 6. c; 7. a; 8. b

LESSON 3

Exercise A

Build and Translate Terms Built from Word Parts

1. **Label:** Figure 3.2, cutane/o; dermat/o; derm/o

2. **Match:** a. -logist, one who studies and treats (specialist, physician); b. -logy, study of; c. path/o, disease; d. -itis, inflammation; e. -y, no meaning

3. **Translate:** a. dermat/o/logy, study of the skin; b. dermat/o/logist, physician who studies and treats disease of the skin; c. dermat/o/path/y, (any) disease of the skin; d. dermat/itis, inflammation of the skin; e. dermat/o/path/o/logist, physician who (microscopically) studies diseases of the skin

4. **Reading Exercise**

5. **Label:** Figure 3.3, dermat/itis

6. **Match:** a. epi-, on, upon, over; b. hypo-, below, deficient, under; c. intra-, within; d. trans-, through, across, beyond; e. -al, -ic, pertaining to

7. **Build:** a. derm/al; b. epi/derm/al; c. intra/derm/al; d. trans/derm/al; e. hypo/derm/ic;

8. **Reading Exercise**

9. **Label:** Figure 3.4, trans/derm/al

10. **Match:** a. per-, through; b. -ous, pertaining to; c. -sub, below, under

11. **Translate:** a. cutane/ous, pertaining to the skin; b. sub/cutane/ous, pertaining to under the skin; c. per/cutane/ous, pertaining to through the skin

12. **Reading Exercise**

13. **Label:** Figure 3.5, hypo/derm/ic, sub/cutane/ous

14. **Label:** Figure 3.6, onych/o

15. **Match:** a. -osis; abnormal condition; b. -lysis; separation; c. myc/o; fungus

16. **Build:** a. onych/osis; b. onych/o/myc/osis; c. onych/o/lysis

17. **Reading Exercise**

18. **Label:** Figure 3.7, onych/o/myc/osis

19. **Term Table: Review of Integumentary System Terms Built from Word Parts**

Exercise B

Pronounce and Spell Terms Built from Word Parts

1. Check responses with the Term Table in Exercise A, #19
2. Check answers with online resources

Exercise C

Build and Translate MORE Terms Built from Word Parts

1. **Label:** Figure 3.8, A. erythr/o; B. xanth/o; C. melan/o; D. leuk/o; E. cyan/o

2. **Match:** a. derm/o, skin; b. -a, no meaning

3. **Translate:** a. leuk/o/derm/a, white skin; b. melan/o/derm/a, black skin; c. erythr/o/derm/a, red skin; d. xanth/o/derm/a, yellow skin

4. **Reading Exercise**

5. **Label:** Figure 3.9, A. leuk/o/derm/a; B. erythr/o/derm/a; C. xanth/o/derm/a

6. **Match:** a. -osis, abnormal condition; b. -oma, tumor; c. acr/o, extremities

7. **Build:** a. xanth/osis; b. cyan/osis; c. acr/o/cyan/osis; d. xanth/oma; e. melan/oma

8. **Reading Exercise**

9. **Label:** Figure 3.10, a. melan/oma; b. cyan/osis

10. **Match:** a. cyt/o, cell(s); b. -e, no meaning

11. **Translate:** a. leuk/o/cyt/e, white (blood) cell; b. erythr/o/cyt/e, red (blood) cell

12. **Reading Exercise**

13. **Label:** Figure 3.11, a. erythr/o/cyt/e(s); b. leuk/o/cyt/e(s)

14. **Term Table: Review of MORE Respiratory System Terms Built from Word Parts**

Exercise D

Pronounce and Spell MORE Terms Built from Word Parts

1. Check responses with the Term Table in Exercise C, #14
2. Check answers with online resources

Exercise E

Label

1. basal cell carcinoma; 2. squamous cell carcinoma; 3. pressure injury; 4. cellulitis; 5. herpes; 6. nevus; 7. impetigo; 8. laceration

Exercise F

Learn Medical Terms NOT Built from Word Parts

1. Lesion; 2. Pressure injuries; 3. abscess; 4. Laceration; 5. Edema;

6. nevus; 7. basal cell carcinoma; squamous cell carcinoma; 8. herpes; 9. Impetigo; 10. cellulitis, erythema; 11. Pallor; 12. Jaundice; 13. Methicillin-resistant *Staphylococcus aureus*.

Exercise G

Pronounce and Spell Terms NOT Built from Word Parts

1. Check responses with the Table for Terms NOT Built from Word Parts
2. Check answers with online resources

Exercise H

Abbreviate Medical Terms

1. a. lac; b. SCC; c. BCC;
2. a. DERM; b. hypo; c. MRSA; d. WBC; e. RBC; f. TD; g. ID; h. subcut

Exercise I

Learn Plural Endings

PLURAL TERM; ENDING

1. thoraces; -aces; 2. appendices; -ices; 3. cervices; -ices; 4. diagnoses; -ses; 5. prognoses; -ses; 6. metastases; -ses; 7. pelves; -es; 8. testes; -es; 9. bronchi; -i; 10. nevi; -i; 11. streptococci; -i; 12. fungi; -i; 13. bacteria; -a; 14. ova; -a; 15. sarcomata; -mata; 16. fibromata; -mata; 17. pharynges; -nges; 18. larynges; -nges; 19. apices; -ices; 20. cortices; -ices; 21. ganglia; -a; 22. spermatozoa; -a; 23. pleurae; -ae; 24. sclerae; -ae; 25. bursae; -ae

Exercise J

Signs and Symptoms

1. edema; 2. lesion; 3. pallor; 4. jaundice; 5. erythema; 6. acrocyanosis; 7. cyanosis; 8. melanoderma; 9. leukoderma; 10. xanthoderma; 11. xanthosis

Exercise K

Diseases and Disorders

1. abscess; 2. cellulitis; 3. pressure injury; 4. laceration; 5. onychosis; 6. dermatopathy; 7. dermatitis; 8. erythroderma; 9. onychomycosis; 10. impetigo; 11. herpes; 12. xanthoma; 13. melanoma; 14. squamous cell carcinoma; 15. basal cell carcinoma; 16. methicillin-resistant *Staphylococcus aureus*; 17. onycholysis

Exercise L

Specialties and Professions

1. dermatology; 2. dermatologist; 3. dermatopathologist

Exercise M

Medical Terms Related to the Integumentary System and Colors

1. erythrocyte; 2. leukocyte; 3. a. cutaneous; b. dermal; 4. epidermal; 5. intradermal; 6. a. hypodermic; b. subcutaneous; 7. a. percutaneous; b. transdermal; 8. nevus

Exercise N

Use Medical Terms in Clinical Statements

1. pressure injury, erythema; 2. lesions, impetigo; 3. erythema, dermatologist, dermatitis; 4. onychomycosis; 5. intradermal; 6. melanoma, metastasis, hypodermic subcutaneous; 7. basal cell carcinoma, squamous cell carcinoma; 8. MRSA, cellulitis, abscess; 9. a. metastases; b. emboli; c. ovum; d. testes; e. lipomata

Exercise O

Apply Medical Terms to Case Study

Answer will vary and may include lesion, nevus, melanoma, biopsy, basal cell carcinoma, squamous cell carcinoma, and dermatologist along with their respective definitions.

Exercise P

Use Medical Language in a Document

1. pathology; 2. melanoma; 3. basal cell carcinoma; 4. nevus; 5. biopsy; 6. proximal; 7. epidermal; 8. anterior; 9. benign; 10. dermatopathologist; 11. b; 12. a. melanoma, S; b. melanomata, P; c. nevi, P; d. nevus, S; e. metastasis, S; f. metastases, P; g. biopsy, S; h. biopsies, P; 13. Research exercise; answers vary.

Exercise Q

Online Review of Lesson Content

Completed with online resources

Exercise R

Lesson Content Quiz

1. b; 2. c; 3. a; 4. c; 5. a; 6. b; 7. c; 8. a; 9. b; 10. b

LESSON 4

Exercise A

Build and Translate Terms Built from Word Parts

1. **Label:** Figure 4.3, (1) sinus/o; (2) nas/o, rhin/o; (3) laryng/o; (4) pharyng/o
2. **Match:** a. -rrhea, flow, discharge; b. -rrhagia, rapid flow of blood; c. -itis, inflammation
3. **Build:** a. rhin/itis; b. rhin/o/rrhea; c. rhin/o/rrhagia
4. **Reading Exercise**
5. **Match:** a. -tomy, cut into, incision; b. -al, -ous, pertaining to; c. muc/o, mucus; d. -itis, inflammation;
6. **Translate:** a. nas/al, pertaining to the nose; b. muc/ous, pertaining to mucus; c. sinus/itis, inflammation of the sinus (membranes); d. sinus/o/tomy, incision of a sinus
7. **Reading Exercise**
8. **Label:** Figure 4.4, sinus/itis
9. **Match:** a. -itis, inflammation; b. -eal, pertaining to; c. -ectomy, surgical removal, excision; d. -scope, instrument used for visual examination; e. -scopy, visual examination
10. **Build:** a. pharyng/itis; b. nas/o/pharyng/itis; c. laryng/itis
11. **Reading Exercise**
12. **Build:** a. pharyng/eal; b. laryng/eal; c. laryng/o/pharyng/eal
13. **Translate:** a. laryng/o/scope, instrument used for visual examination of the larynx; b. laryng/o/scopy, visual examination of the larynx; c. laryng/ectomy, excision of the larynx
14. **Reading Exercise**
15. **Match:** a. a-, an-, absence of, without; b. dys-, difficult, painful, abnormal; c. hyper-, above, excessive; d. hypo-, below, deficient, under; e. -pnea, breathing
16. **Translate:** a. a/pnea, absence of breathing; b. dys/pnea, difficult breathing; c. hypo/pnea, deficient breathing; d. hyper/pnea, excessive breathing
17. **Reading Exercise**
18. **Match:** a. -ia, condition of; b. -meter, instrument used to measure; c. hyper-, excessive, above; d. hypo-, below, deficient, under;

e. capn/o, carbon dioxide; f. ox/i, oxygen; g. spir/o, breathing
19. **Build:** a. hyper/ox/ia; b. hyper/capn/ia; c. hypo/capn/ia; d. hyp/ox/ia [the **o** from the prefix **hypo-** has been dropped]
20. **Reading Exercise**
21. **Translate:** a. capn/o/meter, instrument used to measure carbon dioxide; b. ox/i/meter, instrument used to measure oxygen; c. spir/o/meter, instrument used to measure breathing
22. **Reading Exercise**
23. **Label:** Figure 4.5, A. pulse ox/i/meter; B. capn/o/meter; C. spir/o/meter
24. **Term Table: Review of Respiratory System Terms Built from Word Parts**

Exercise B

Pronounce and Spell Terms Built from Word Parts
1. Check responses with the Term Table in Exercise A, #24
2. Check answers with online resources

Exercise C

Build and Translate MORE Medical Terms Built from Word Parts
1. **Label:** Figure 4.6, (1) trache/o; (2) bronch/o; (3) pneum/o, pneumon/o, pulmon/o; (4) thorac/o, -thorax
2. **Match:** a. -stomy, creation of an artificial opening; b. -tomy, cut into, incision; c. endo-, within; d. -al, pertaining to; e. -scope, instrument used for visual examination
3. **Translate:** a. trache/o/tomy, incision of the trachea; b. trache/o/stomy, creation of an artificial opening into the trachea; c. endo/trache/al, pertaining to within the trachea
4. **Reading Exercise**
5. **Label:** Figure 4.7, endo/trache/al, laryng/o/scope
6. **Reading Exercise**
7. **Label** Figure 4.8, trache/o/stomy
8. **Match:** a. -scope, instrument used for visual examination; b. -scopy, visual examination; c. -itis, inflammation
9. **Build:** a. bronch/itis; b. bronch/o/scope; c. bronch/o/scopy
10. **Reading Exercise**
11. **Label:** Figure 4.9, bronch/o/scopy

12. **Match:** a. -ia, diseased state, condition of; b. -ectomy, surgical removal, excision; c. -ary, pertaining to; d. -logy, study of; e. -logist, one who studies and treats (specialist, physician)
13. **Translate:** a. pulmon/ary, pertaining to the lung; b. pulmon/o/logy, study of the lung; c. pulmon/o/logist, physician who studies and treats diseases of the lung
14. **Reading Exercise**
15. **Build:** a. pneumon/ia; b. bronch/o/pneumon/ia; c. pneumon/ectomy
16. **Reading Exercise**
17. **Match:** a. -tomy, cut into, incision; b. -centesis, surgical puncture to remove fluid (with a sterile needle); c. -thorax, thorac/o; chest, chest cavity; d. pneum/o, lung, air
18. **Build:** a. pneum/o/thorax; b. thorac/o/tomy; c. thora/centesis
19. **Label:** Figure 4.10, pneum/o/thorax
20. **Reading Exercise**
21. **Label:** Figure 4.11, thora/centesis
22. **Match:** a. thorac/o, chest, chest cavity; b. endo-, within; c. -scope, instrument for visual examination; d. -scopy, visual examination; e. -scopic, pertaining to visual examination; f. -ic, pertaining to
23. **Translate:** a. endo/scope, instrument used for visual examination within; b. endo/scopic, pertaining to visual examination within; c. endo/scopy, visual examination within
24. **Reading Exercise**
25. **Build:** a. thorac/ic; b. thorac/o/scopy; c. thorac/o/scope; d. thorac/o/scopic
26. **Reading Exercise**
27. **Label:** Figure 4.12, thorac/o/scopic
28. **Match:** a. -graphy, process of recording; b. -gram, record; c. poly-, many; d. somn/o, sleep
29. **Translate:** a. poly/somn/o/graphy, process of recording many sleep (tests); b. poly/somn/o/gram, record of many sleep (tests)
30. **Reading Exercise**
31. **Label:** Figure 4.13, A. poly/somn/o/graphy; B. poly/somn/o/gram
32. **Term Table: Review of MORE Terms Built from Word Parts**

Exercise D

Pronounce and Spell Medical Terms Built from Word Parts
1. Check responses with the Term Table in Exercise C, #32

2. Check answers with the online resources

Exercise E

Label
1. computed tomography; 2. radiograph; 3. obstructive sleep apnea; 4. emphysema; 5. upper respiratory infection; 6. culture and sensitivity

Exercise F

Learn Medical Terms NOT Built from Word Parts
1. chronic obstructive pulmonary disease; radiograph; 2. asthma; 3. upper respiratory infection; influenza; 4. tuberculosis; sputum; culture and sensitivity; 5. emphysema; 6. computed tomography; 7. obstructive sleep apnea; OSA

Exercise G

Pronounce and Spell Medical NOT Terms Built from Word Parts
1. Check responses with the Table for Terms NOT Built from Word Parts
2. Check answers with online resources

Exercise H

Abbreviate Medical Terms
1. Sign and Symptom
   SOB
2. Diseases and disorders
   a. TB; b. COPD; c. flu; d. URI; e. OSA
3. Diagnostic tests and equipment
   a. C&S; b. CT; c. CXR; d. V/Q scan; e. PSG; f. PFTs; g. ABGs
4. Profession
   RT
5. Related Terms
   a. CPAP; b. CO_2; c. ET; d. O_2

Exercise I

Signs and Symptoms
1. apnea; 2. dyspnea; 3. hyperpnea; 4. hypopnea; 5. hyperoxia; 6. hypoxia; 7. hypocapnia; 8. hypercapnia; 9. rhinitis; 10. rhinorrhagia; 11. rhinorrhea

Exercise J

Diseases and Disorders
1. sinusitis; 2. laryngitis; 3. pharyngitis; 4. nasopharyngitis; 5. upper respiratory infection; 6. influenza; 7. tuberculosis; 8. pneumothorax; 9. pneumonia; 10. bronchopneumonia;

11. bronchitis; 12. emphysema;
13. chronic obstructive pulmonary
disease; 14. obstructive sleep apnea;
15. asthma

Exercise K

Diagnostic Tests and Equipment
1. capnometer; 2. oximeter;
3. spirometer; 4. endoscopic;
5. thoracoscopy; 6. laryngoscopy;
7. bronchoscopy; 8. endoscope;
9. laryngoscope; 10. bronchoscope;
11. thoracoscope; 12. endoscopy;
13. thoracoscopic; 14. radiograph;
15. computed tomography; 16. culture
and sensitivity; 17. polysomnography;
18. polysomnogram

Exercise L

Surgical Procedures
1. thoracentesis; 2. thoracotomy;
3. sinusotomy; 4. tracheotomy;
5. tracheostomy; 6. laryngectomy;
7. pneumonectomy

Exercise M

Specialties and Professions
1. pulmonology; 2. pulmonologist

Exercise N

*Medical Terms Related to the
Respiratory System*
1. thoracic; 2. pulmonary; 3. nasal;
4. laryngeal; 5. pharyngeal;
6. endotracheal; 7. mucous; 8. sputum

Exercise O

*Use Medical Terms in Clinical
Statements*
1. hypopnea; apnea; acrocyanosis
2. bronchoscopy; carcinoma, metastasis;
thoracentesis; pneumonectomy
3. dyspnea; pneumothorax; thoracotomy
4. Sinusitis; rhinitis; rhinorrhea;
Endoscopic; 5. radiograph; tuberculosis;
pneumonia; COPD; pulmonary;
6. oximeter; radiograph; computed
tomography; emphysema; Hypercapnia
7. rhinorrhagia; 8. pharyngitis; 9. V/Q
scan; pulmonary; 10. polysomnography,
polysomnogram, pulmonologist

Exercise P

Apply Medical Terms to Case Study
Answer will vary and may include
dyspnea, pharyngitis, rhinorrhea, upper
respiratory infection, and/or sputum along
with their respective definitions.

Exercise Q

Use Medical Language in Documents
1. dyspnea; 2. sputum; 3. rhinorrhea;
4. nasal; 5. edema; 6. cyanosis;
7. radiographs; 8. pneumonia; 9. upper
respiratory infection; 10. mucus;
resembling; resembling mucus;
11. oximeter; radiographs;
12. posteroanterior; back to the front;
13. Research exercise; answers vary.

Exercise R

*Use Medical Language in Online
Electronic Health Records*
Completed with online resources.

Exercise S

Online Review of Lesson Content
Completed with online resources.

Exercise T

Lesson Content Quiz
   1. b; 2. a; 3. a; 4. a; 5. b; 6. c; 7. b;
   8. a; 9. c; 10. a

LESSON 5

Exercise A

*Build and Translate Medical Terms Built
from Word Parts*
1. **Label:** Figure 5.3, (1) cyst/o;
   (2) urethr/o
2. **Match:** a. -gram; record, radiographic
   image; b. -graphy; process of
   recording, radiographic imaging; c. -itis;
   inflammation; d. -iasis; condition;
   e. lith/o; stone(s), calculus (*pl.* calculi)
3. **Build:** a. cyst/itis; b. cyst/o/graphy;
   c. cyst/o/gram; d. cyst/o/lith/iasis
4. **Reading exercise**
5. **Label:** Figure 5.4, A. cyst/o/gram;
   B. cyst/o/lith/iasis
6. **Match:** a. -stomy; creation of an
   artificial opening; b. -scope;
   instrument used for visual
   examination; c. -scopy; visual
   examination; d. -tomy; cut into,
   incision; e. -plasty; surgical repair;
   f. lith/o; stone(s), calculus (*pl.*
   calculi)
7. **Translate:** a. cyst/o/stomy; creation
   of an artificial opening into the
   bladder; b. cyst/o/scope; instrument
   used for visual examination of the
   bladder; c. cyst/o/scopy; visual
   examination of the bladder; d. cyst/o/
   lith/o/tomy; incision into the bladder to
   remove stone(s)

8. **Reading Exercise**
9. **Build:** a. urethr/o/scope; b. urethr/o/
   cyst/itis; c. cyst/o/urethr/o/graphy;
   d. urethr/o/plasty
10. **Reading Exercise**
11. **Label:** Figure 5.5, cyst/o/urethr/o/
    graphy
12. **Match:** a. ur/o; urine, urination,
    urinary tract; b. hem/o, hemat/o;
    blood; c. py/o; pus; d. dys-; difficult
    or painful; e. -ia; diseased state,
    condition of
13. **Translate:** a. hemat/ur/ia; condition
    of blood in the urine; b. py/ur/ia;
    condition of pus in the urine; c. dys/
    ur/ia; condition of difficult or painful
    urination
14. **Reading Exercise**
15. **Match:** a. a-, an-; absence of,
    without; b. noct/i; night; c. olig/o;
    few, scanty; d. -emia; blood condition;
    e. ur/o; urine, urination, urinary tract
16. **Build:** a. an/ur/ia; b. noct/ur/ia;
    c. olig/ur/ia; d. ur/emia
17. **Reading Exercise**
18. **Label:** Figure 5.6, (1) nephr/o, ren/o;
    (2) pyel/o
19. **Match:** a. lith/o; stone(s), calculus (*pl.*
    calculi); b. nephr/o; kidney; c. pyel/o;
    renal pelvis; d. -tripsy; surgical
    crushing; e. -iasis; condition
20. **Translate:** a. lith/o/tripsy; surgical
    crushing of stone(s); b. nephr/o/lith/
    iasis; condition of stone(s) in the
    kidney; c. pyel/o/lith/o/tomy; incision
    into the renal pelvis to remove stone(s)
21. **Reading Exercise**
22. **Label:** Figure 5.7, pyel/o/lith/o/tomy
23. **Term Table: Review of Urinary
    System Terms Built from
    Word Parts**

Exercise B

*Pronounce and Spell Medical Terms
Built from Word Parts*
1. Check responses with the Term Table
   in Exercise A, #23
2. Check answers with online resources

Exercise C

*Build and Translate MORE Medical
Terms Built from Word Parts*
1. **Label:** Figure 5.8, 1. ureter/o; 2. meat/o
2. **Match:** a. -itis; inflammation;
   b. -osis; abnormal condition;
   c. -al; pertaining to; d. hydr/o; water;
   e. pyel/o; renal pelvis

3. **Translate:** a. nephr/itis; inflammation of the kidney; b. ren/al; pertaining to the kidney; c. hydr/o/nephr/osis; abnormal condition of water (urine) in the kidney; d. pyel/o/nephr/itis; inflammation of the renal pelvis and kidney
4. **Reading Exercise**
5. **Label:** Figure 5.9, pyel/o/nephr/itis
6. **Reading Exercise**
7. **Label:** Figure 5.10, hydr/o/nephr/osis
8. **Match:** a. pyel/o; renal pelvis; b. -ectomy; surgical removal, excision; c. -stomy; creation of an artificial opening; d. -tomy; cut into, incision
9. **Build:** a. nephr/ectomy; b. nephr/o/stomy; c. nephr/o/tomy
10. **Reading Exercise**
11. **Label:** Figure 5.11, nephr/o/stomy
12. **Match:** a. -itis; inflammation; b. -tomy; cut into, incision; c. -iasis; condition; d. -plasty; surgical repair; e. lith/o; stone(s), calculus (*pl.* calculi)
13. **Translate:** a. ureter/o/lith/iasis; condition of stone(s) in the ureter; b. ureter/o/pyel/o/nephr/itis; inflammation of the ureter, renal pelvis, and kidney; c. ureter/o/lith/o/tomy; incision into the ureter to remove stone(s)
14. **Reading Exercise**
15. **Build:** a. ureter/ectomy; b. ureter/o/plasty
16. **Reading Exercise**
17. **Label:** Figure 5.12, ureter/o/plasty
18. **Match:** a. -al; pertaining to; b. -scopy; visual examination; c. -tomy; cut into, incision
19. **Translate:** a. meat/al; pertaining to the meatus; b. meat/o/scopy; visual examination of the meatus; c. meat/o/tomy; incision into the meatus (to enlarge it)
20. **Reading Exercise**
21. **Match:** a. -gram; record, radiographic image; b. -logist; one who studies and treats (specialist, physician); c. -logy; study of; d. -stomy; creation of an artificial opening
22. **Build:** a. ur/o/gram; b. ur/o/logist; c. ur/o/logy; d. ur/o/stomy
23. **Reading Exercise**
24. **Label:** Figure 5.13, ur/o/gram
25. **Translate:** a. nephr/o/logist; physician who studies and treats diseases of the kidney; b. nephr/o/logy; study of the kidney

26. **Reading Exercise**
27. **Term Table: Review of MORE Urinary System Terms Built from Word Parts**

Exercise D
Pronounce and Spell Terms Built from Word Parts
1. Check responses with the Term Table in Exercise C, #27
2. Check answers with the online resources

Exercise E
Label
1. urinary catheterization;
2. extracorporeal shock wave lithotripsy;
3. dialysis; 4. renal calculi; 5. urinalysis;
6. renal transplant

Exercise F
Learn Medical Terms NOT Built from Word Parts
1. incontinence; void; urinary tract infection; urinalysis; urinary catheterization
2. chronic kidney disease; renal failure
3. dialysis
4. renal calculi; extracorporeal shock wave lithotripsy

Exercise G
Pronounce and Spell Medical Terms NOT Built from Word Parts
1. Check responses with the Table for Terms NOT Built from Word Parts
2. Check answers with the online resources

Exercise H
Write abbreviations
1. Diseases and Disorders:
   a. CKD; b. UTI; c. PKD; d. OAB
2. Diagnostic Tests:
   a. UA; b. VCUG
3. Surgical Procdures:
   a. ESWL; b. HD
4. Specialties and Professions: PCT
5. Related Term: cath

Exercise I
Signs and Symptoms
1. anuria; 2. dysuria; 3. hematuria;
4. nocturia; 5. oliguria; 6. pyuria;
7. incontinence

Exercise J
Diseases and Disorders
1. cystitis; 2. cystolithiasis;
3. hydronephrosis; 4. nephrolithiasis (or renal calculi); 5. nephritis;
6. pyelonephritis; 7. urethrocystitis;
8. renal calculi (or nephrolithiasis);
9. renal failure; 10. urinary tract infection;
11. uremia; 12. ureterolithiasis;
13. ureteropyelonephritis;
14. chronic kidney disease

Exercise K
Diagnostic Tests and Equipment
1. cystogram; 2. cystography;
3. cystoscope; 4. cystoscopy;
5. cystourethrography; 6. meatoscopy;
7. urethroscope; 8. urinalysis;
9. urogram

Exercise L
Surgical Procedures
1. cystolithotomy; 2. cystostomy;
3. extracorporeal shock wave lithotripsy;
4. lithotripsy; 5. meatotomy;
6. nephrectomy; 7. ureteroplasty;
8. nephrostomy; 9. nephrotomy;
10. pyelolithotomy; 11. renal transplant;
12. ureterectomy; 13. urostomy;
14. ureterolithotomy;
15. urethroplasty

Exercise M
Specialties and Professions
1. nephrology; 2. nephrologist;
3. urology; 4. urologist

Exercise N
Medical Terms related to the Urinary System
1. meatal; 2. renal; 3. dialysis;
4. urinary catheterization; 5. void

Exercise O
Use Medical Terms in Clinical Statements
1. nephrectomy; renal; nephritis
2. dysuria; hematuria; urinalysis; pyuria; cystitis
3. cystitis; cystogram; cystoscopy
4. Lithotripsy; ureterolithiasis
5. incontinence; urologist; urethroplasty
6. cystourethrography; urinary tract infection
7. nephrologist; CKD (chronic kidney disease); dialysis; incontinence

Exercise P

Apply Medical Terms to the Case Study
Answers will vary and may include hematuria, urinary tract infection, dysuria, nephrolithiasis and/or renal calculi along with their respective definitions.

Exercise Q

Use Medical Terms in a Document
1. hematuria; 2. nephrolithiasis or renal calculi; 3. urinary tract infection; 4. renal; 5. dialysis; 6. urinalysis; 7. pyuria; 8. ureterolithiasis; 9. hydronephrosis
10. urine, urination, urinary tract; diseased state, condition of; blood; condition of blood in the urine
11. may include pyuria, nocturia, oliguria, anuria, dysuria
12. chronic kidney disease
13. pertaining to away; ureter (Away means far from the kidney in this case)
14. Dictionary and use of online resources exercise; answers vary

Exercise R

Use Medical Language in Electronic Health Records Online
Completed with online resources.

Exercise S

Online Review of Lesson Content
Completed with online resources.

Exercise T

Lesson Content Quiz
1. b; 2. a; 3. c; 4. a; 5. c; 6. b; 7. a; 8. b; 9. c; 10. b

LESSON 6

Exercise A

Build and Translate Terms Built from Word Parts
1. **Label:** Figure 6.2, A. (1) oophor/o, (2) salping/o, (3) endometri/o, (4) cervic/o
   B. (1) colp/o, vagin/o; (2) hyster/o
2. **Match:** a. -al, pertaining to; b. -itis, inflammation; c. -osis, abnormal condition
3. **Build:** a. vagin/itis; b. salping/itis; c. oophor/itis; d. cervic/itis
4. **Translate:** a. vagin/al, pertaining to the vagina; b. cervic/al, pertaining to

the cervix; c. endometri/al, pertaining to the endometrium; d. endometr/itis, inflammation of the endometrium; e. endometri/osis, abnormal condition of the endometrium (growth of endometrial tissue outside of the uterus)
5. **Reading exercise**
6. **Label:** Figure 6.3, (1) endometr/itis, (2) cervic/itis, (3) vagin/itis, (4) salping/itis
7. **Reading exercise**
8. **Label:** Figure 6.4, endometri/osis
9. **Match:** a. -logy, study of; b.-logist, one who studies and treats (physician, specialist); c. -scope, instrument used for visual examination; d. -scopy, visual examination; e. gynec/o, woman (women)
10. **Build:** a. colp/o/scope; b. colp/o/scopy; c. gynec/o/logy; d. gynec/o/logist
11. **Reading exercise**
12. **Match:** a. -cele, hernia, protrusion; b. -pexy, surgical fixation
13. **Translate:** a. cyst/o/cele, protrusion of the (urinary) bladder (through anterior vaginal wall); b. hyster/o/pexy, surgical fixation of the uterus
14. **Reading exercise**
15. **Label:** Figure 6.5, cyst/o/cele
16. **Match:** a. -gram, record, radiographic image; b. -pexy, surgical fixation; c. -ectomy, surgical removal, excision; d. -rrhexis, rupture; e. -rrhaphy, suturing, repairing
17. **Build:** a. hyster/ectomy; b. oophor/o/pexy; c. hyster/o/rrhexis; d. hyster/o/rrhaphy
18. **Reading exercise**
19. **Translate:** a. cervic/ectomy, excision of the cervix; b. oophor/ectomy, excision of the ovary; c. hyster/o/salping/o/-oophor/ectomy, excision of the uterus, uterine tube(s), and ovaries; d. hyster/o/salping/o/gram, radiographic image of the uterus and uterine tubes
20. **Reading exercise**
21. **Label:** Figure 6.6, hyster/o/salping/o/gram
22. **Reading exercise**
23. **Label:** Figure 6.7, A. hyster/ectomy, B. oophor/ectomy, C. hyster/o/salping/o/-oophor/ectomy
24. **Match:** a. a-, without, absence of; b. dys-, difficult, painful, abnormal; c. men/o, menstruation, menstrual;

d. -rrhea, flow, discharge; e. -rrhagia, rapid flow of blood; excessive bleeding
25. **Translate:** a. a/men/o/rrhea, without menstrual flow; b. dys/men/o/rrhea, painful menstrual flow; c. men/o/rrhea, flow at menstruation; d. men/o/rrhagia, rapid flow of blood at menstruation
26. **Reading exercise**
27. **Match:** a. -gram, record, radiographic image; b. -graphy, process of recording, radiographic imaging; c. -plasty, surgical repair; d. -ectomy, surgical removal, excision; e. mamm/o, mast/o, breast; f. son/o, sound; g. -pexy, surgical fixation
28. **Build:** a. mast/ectomy; b. mast/o/pexy; c. mamm/o/gram; d. mamm/o/graphy; e. mamm/o/plasty; f. son/o/graphy
29. **Reading exercise**
30. **Label:** Figure 6.8, A. mamm/o/graphy, B. mamm/o/gram
31. **Review of Female Reproductive System Terms Built from Word Parts**

Exercise B

Pronounce and Spell Terms Built from Word Parts
1. Check responses with the Term Table in Exercise A, #31
2. Check answers with the online resources

Exercise C

Build and Translate MORE Medical Terms Built from Word Parts
1. **Label:** Figure 6.9, 1. prostat/o, 2. scrot/o, 3. orchi/o
2. **Match:** a. cyst/o, bladder, sac; b. lith/o, stone(s), calculus (*pl.* calculi); c. -itis, inflammation; d. -ectomy, surgical removal, excision; e. -ic, pertaining to
3. **Translate:** a. prostat/itis, inflammation of the prostate gland; b. prostat/o/cyst/itis, inflammation of the prostate gland and the (urinary) bladder; c. prostat/ic, pertaining to the prostate gland; d. prostat/o/lith, stone(s) in the prostate gland; e. prostat/ectomy, excision of the prostate gland
4. **Reading exercise**
5. **Label:** Figure 6.10, prostat/ic
6. **Match:** a. -itis, inflammation; b. -ectomy, surgical removal, excision;

c. -pexy, surgical fixation; d. -al, pertaining to; e. -plasty, surgical repair
7. **Build:** a. orch/itis [the i from the the combining form orchi/o has been dropped], b. orchi/o/pexy, c. orchi/ectomy; d. scrot/al; e. scrot/o/plasty
8. **Reading Exercise**
9. **Match:** a. vas/o, vessel, duct, b. -ectomy, surgical removal, excision, c. -stomy, creation of an artificial opening
10. **Translate:** a. vas/ectomy, excision of the duct (vas deferens); b. creation of an artificial opening between ducts
11. **Reading Exercise**
12. **Label:** 6.11, vas/ectomy
13. **Review of Male Reproductive System Terms Built from Word Parts**

Exercise D
Pronounce and Spell MORE Terms Built from Word Parts
1. Check responses with the Term Table in Exercise C, #13
2. Check answers with the online resources

Exercise E
Label
1. dilation and curettage; 2. uterine fibroid; 3. benign prostatic hyperplasia; 4. pelvic inflammatory disease; 5. transurethral resection of the prostate gland; 6. circumcision; 7. Pap test

Exercise F
Learn Medical Terms NOT Built from Word Parts
1. Pap test; 2. sexually transmitted infection; 3. uterine fibroids; 4. pelvic inflammatory disease; 5. dilation and curettage; 6. prostate-specific antigen assay; digital rectal examination; 7. benign prostatic hyperplasia; transurethral resection of the prostate gland; 8. erectile dysfunction; 9. circumcision; 10. semen analysis; 11. obstetrics; 12. uterovaginal prolapse

Exercise G
Pronounce and Spell Medical NOT Terms Built from Word Parts
1. Check responses with the Table for Terms NOT Built from Word Parts

2. Check answers with the online resources.

Exercise H
Write Abbreviations
1. Diseases and Disorders: a. STI; b. STD; c. PID; d. BPH; e. HPV; f. ED
2. Diagnostic Tests: a. DRE; b. PSA; c. HSG; d. TRUS
3. Surgical Procedures: a. D&C; b. TURP; c. TAH/BSO; d. RP
4. Specialties and Professions: a. OB-GYN
5. Related Terms: Cx

Exercise I
Signs and Symptoms
1. menorrhagia; 2. amenorrhea; 3. dysmenorrhea

Exercise J
Diseases and Disorders
1. benign prostatic hyperplasia; 2. erectile dysfunction; 3. sexually transmitted infection; 4. cervicitis; 5. cystocele; 6. endometritis; 7. endometriosis; 8. uterovaginal prolapse; 9. mastitis; 10. oophoritis; 11. salpingitis; 12. vaginitis; 13. orchitis; 14. prostatitis; 15. prostatocystitis; 16. prostatolith; 17. pelvic inflammatory disease; 18. uterine fibroid

Exercise K
Surgical Procedures
1. orchiectomy; 2. orchiopexy; 3. prostatectomy; 4. scrotoplasty; 5. vasectomy; 6. vasovasostomy; 7. cervicectomy; 8. hysterectomy; 9. hysteropexy; 10. hysterorrhaphy; 11. hysterorrhexis; 12. hysterosalpingo-oophorectomy; 13. mammoplasty; 14. mastectomy; 15. oophorectomy; 16. oophoropexy; 17. transurethral resection of the prostate gland; 18. dilation and curettage; 19. mastopexy

Exercise L
Diagnostic Tests and Equipment
1. colposcope; 2. colposcopy; 3. hysterosalpingogram; 4. mammogram; 5. mammography; 6. Pap test; 7. digital rectal examination; 8. prostate-specific antigen assay; 9. semen analysis; 10. sonography

Exercise M
Specialties and Professions
1. gynecology; 2. gynecologist; 3. obstetrics

Exercise N
Medical Terms Related to the Reproductive Systems
1. menorrhea; 2. vaginal; 3. cervical; 4. endometrial; 5. scrotal; 6. prostatic

Exercise O
Use Medical Terms in Clinical Statements
1. colposcopy; Pap test
2. vaginal; vaginitis
3. mammography; mammogram; mastectomy; mammoplasty
4. BPH; prostatitis; prostatic; prostatectomy
5. scrotal; orchiectomy, orchiopexy

Exercise P
Apply Medical Terms to Case Study
Answers will vary, and may include menorrhea, dysmenorrhea, menorrhagia, sexually transmitted infection, orchiopexy, and corresponding definitions.

Exercise Q
Use Medical Terms in a Document
1. orchiopexy; 2. menorrhea; 3. dysmenorrhea; 4. menorrhagia; 5. Pap test; 6. prostatitis; 7. sexually transmitted infections; 8. cervicitis; 9. pelvic inflammatory disease 10. semen analysis 11. hysterosalpingogram 12. scrot/o, scrotum; -cele, hernia, protrusion; scrotocele, hernia of the scrotum 13. DRE, digital rectal examination; BPH, benign prostatic hyperplasia 14. Dictionary exercise; answers will vary

Exercise R
Use Medical Language in Electronic Health Records Online
Completed with online resources.

Exercise S
Online Review of Lesson Content
Completed with online resources.

Exercise T

Lesson Content Quiz

1. b; 2. a; 3. c; 4. a; 5. a; 6. c; 7. b;
8. a; 9. b; 10. c

LESSON 7

Exercise A

Build and Translate Medical Terms Built from Word Parts

1. **Label:** Figure 7.5, (1) arteri/o;
(2) cardi/o; (3) angi/o
2. **Match:** a. -logist; one who studies and treats (specialist, physician);
b. -logy; study of; c. -ac; pertaining to; d. -megaly; enlargement
3. **Build:** a. cardi/ac; b. cardi/o/logy;
c. cardi/o/logist; d. cardi/o/megaly
4. **Reading Exercise**
5. **Match:** a. -gram; record, radiographic image; b. -graph; instrument used to record; c. -graphy; process of recording, radiographic imaging
6. **Translate:** a. electr/o/cardi/o/gram, record of the electrical activity of the heart; b. electr/o/cardi/o/graph, instrument used to record the electrical activity of the heart;
c. electr/o/cardi/o/graphy, process of recording the electrical activity of the heart
7. **Reading Exercise**
8. **Label:** Figure 7.6, electr/o/cardi/o/gram
9. **Match:** a. my/o; muscle; b. ech/o; sound; c. tachy-; rapid, fast;
d. brady-; slow; e. -pnea; breathing;
f. path/o; disease; g. -a, -y; no meaning
10. **Build:** a. ech/o/cardi/o/gram;
b. brady/cardi/a;
c. cardi/o/my/o/path/y
11. **Reading Exercise**
12. **Label:** Figure 7.7, ech/o/cardi/o/gram
13. **Translate:** a. my/o/cardi/al, pertaining to the muscle of the heart;
b. tachy/cardi/a, rapid heart rate;
c. tachy/pnea, rapid breathing
14. **Reading Exercise**
15. **Match:** a. -ectomy; surgical removal, excision; b. -al; pertaining to; c. -gram; record, radiographic image;
d. -sclerosis; hardening; e. endo-; within
16. **Build:** a. end/arter/ectomy [the o from the prefix endo- has been dropped];
b. arteri/al; c. arteri/o/sclerosis;
d. arteri/o/gram

17. **Reading Exercise**
18. **Label:** Figure 7.8, arteri/o/gram;
Figure 7.9, end/arter/ectomy [the o from the prefix endo- has been dropped]
19. **Match:** a. -graphy; process of recording, radiographic imaging;
b. -plasty; surgical repair
20. **Translate:** a. angi/o/graphy, radiographic imaging of the blood vessels; b. angi/o/plasty, surgical repair of the blood vessels
21. **Reading Exercise**
22. **Label:** Figure 7.10, angi/o/plasty
23. **Term Table: Review of Cardiovascular and Lymphatic System Terms Built from Word Parts**

Exercise B

Pronounce and Spell Terms Built from Word Parts

1. Check responses with the Term Table in Exercise A, #23
2. Check answers with online resources

Exercise C

Build and Translate MORE Medical Terms Built from Word Parts

1. **Label:** Figure 7.11, phleb/o, ven/o
2. **Match:** a. -ous; pertaining to;
b. -gram; record, radiographic image;
c. -intra; within
3. **Build:** a. intra/ven/ous; b. ven/o/gram
4. **Reading Exercise**
5. **Label:** Figure 7.12 A. ven/o/gram;
B. intra/ven/ous
6. **Match:** a. -itis; inflammation;
b. -tomy; cut into, incision;
c. thromb/o; blood clot;
d. -osis; abnormal condition
7. **Translate:** a. phleb/itis, inflammation of the veins; b. phleb/o/tomy, incision into the vein (with a needle to remove or instill fluid); c. thromb/osis, abnormal condition of a blood clot;
d. thromb/o/phlebitis, inflammation of the veins associated with blood clots
8. **Reading Exercise**
9. **Label:** Figure 7.13, thromb/osis
10. **Match:** a. cyt/o; cell; b. -e; no meaning; c. -penia; abnormal reduction (in number); d. leuk/o; white; e. thromb/o; blood clot
11. **Translate:** a. thromb/o/cyt/e, blood clotting cell; b. thromb/o/cyt/o/penia, abnormal reduction of blood clotting

cells; c. leuk/o/cyt/o/penia, abnormal reduction of white blood cells
12. **Reading Exercise**
13. **Label:** Figure 7.14, (1) lymph/o;
(2) splen/o
14. **Match:** a. -ectomy; surgical removal, excision; b. -megaly; enlargement
15. **Build:** a. splen/o/megaly;
b. splen/ectomy
16. **Reading Exercise**
17. **Match:** a. -itis; inflammation;
b. path/o; disease; c. -oma; tumor;
d. aden/o; gland(s); node(s); e. -y; no meaning
18. **Translate:** a. lymph/aden/o/path/y, disease of the lymph nodes;
b. lymph/aden/itis, inflammation of the lymph nodes; c. lymph/oma, tumor of lymphatic tissue
19. **Reading Exercise**
20. **Match:** a. -logist; one who studies and treats (specialist, physician);
b. -logy; study of; c. -oma; tumor;
d. -stasis; control, stop; e. -lysis; dissolution, separating
21. **Build:** a. hemat/o/logy;
b. hemat/o/logist; c. hemat/oma;
d. hem/o/stasis; e. hem/o/lysis
22. **Reading Exercise**
23. **Label:** Figure 7.15, hemat/oma
24. **Term Table: Review of MORE Cardiovascular and Lymphatic System Terms Built from Word Parts**

Exercise D

Pronounce and Spell MORE Terms Built from Word Parts

1. Check responses with the Term Table in Exercise C, #24
2. Check answers with the online resources

Exercise E

Label

1. cardiac catheterization; 2. coronary artery bypass graft; 3. varicose veins;
4. complete blood count; 5. aneurysm;
6. cardiopulmonary resuscitation;
7. stethoscope; 8. blood pressure

Exercise F

Learn Medical Terms NOT Built from Word Parts

1. complete blood count; CBC; 2. blood pressure; BP; pulse; P; 3. stethoscope;

sphygmomanometer; hypertension; HTN; hypotension; 4. coronary artery disease; CAD; myocardial infarction; MI; cardiac catheterization; 5. aneurysm; 6. anemia; hemorrhage; leukemia; 7. heart failure; HF; cardiopulmonary resuscitation; CPR; 8. embolus; coronary artery bypass graft; CABG; 9. varicose veins

Exercise G

Pronounce and Spell Terms NOT Built from Word Parts

1. Check responses with the Table for Terms NOT Built from Word Parts
2. Check answers with the online resources

Exercise H

Abbreviate Medical Terms

1. Diseases and Disorders:
   a. CAD; b. HF; c. MI; d. HTN; e. PAD; f. HHD; g. DVT
2. Diagnostic Tests and Equipment:
   a. BP; b. CBC; c. ECHO; d. ECG, EKG; e. VS; f. P; g. DSA
3. Surgical Procedures: a. CABG; b. PTCA
4. Related Terms: a. CPR; b. IV

Exercise I

Signs and Symptoms

1. bradycardia; 2. cardiomegaly; 3. hemorrhage; 4. hypertension; 5. hypotension; 6. splenomegaly; 7. tachycardia; 8. tachypnea

Exercise J

Diseases and Disorders

1. anemia; 2. aneurysm; 3. arteriosclerosis; 4. cardiomyopathy; 5. coronary artery disease; 6. embolus; 7. heart failure; 8. hematoma; 9. hemolysis; 10. leukemia; 11. leukocytopenia; 12. lymphadenitis; 13. lymphadenopathy; 14. lymphoma; 15. myocardial infarction; 16. phlebitis; 17. thrombocytopenia; 18. thrombophlebitis; 19. thrombosis; 20. varicose veins

Exercise K

Diagnostic Tests and Equipment

1. angiography; 2. arteriogram; 3. blood pressure; 4. cardiac catheterization; 5. complete blood count; 6. echocardiogram; 7. electrocardiogram; 8. electrocardiograph;

9. electrocardiography; 10. pulse; 11. sphygmomanometer; 12. stethoscope; 13. venogram

Exercise L

Surgical Procedures

1. angioplasty; 2. coronary artery bypass graft; 3. endarterectomy; 4. phlebotomy; 5. splenectomy

Exercise M

Specialties and Professions

1. cardiologist; 2. cardiology; 3. hematologist; 4. hematology

Exercise N

Medical Terms related to Cardiovascular and Lymphatic Systems

1. arterial; 2. cardiac; 3. cardiopulmonary resuscitation; 4. hemostasis; 5. intravenous; 6. myocardial; 7. thrombocyte

Exercise O

Use Medical Terms in Clinical Statements

1. heart failure; electrocardiography; cardiac
2. thrombophlebitis; embolus
3. Thrombocytopenia; hemorrhage; hemostasis; anemia
4. Tachycardia; pulse; hypotension
5. Arteriosclerosis; arterial
6. complete blood count; leukemia; hematologist
7. Coronary artery disease; angioplasty; coronary artery bypass graft

Exercise P

Apply Medical Terms to the Case Study

Answers will vary and may include blood pressure, hypertension, tachycardia, and tachypnea, along with their corresponding definitions.

Exercise Q

Use Medical Terms in a Document

1. hypertension; 2. varicose veins; 3. cardiologist; 4. coronary artery bypass graft (CABG); 5. aneurysm; 6. Phlebotomy; 7. Electrocardiogram (ECG, EKG); 8. myocardial infarction (MI); 9. Cardiac catheterization; 10. fatty plaque; vessel wall; producing, originating, causing; causing a fatty plaque deposit on a vessel wall;

11. HF; 12. coronary; 13. Dictionary and use of online references

Exercise R

Use Medical Language in Electronic Health Records Online

Complete with online resources

Exercise S

Online Review of Lesson Content

Complete with online resources

Exercise T

Lesson Content Quiz

1. a; 2. c; 3. b; 4. c; 5. c; 6. b; 7. a; 8. c; 9. a; 10. c

LESSON 8

Exercise A

Build and Translate Medical Terms Built from Word Parts

1. **Label:** Figure 8.3, (1) gloss/o; lingu/o; (2) gingiv/o; (3) or/o; (4) esophag/o; (5) gastr/o
2. **Match:** a. -algia; pain; b. -itis; inflammation
3. **Build:** a. gingiv/algia; b. gingiv/itis
4. **Reading Exercise**
5. **Label:** Figure 8.4, gingiv/itis
6. **Match:** a. -itis; inflammation; b. -al; pertaining to; c. sub-; below, under
7. **Translate:** a. gloss/itis; inflammation of the tongue; b. sub/lingu/al; pertaining to under the tongue
8. **Build:** or/al
9. **Reading Exercise**
10. **Label:** Figure 8.5, sub/lingu/al
11. **Match:** a. peps/o; digestion; b. phag/o; swallowing, eating; c. enter/o; intestines (the small intestine); d. -ia; diseased state, condition of; e. -y; no meaning; f. a-; without
12. **Build:** a. dys/enter/y; b. dys/peps/ia; c. dys/phag/ia
13. **Translate:** a/phag/ia; condition of without swallowing
14. **Reading Exercise**
15. **Match:** a. -eal; pertaining to; b. -itis; inflammation
16. **Build:** a. esophag/eal; b. esophag/itis
17. **Reading Exercise**
18. **Label:** Figure 8.6, esophag/itis
19. **Match:** a. enter/o; intestines (the small intestine); b. -itis; inflammation;

c. -logist; one who studies and treats (specialist, physician); d. -logy; study of
20. **Build:** a. gastr/o/enter/o/logist; b. gastr/o/enter/o/logy; c. gastr/o/enter/itis
21. **Match:** a. -ectomy; excision; b. -itis; inflammation; c. -eal, -ic; pertaining to; d. esophag/o; esophagus
22. **Translate:** a. gastr/itis; inflammation of the stomach; b. gastr/ic; pertaining to the stomach; c. gastr/ectomy; excision of the stomach; d. gastr/o/esophag/eal; pertaining to the stomach and esophagus
23. **Reading Exercise**
24. **Label:** Figure 8.7, gastr/ectomy
25. **Match:** a. -scope; instrument used for visual examination; b. -stomy; creation of an artificial opening; c. -scopy; visual examination
26. **Build:** a. gastr/o/scope; b. gastr/o/scopy; c. gastr/o/stomy
27. **Reading Exercise**
28. **Label:** Figure 8.8, A. gastr/o/scopy; B. gastr/o/scope
29. **Match:** a. -scope; instrument used for visual examination; b. -scopic; pertaining to visual examination; c. -scopy; visual examination; d. abdomin/o, lapar/o; abdomen, abdominal cavity
30. **Translate:** a. lapar/o/scope; instrument used for visual examination of the abdominal cavity; b. lapar/o/scopic; pertaining to visual examination of the abdominal cavity; c. lapar/o/scopy; visual examination of the abdominal cavity
31. **Reading Exercise**
32. **Label:** Figure 8.9, Lapar/o/scopic
33. **Match:** a. -centesis; surgical puncture to remove fluid; b. -tomy; incision
34. **Translate:** a. abdomin/o/centesis; surgical puncture to remove fluid from the abdominal cavity; b. lapar/o/tomy; incision into the abdominal cavity
35. **Reading Exercise**
36. **Term Table: Review of the Digestive System Terms Built from Word Parts**

Exercise B

Pronounce and Spell Terms Built from Word Parts
1. Check responses with the Term Table in Exercise A, #36

2. Check answers with the online resources

Exercise C

Build and Translate MORE Medical Terms Built from Word Parts
1. **Label:** Figure 8.10, (1) chol/e, cyst/o; (2) duoden/o; (3) ile/o; (4) append/o, appendic/o; (5) proct/o, rect/o; (6) hepat/o; (7) pancreat/o; (8) col/o, colon/o; (9) jejun/o; (10) sigmoid/o; (11) an/o
2. **Match:** a. duoden/o; duodenum; b. -al; pertaining to; c. esophag/o; esophagus; d. gastr/o; stomach; e. -scopy; visual examination
3. **Translate:** a. esophag/o/gastr/o/duoden/o/scopy; visual examination of the esophagus, stomach, and duodenum; b. duoden/al; pertaining to the duodenum
4. **Reading Exercise**
5. **Match:** a. -stomy; creation of an artificial opening; b. jejun/o; jejunum; c. ile/o; ileum
6. **Build:** a. ile/o/stomy; b. jejun/o/stomy
7. **Reading Exercise**
8. **Match:** a. -oma; tumor; b. -itis; inflammation; c. -megaly; enlargement
9. **Translate:** a. hepat/itis; inflammation of the liver; b. hepat/oma; tumor of the liver; c. hepat/o/megaly; enlargement of the liver
10. **Reading Exercise**
11. **Label:** Figure 8.11, hepat/oma
12. **Match:** a. -itis; inflammation; b. -ectomy; excision; c. cyst/o; bladder, sac; d. lith/o; stone(s), calculus (*pl.* calculi)
13. **Translate:** a. chol/e/cyst/itis; inflammation of the gallbladder; b. chol/e/cyst/ectomy; excision of the gallbladder; c. chol/e/lith/iasis; condition of gallstone(s)
14. **Reading Exercise**
15. **Label:** Figure 8.12, chol/e/lith/iasis
16. **Match:** a. -ic; pertaining to; b. -itis; inflammation
17. **Build:** a. pancreat/ic; b. pancreat/itis
18. **Reading Exercise**
19. **Match:** a. -itis; inflammation; b. -ectomy; excision
20. **Translate:** a. append/ectomy; excision of the appendix; b. appendic/itis; inflammation of the appendix

21. **Reading Exercise**
22. **Label:** Figure 8.13, appendic/itis
23. **Match:** a. -itis; inflammation; b. -stomy; creation of an artificial opening; c. -ectomy; excision; d. -graphy; process of recording, radiographic imaging; e. -scopy; visual examination
24. **Build:** a. colon/o/scopy; b. CT colon/o/graphy
25. **Reading Exercise**
26. **Label:** Figure 8.14, colon/o/graphy
27. **Build:** a. col/itis; b. col/o/stomy; c. col/ectomy
28. **Reading Exercise**
29. **Label:** Figure 8.15, Col/o/stomy
30. **Match:** a. -scopy; visual examination; b. sigmoid/o; sigmoid colon; c. proct/o; rectum; d. -scope; instrument used for visual examination
31. **Translate:** a. sigmoid/o/scopy; visual examination of the sigmoid colon; b. proct/o/scope; instrument used for visual examination of the rectum; c. proct/o/scopy; visual examination of the rectum
32. **Reading Exercise**
33. **Label:** Figure 8.16, Sigmoid/o/scopy
34. **Match:** a. an/o; anus; b. rect/o; rectum; c. -cele; hernia, protrusion; d. -al; pertaining to
35. **Build:** a. rect/o/cele; b. rect/al
36. **Translate:** an/al; pertaining to the anus
37. **Reading Exercise**
38. **Term Table: Review of MORE Digestive System Terms Built from Word Parts**

Exercise D

Pronounce and Spell MORE Terms Built from Word Parts
1. Check responses with the Term Table in Exercise C, #38
2. Check answers with online resources.

Exercise E

Label
1. endoscopic retrograde cholangiopancreatography; 2. peptic ulcer; 3. gastroesophageal reflux disease; 4. barium enema; 5. polyp; 6. stoma; 7. bariatric surgery; 8. hemorrhoids

Exercise F

Learn Medical Terms NOT Built from Word Parts

1. gastroesophageal reflux disease; GERD; 2. irritable bowel syndrome; IBS; constipation; diarrhea; 3. polyp; barium enema; 4. endoscopic retrograde cholangiopancreatography; 5. ulcerative colitis; stoma; Crohn disease; 6. cirrhosis; 7. peptic ulcer; upper GI series; 8. celiac disease; parenteral

Exercise G

Pronounce and Spell Terms NOT Built from Word Parts

1. Check responses with the Table for Terms NOT Built from Word Parts
2. Check answers with online resources.

Exercise H

Abbreviate Medical Terms

1. Diseases and disorders:
   a. GERD; b. IBS; c. UC
2. Diagnostic tests and equipment;
   a. BE; b. EGD; c. ERCP; d. UGI series
3. Surgical procedures: PEG
4. Related terms: a. BM; b. GI; c. TPN

Exercise I

Signs and Symptoms

1. aphagia; 2. constipation; 3. diarrhea; 4. dyspepsia; 5. dysphagia; 6. gingivalgia; 7. hepatomegaly

Exercise J

Diseases and Disorders

1. appendicitis; 2. cholecystitis; 3. cholelithiasis; 4. colitis; 5. Crohn disease; 6. dysentery; 7. esophagitis; 8. gastritis; 9. gastroenteritis; 10. gastroesophageal reflux disease; 11. gingivitis; 12. glossitis; 13. hemorrhoids; 14. hepatitis; 15. hepatoma; 16. celiac disease; 17. irritable bowel syndrome; 18. pancreatitis; 19. peptic ulcer; 20. polyp; 21. rectocele; 22. ulcerative colitis; 23. cirrhosis

Exercise K

Diagnostic Tests and Equipment

1. barium enema; 2. colonoscopy; 3. CT colonography; 4. endoscopic retrograde cholangiopancreatography;

5. esophagogastroduodenoscopy; 6. gastroscope; 7. gastroscopy; 8. laparoscope; 9. laparoscopic; 10. laparoscopy; 11. proctoscope; 12. proctoscopy; 13. sigmoidoscopy; 14. upper GI series

Exercise L

Surgical Procedures

1. abdominocentesis; 2. appendectomy; 3. bariatric surgery; 4. cholecystectomy; 5. colectomy; 6. colostomy; 7. gastrectomy; 8. gastrostomy; 9. ileostomy; 10. jejunostomy; 11. laparotomy

Exercise M

Specialties and Professions

1. gastroenterologist; 2. gastroenterology

Exercise N

Medical Terms Related to the Digestive System

1. anal; 2. duodenal; 3. esophageal; 4. gastric; 5. gastroesophageal; 6. oral; 7. pancreatic; 8. rectal; 9. sublingual; 10. parenteral; 11. stoma

Exercise O

Use Medical Terms in Clinical Statements

1. cholecystitis; laparoscopy; cholecystectomy; 2. gastrostomy; esophageal; 3. esophagogastroduodenoscopy; gastroenterologist; peptic ulcer; 4. Hepatomegaly; hepatitis; hepatoma; cirrhosis; 5. GERD, gastroesophageal; dysphagia; esophagitis; 6. oral; gingivitis; glossitis; sublingual; 7. Ulcerative colitis; colectomy; ileostomy

Exercise P

Apply Medical Terms to the Case Study

Answers will vary and may include gastric, dyspepsia, gastroesophageal reflux disease, dysphagia, and gastroenterologist, along with their respective definitions.

Exercise Q

Use Medical Terms in a Document

1. dyspepsia; 2. esophagogastroduodenoscopy; 3. intravenous; 4. lateral; 5. gastroscope; 6. gastric; 7. distal; 8. gastritis; 9. duodenal; 10. blood;

vomiting; vomiting blood; 11. causing (producing, originating) ulcers; 12. dictionary/online exercise

Exercise R

Use Medical Language in Electronic Health Records Online

Completed with online resources.

Exercise S

Online Review of Lesson Content

Completed with online resources.

Exercise T

Lesson Content Quiz

1. a; 2. a; 3. b; 4. a; 5. c; 6. b; 7. b; 8. c; 9. a; 10. c

LESSON 9

Exercise A

Build and Translate Terms Built from Word Parts

1. **Label:** Figure 9.5, A. (1) ophthalm/o, (2) blephar/o, (3) scler/o, (4) ir/o, irid/o; B. (1) kerat/o, (2) retin/o
2. **Match:** a. -logy, study of; b. -scope, instrument used for visual examination; c. -logist, one who studies and treats (specialist, physician); d. -meter, instrument used to measure; e. -itis, inflammation
3. **Build:** a. ophthalm/o/logy; b. ophthalm/o/logist
4. **Translate:** A. ophthalm/o/scope, instrument used for visual examination of the eye; B. kerat/o/meter, instrument used to measure (the curvature of) the cornea
5. **Reading exercise**
6. **Label:** Figure 9.6, ophthalm/o/scope
7. **Translate:** a. blephar/itis, inflammation of the eyelid; b. ir/itis, inflammation of the iris; c. retin/itis, inflammation of the retina; d. scler/itis, inflammation of the sclera
8. **Reading exercise**
9. **Label:** Figure 9.7, A. scler/itis, B. blephar/itis
10. **Match:** a. -ptosis, drooping, sagging, prolapse; b. -plegia, paralysis; c. -ectomy, excision; d. -plasty, surgical repair
11. **Build:** a. irid/ectomy; b. blephar/o/plasty; c. kerat/o/plasty

12. **Translate:** a. irid/o/plegia, paralysis of the iris; b. blephar/o/ptosis, drooping of the eyelid
13. **Label:** Figure 9.8, blephar/o/ptosis
14. **Reading exercise**
15. **Match:** a. -al, -ic, pertaining to; b. -metry, measurement; c. opt/o, vision
16. **Build:** a. opt/o/metry; b. opt/ic; c. ophthalm/ic
17. **Translate:** a. scler/al, pertaining to the sclera; b. retin/al, pertaining to the retina
18. **Reading exercise**
19. **Review of Eye Terms Built from Word Parts**

Exercise B

Pronounce and Spell Terms Built from Word Parts

1. Check responses with the Term Table in Exercise A, #19
2. Check answers with the online resources

Exercise C

Build and Translate MORE Medical Terms Built from Word Parts

1. **Label:** Figure 9.9. 1. ot/o; 2. myring/o; 3. tympan/o
2. **Match:** a. -rrhea, flow, discharge; b. -plasty, surgical repair; c. -scope, instrument used for visual examination; d. -itis, inflammation
3. **Translate:** a. ot/o/rrhea, discharge from the ear; b. ot/o/scope, instrument used for visual examination of the ear; c. ot/o/plasty, surgical repair of the (outer) ear
4. **Label:** Figure 9.10, ot/o/scope
5. **Build:** a. ot/itis, b. myring/itis
6. **Reading exercise**
7. **Label:** Figure 9.11, ot/itis
8. **Match:** a. -ic, pertaining to, b. -tomy, incision; c. -plasty, surgical repair; d. -logy, study of; e. -logist, one who studies and treats (specialist, physician); f. laryng/o, larynx (voice box)
9. **Build:** a. tympan/ic; b. tympan/o/plasty
10. **Translate:** a. myring/o/tomy, incision of the eardrum; b. myring/o/plasty, surgical repair of the eardrum
11. **Reading exercise**
12. **Label:** Figure 9.12, myring/o/tomy

13. **Build:** a. ot/o/laryng/o/logy, b. ot/o/laryng/o/logist
14. **Reading exercise**
15. **Match:** a. audi/o, hearing; b. -logy, study of; c. -logist, one who studies and treats (specialist, physician); d. -meter, instrument used to measure; e. -metry, measurement
16. **Translate:** a. audi/o/logy, study of hearing; b. audi/o/logist, specialist who studies and treats (impaired) hearing; c. audi/o/meter, instrument used to measure hearing; d. audi/o/metry, measurement of hearing
17. **Reading exercise**
18. **Label:** Figure 9.13, audi/o/meter
19. **Review of Ear Terms Built from Word Parts**

Exercise D

Pronounce and Spell MORE Terms Built from Word Parts

1. Check responses with the Term Table in Exercise C, #19
2. Check answers with the online resources

Exercise E

Label

1. cataract; 2. retinal detachment; 3. macular degeneration; 4. LASIK; 5. optometrist; 6. tinnitus; 7. A. presbyopia; B. presbycusis

Exercise F

Learn Medical Terms NOT Built from Word Parts

1. LASIK; astigmatism; hyperopia; myopia; 2. glaucoma; 3. cataract; optometrist; 4. macular degeneration; age-related; 5. retinal detachment; 6. otitis media; 7. tinnitus; 8. presbyopia; presbycusis

Exercise G

Pronounce and Spell Terms NOT Built from Word Parts

1. Check responses with the Table for Terms NOT Built from Word Parts
2. Check answers with the online resources

Exercise H

Abbreviate medical terms.

1. Signs and Symptoms: a. IOP; b. HOH
2. Diseases and Disorders: a. OM; b. AST; c. ARMD

3. Diagnostic Test: VA
4. Specialties and Professions: a. Ophth, b. ENT
5. Related: ENT

Exercise I

Signs and Symptoms

1. otorrhea; 2. tinnitus

Exercise J

Diseases and Disorders

1. astigmatism; 2. otitis media; 3. myopia; 4. hyperopia; 5. cataract; 6. macular degeneration; 7. retinal detachment; 8. glaucoma; 9. presbycusis; 10. presbyopia; 11. blepharitis; 12. blepharoptosis; 13. iridoplegia; 14. iritis; 15. scleritis; 16. retinitis; 17. myringitis; 18. otitis

Exercise K

Diagnostic Tests and Equipment

1. ophthalmoscope; 2. keratometer; 3. audiometer; 4. otoscope; 5. audiometry

Exercise L

Surgical Procedures

1. blepharoplasty; 2. iridectomy; 3. keratoplasty; 4. LASIK; 5. myringoplasty; 6. myringotomy; 7. otoplasty; 8. tympanoplasty

Exercise M

Specialties and Professions

1. ophthalmologist; 2. ophthalmology; 3. optometry; 4. optometrist; 5. audiologist; 6. audiology; 7. otolaryngologist; 8. otolaryngology

Exercise N

Medical Terms Related to the Eye and Ear

1. ophthalmic; 2. optic; 3. retinal; 4. scleral; 5. tympanic

Exercise O

Use Medical Terms in Clinical Statements

1. ophthalmologist
2. LASIK; hyperopia
3. iridectomy; glaucoma
4. blepharoplasty; blepharoptosis
5. keratometer
6. Presbyopia; optometrist
7. otoscope; audiometer
8. otolaryngologist; myringotomy

9. Myringoplasty; tympanoplasty
10. Presbycusis; audiologist

Exercise P

Apply Medical Terms to Case Study
Answers will vary and may include
  presbyopia, presbycusis, glaucoma,
  ophthalmologist, otolaryngologist, and
  otitis media along with corresponding
  definitions.

Exercise Q

Use Medical Terms in a Document
  1. ENT; 2. tinnitus; 3. otitis media;
  4. tympanoplasty; 5. glaucoma;
  6. ophthalmologist; 7. optometrist;
  8. otoscope; 9. tympanic; 10. otorrhea;
  11. audiologist; 12. otitis; 13. audiology;
  14. otolaryngologist;
  15. ocul/o, eye; -ar, pertaining to; ocul/ar,
    pertaining to the eye;
  16. any visible change in tissue resulting
    from injury or disease;
  17. Research activity. Answers will vary.

Exercise R

*Use Medical Language in Electronic
Health Records Online*
Completed with online resources.

Exercise S

Online Review of Lesson Content
Completed with online resources.

Exercise T

Lesson Content Quiz
  1. a; 2. c; 3. b; 4. c; 5. b; 6. c; 7. b;
  8. a; 9. a; 10. c

LESSON 10

Exercise A

*Build and Translate Medical Terms Built
from Word Parts*
  1. **Label:** Figure 10.2, (1) rachi/o,
    spondyl/o, vertebr/o; (2) carp/o;
    (3) phalang/o
  2. **Match:** a. -al; pertaining to;
    b. -ectomy; excision; c. -plasty;
    surgical repair; d. inter-; between
  3. **Build:** a. vertebr/al; b. inter/vertebr/al;
    c. vertebr/ectomy; d. vertebr/o/plasty
  4. **Label:** Figure 10.3: inter/vertebr/al
  5. **Reading Exercise**

  6. **Match:** a. -schisis; split, fissure;
    b. -tomy; incision; c. -itis;
    inflammation; d. arthr/o; joint(s)
  7. **Translate:** a. rachi/schisis; fissure of
    the vertebral column; b. rachi/o/tomy;
    incision into the vertebral column
  8. **Build:** a. spondyl/arthr/itis
  9. **Reading Exercise**
  10. **Match:** a. -osis; abnormal condition;
    b. kyph/o; hump (thoracic spine);
    c. lord/o; bent forward (lumbar spine);
    d. scoli/o; crooked, curved (spine)
  11. **Translate:** a. scoli/osis; abnormal
    condition of crooked, curved (spine);
    b. kyph/osis; abnormal condition of
    a hump (thoracic spine); c. lord/osis;
    abnormal condition of bent forward
    (lumbar spine)
  12. **Label:** Figure 10.5, A. lord/osis;
    B. kyph/osis; C. scoli/osis
  13. **Match:** a. -al, -eal; pertaining to;
    b. -ectomy; excision
  14. **Build:** a. carp/al; b. carp/ectomy
  15. **Reading Exercise**
  16. **Translate:** a. phalang/eal; pertaining
    to a phalanx; b. phalang/ectomy;
    excision of a phalanx
  17. **Reading Exercise**
  18. **Match:** a. a-; absence of, without;
    b. dys-; difficult, painful, abnormal;
    c. hyper-; above, excessive;
    d. -y; no meaning; e. -ic; pertaining to
  19. **Build:** a. dys/troph/y; b. a/troph/y;
    c. hyper/troph/y; d. hyper/troph/ic
  20. **Reading Exercise**
  21. **Label:** Figure 10.7, hyper/troph/ic
  22. **Label:** Figure 10.8, burs/o
  23. **Match:** a. -itis; inflammation;
    b. -ectomy; excision; c. -tomy;
    incision
  24. **Translate:** a. burs/ectomy; excision
    of a bursa; b. burs/itis; inflammation
    of the bursa; c. burs/o/tomy; incision
    into a bursa
  25. **Reading Exercise**
  26. **Label:** Figure 10.9, burs/itis
  27. **Label:** Figure 10.10, (1) ili/o; (2)
    pub/o; (3) ischi/o
  28. **Match:** a. -al, -ac; pertaining to;
    b. femor/o; femur
  29. **Translate:** a. ili/ac; pertaining to the
    ilium; b. femor/al; pertaining to the
    femur; c. ili/o/femor/al; pertaining to
    the ilium and the femur; d. ischi/al;
    pertaining to the ischium; e. ischi/o/
    pub/ic; pertaining to the ischium
    and the pubis

  30. **Reading Exercise**
  31. **Match:** a. -algia; pain; b. -asthenia;
    weakness; c. -gram; record,
    radiographic image; d. electr/o;
    electrical activity; e. my/o, muscle
  32. **Build:** a. my/algia; b. my/asthenia;
    c. electr/o/my/o/gram
  33. **Reading Exercise**
  34. **Label:** Figure 10.11,
    electr/o/my/o/gram
  35. **Match:** a. -brady-; slow; b. dys-;
    difficult, painful, abnormal; c. -a; no
    meaning
  36. **Build:** a. brady/kinesi/a; b. dys/
    kinesi/a
  37. **Reading Exercise**
  38. **Term Table: Review of the
    Musculoskeletal System Terms
    Built from Word Parts**

Exercise B

*Pronounce and Spell Medical Terms
Built from Word Parts*
  1. Check responses with the Term Table
    in Exercise A, #38
  2. Check answers with the online
    resources

Exercise C

*Build and Translate MORE Medical
Terms Built from Word Parts*
  1. **Label:** Figure 10.12, (1) crani/o;
    (2) stern/o; (3) cost/o
  2. **Match:** a. -tomy; incision;
    b. intra-; within; c. -schisis; split,
    fissure; d. -malacia; softening;
    e. -al; pertaining to; f. -ia; diseased
    state, condition of
  3. **Build:** a. intra/crani/al;
    b. crani/o/schisis; c. crani/o/tomy;
    d. crani/o/malacia
  4. **Reading Exercise**
  5. **Label:** Figure 10.13, intra/crani/al
  6. **Match:** a. -al; pertaining to; b. inter-;
    between; c. sub-; below, under
  7. **Translate:** a. stern/al; pertaining to
    the sternum; b. stern/o/cost/al;
    pertaining to the sternum and
    the ribs
  8. **Reading Exercise**
  9. **Label:** Figure 10.14, stern/al
  10. **Build:** a. inter/cost/al; b. sub/cost/al
  11. **Reading Exercise**
  12. **Label:** Figure 10.15, (1) oste/o;
    (2) ten/o, tendin/o; (3) arthr/o;
    (4) chondr/o

13. **Match:** a. -itis; inflammation; b. -ectomy; excision; c. -malacia; softening; d. -al; pertaining to
14. **Translate:** a. cost/o/chondr/al; pertaining to the ribs and cartilage; b. chondr/itis; inflammation of cartilage; c. chondr/ectomy; excision of cartilage; d. chondr/o/malacia; softening of cartilage
15. **Reading Exercise**
16. **Label:** Figure 10.16, cost/o/chondr/al
17. **Match:** a. -osis; abnormal condition; b. -itis; inflammation; c. necr/o; death
18. **Build:** a. necr/osis; b. oste/o/necr/osis; c. oste/o/chondr/itis
19. **Reading Exercise**
20. **Match:** a. path/o; disease; b. -malacia; softening; c. -penia; abnormal reduction; d. -y; no meaning
21. **Translate:** a. oste/o/path/y; disease of the bone; b. oste/o/penia; abnormal reduction of bone mass; c. oste/o/malacia; softening of the bone
22. **Reading Exercise**
23. **Match:** a. sarc/o; flesh, connective tissue; b. -oma; tumor; c. -itis; inflammation
24. **Build:** a. oste/o/arthr/itis; b. oste/o/sarc/oma
25. **Reading Exercise**
26. **Label:** Figure 10.17, oste/o/sarc/oma
27. **Match:** a. -algia; pain; b. -desis; surgical fixation, fusion; c. -plasty; surgical repair; d. -itis; inflammation
28. **Translate:** a. arthr/algia; pain in the joint; b. arthr/itis; inflammation of the joint(s); c. arthr/o/desis; surgical fixation (fusion) of a joint; d. arthr/o/plasty; surgical repair of a joint
29. **Reading Exercise**
30. **Match:** a. -centesis; surgical puncture to remove fluid; b. -gram; record, radiographic image; c. -scopy; visual examination; d. -scopic; pertaining to visual examination
31. **Build:** a. arthr/o/centesis; b. arthr/o/gram; c. arthr/o/scopy; d. arthr/o/scopic
32. **Label:** Figure 10.18, arthr/o/scopy, arthr/o/scopic
33. **Match:** a. -desis; surgical fixation, fusion; b. -itis; inflammation; c. -plasty; surgical repair
34. **Translate:** a. tendin/itis; inflammation of the tendon(s); b. ten/o/plasty;

surgical repair of a tendon; c. ten/o/desis; surgical fixation (fusion) of a tendon
35. **Reading Exercise**
36. **Term Table: Review of MORE Musculoskeletal Terms Built from Word Parts**

Exercise D

Pronounce and Spell Medical Terms Built from Word Parts

1. Check responses with the Term Table in Exercise C, #36
2. Check answers with the online resources

Exercise E

Label

1. Lyme disease; 2. carpal tunnel syndrome; 3. fracture; 4. gout; 5. osteoporosis; 6. herniated disk; 7. spinal stenosis; 8. plantar fasciitis; 9. nuclear medicine; 10. magnetic resonance imaging; 11. rheumatoid arthritis

Exercise F

Learn Medical Terms NOT Built from Word Parts

1. Orthopedics; orthopedist; fracture; herniated disk; spinal stenosis; 2. rheumatoid arthritis; 3. Gout; 4. muscular dystrophy; 5. carpal tunnel syndrome; plantar fasciitis; 6. magnetic resonance imaging; 7. nuclear medicine; 8. osteoporosis; 9. hernia; 10. chiropractic; 11. Lyme disease

Exercise G

Pronounce and Spell Medical Terms NOT Built from Word Parts

1. Check responses with the Table for Terms NOT Built from Word Parts
2. Check answers with the online resources

Exercise H

Abbreviate Medical Terms

1. Diseases and Disorders: a. CTS; b. Fx; c. MD; d. OA; e. RA
2. Diagnostic tests and equipment: a. EMG; b. MR; c. MRI; d. NM
3. Surgical Procedures: a. TKA; b. THA
4. Specialties and Professions: a. ortho; b. PT; c. DO; d. OT; e. DC

5. Related Terms: a. C1-C7; b. L1-L5; c. T1-T12; d. ROM

Exercise I

Signs and Symptoms

1. arthralgia; 2. atrophy; 3. bradykinesia; 4. dyskinesia; 5. dystrophy; 6. hypertrophy; 7. myalgia; 8. myasthenia; 9. hernia

Exercise J

Diseases and Disorders

1. arthritis; 2. plantar fasciitis; 3. bursitis; 4. carpal tunnel syndrome; 5. chondritis; 6. chondromalacia; 7. craniomalacia; 8. cranioschisis; 9. fracture; 10. gout; 11. herniated disk; 12. kyphosis; 13. lordosis; 14. muscular dystrophy; 15. necrosis; 16. osteoarthritis; 17. osteochondritis; 18. osteomalacia; 19. osteonecrosis; 20. osteopathy; 21. osteopenia; 22. osteoporosis; 23. osteosarcoma; 24. rachischisis; 25. rheumatoid arthritis; 26. scoliosis; 27. spondylarthritis; 28. tendinitis; 29. spinal stenosis; 30. Lyme disease

Exercise K

Diagnostic Tests and Equipment

1. arthrogram; 2. arthroscopic; 3. arthroscopy; 4. electromyogram; 5. magnetic resonance imaging; 6. nuclear medicine

Exercise L

Surgical Procedures

1. arthrocentesis; 2. arthrodesis; 3. arthroplasty; 4. bursectomy; 5. bursotomy; 6. carpectomy; 7. chondrectomy; 8. craniotomy; 9. phalangectomy; 10. rachiotomy; 11. tenodesis; 12. tenoplasty; 13. vertebrectomy; 14. vertebroplasty

Exercise M

Specialties and Professions

1. orthopedics; 2. orthopedist; 3. chiropractic

Exercise N

Medical Terms related to the Musculoskeletal System

1. carpal; 2. costochondral; 3. femoral; 4. hypertrophic; 5. iliac; 6. iliofemoral;

7. intercostal; 8. intervertebral;
9. intracranial; 10. ischial; 11.
ischiopubic; 12. phalangeal; 13. sternal;
14. sternocostal; 15. subcostal;
16. vertebral

Exercise O

Use Medical Terms in Clinical Statements

1. arthritis; fracture; arthrodesis
2. arthrogram; arthroscopy; arthroscopic
3. arthroplasty; osteoarthritis
4. scoliosis; lordosis; kyphosis; osteoporosis
5. muscular dystrophy; electromyogram
6. orthopedist; tendinitis; tenoplasty
7. Bursitis; arthritis; bursotomy
8. Chondromalacia; Osteomalacia
9. Hypertrophy; atrophy
10. chiropractic; spinal stenosis
11. intracranial; intercostal; subcostal; ischiopubic; iliac; sternocostal; vertebral; femoral; sternal

Exercise P

Apply Medical Terms to A Case Study

Answers will vary and may include
phalangeal, carpal, iliac, myalgia, and
contusion, along with their respective
definitions.

Exercise Q

Use Medical Terms in a Document

1. orthopedics; 2. fracture;
3. myalgia; 4. kyphosis;
5. vertebral; 6. iliac;
7. carpal; 8. phalangeal;
9. osteoporosis
10. a. radi/al;
    b. uln/ar
11. student exercise; 12. bruise
13. dictionary/online exercise

Exercise R

Use Medical Language in Electronic Health Records Online

Complete with online resources

Exercise S

Online Review of Lesson Content

Complete with online resources

Exercise T

Lesson Content Quiz

1. b; 2. a; 3. b; 4. c; 5. a; 6. b; 7. c;
8. b; 9. a; 10. c

LESSON 11

Exercise A

Build and Translate Medical Terms Built from Word Parts

1. **Label:** Figure 11.3, 1. cerebr/o;
   2. encephal/o
2. **Match:** a. -al; pertaining to; b. angi/o; blood vessel(s); c. -graphy; process of recording, radiographic imaging; d. thromb/o; blood clot; e. -osis; abnormal condition
3. **Build:** a. cerebr/al; b. cerebral angi/o/graphy; c. cerebral thromb/osis
4. **Reading Exercise**
5. **Label:** Figure 11.4, cerebr/al angi/o/graphy
6. **Match:** a. -itis; inflammation; b. -y; no meaning; c. path/o; disease
7. **Build:** a. encephal/o/path/y; b. encephal/itis
8. **Reading Exercise**
9. **Match:** a. electr/o; electrical activity; b. -graphy; process of recording, radiographic imaging; c. -graph; instrument used to record; d. -gram; record, radiographic image
10. **Translate:** a. electr/o/encephal/o/gram; record of electrical activity of the brain; b. electr/o/encephal/o/graph; instrument used to record electrical activity of the brain; c. electr/o/encephal/o/graphy; process of recording the electrical activity of the brain
11. **Reading Exercise**
12. **Label:** Figure 11.5, electr/o/encephal/o/graphy
13. **Match:** a. -al; pertaining to; b. -algia; pain
14. **Build:** a. neur/al; b. neur/algia
15. **Reading Exercise**
16. **Label:** Figure 11.6, neur/algia
17. **Match:** a. -logist; one who studies and treats (specialist, physician); b. -logy; study of; c. path/o; disease; d. -y; no meaning
18. **Translate:** a. neur/o/logist; physician who studies and treats diseases of the nervous system; b. neur/o/logy: study of the nerves (nervous system); c. neur/o/path/y; disease of the nerves (nervous system)
19. **Reading Exercise**
20. **Match:** a. -itis; inflammation; b. -algia; pain; c. arthr/o; joint(s); d. my/o; muscle(s); e. neur/o; nerve(s)

21. **Build:** a. poly/my/algia; b. poly/arthr/itis; c. poly/neur/itis
22. **Reading Exercise**
23. **Term Table: Review of the Nervous System and Behavioral Health Terms Built from Word Parts**

Exercise B

Pronounce and Spell Medical Terms Built from Word Parts

1. Check responses with the Term Table in Exercise A, #23
2. Check answers with online resources

Exercise C

Build and Translate MORE Medical Terms Built from Word Parts

1. **Label:** Figure 11.7, 1. myel/o; 2. mening/o, meningi/o
2. **Match:** a. -oma; tumor; b. -itis; inflammation; c. -cele; hernia, protrusion
3. **Build:** a. mening/o/cele; b. mening/itis; c. meningi/oma
4. **Reading Exercise**
5. **Label:** Figure 11.8, meningi/oma
6. **Match:** a. -itis; inflammation; b. poli/o; gray matter
7. **Translate:** a. mening/o/myel/itis; inflammation of the meninges and spinal cord; b. poli/o/myel/itis; inflammation of the gray matter of the spinal cord
8. **Reading Exercise**
9. **Match:** a. -graphy; process of recording, radiographic imaging; b. -gram; record, radiographic image
10. **Build:** a. myel/o/gram; b. myel/o/graphy
11. **Reading Exercise**
12. **Label:** Figure 11.9, myel/o/graphy
13. **Match:** a. -algia; pain; b. -us; no meaning; c. hydr/o; water d. micro-; small
14. **Translate:** a. micro/cephal/us; small head; b. hydr/o/cephal/us; water (cerebrospinal fluid) in the head (brain); c. ceph/algia pain in the head (headache) *NOTE: the **al** is dropped from the combining form cephal/o.*
15. **Reading Exercise**
16. **Match:** a. a-; absence of, without; b. dys-; difficult, painful, abnormal; c. hemi-; half; d. quadr/i; four; e. -ia; diseased state, condition of

17. **Build:** a. a/phas/ia; b. dys/phas/ia
18. **Reading Exercise**
19. **Translate:** a. hemi/pleg/ia; condition of paralysis of half (right or left side of the body); b. quadr/i/pleg/ia; condition of paralysis of four (limbs)
20. **Reading Exercise**
21. **Label:** Figure 11.10, A. hemi/pleg/ia; C. quadr/i/pleg/ia
22. **Match:** a. -genic; producing, originating, causing; b. path/o; disease; c. -y; no meaning; d. -osis; abnormal condition
23. **Build:** a. psych/o/genic; b. psych/o/path/y; c. psych/osis
24. **Reading Exercise**
25. **Match:** a. -logist; one who studies and treats (specialist, physician); b. -logy; study of
26. **Translate:** a. psych/o/logist; specialist who studies and treats the mind; b. psych/o/logy; study of the mind
27. **Reading Exercise**
28. **Term Table: Review of MORE Nervous System and Behavioral Health Terms Built from Word Parts**

Exercise D
Pronounce and Spell MORE Terms Built from Word Parts
1. Check responses with the Term Table in Exercise C, #28
2. Check answers with online resources

Exercise E
Label
1. transient ischemic attack; 2. stroke;
3. subarachnoid hemorrhage;
4. dementia; 5. Alzheimer disease;
6. lumbar puncture; 7. paraplegia;
8. sciatica; 9. migraine; 10. psychiatrist

Exercise F
Learn Medical Terms NOT Built from Word Parts
1. multiple sclerosis; MS; 2. Parkinson disease; PD; 3. dementia; Alzheimer disease; 4. concussion; seizure;
5. sciatica; epidural nerve block;
6. migraine; 7. lumbar puncture; LP;
8. stroke; CVA; 9. subarachnoid hemorrhage; 10. transient ischemic

attack; TIA; syncope; 11. paraplegia;
12. anxiety disorder; 13. depression;
14. bipolar disorder; 15. psychiatrist

Exercise G
Pronounce and Spell Terms NOT Built from Word Parts
1. Check responses with the Table for Terms NOT Built from Word Parts
2. Check answers with online resources

Exercise H
Abbreviate Medical Terms
1. Diseases and Disorders:
   a. AD; b. CVA; c. MS; d. PD;
   e. SAH; f. TIA
2. Diagnostic Tests and Equipment:
   a. EEG; b. LP
3. Related Terms:
   a. CNS; b. CSF; c. PNS;
   d. ADL, ADLs

Exercise I
Signs and Symptoms
1. aphasia; 2. cephalgia;
3. dysphasia; 4. neuralgia;
5. polyarthritis; 6. polymyalgia;
7. polyneuritis; 8. seizure;
9. syncope

Exercise J
Diseases and Disorders
1. Alzheimer disease; 2. anxiety disorder; 3. bipolar disorder; 4. cerebral thrombosis; 5. concussion; 6. dementia;
7. depression; 8. encephalitis;
9. encephalopathy; 10. hemiplegia;
11. hydrocephalus; 12. meningioma;
13. meningitis; 14. meningocele;
15. meningomyelitis; 16. migraine;
17. multiple sclerosis; 18. neuropathy;
19. paraplegia; 20. Parkinson disease;
21. poliomyelitis; 22. psychopathy;
23. psychosis; 24. quadriplegia;
25. sciatica; 26. stroke (cerebrovascular accident); 27. subarachnoid hemorrhage;
28. transient ischemic attack;
29. microcephalus

Exercise K
Diagnostic Tests and Equipment
1. cerebral angiography
2. electroencephalogram
3. electroencephalograph

4. electroencephalography
5. lumbar puncture
6. myelogram
7. myelography

Exercise L
Surgical Procedure
epidural nerve block

Exercise M
Specialties and Professions
1. neurologist; 2. neurology;
3. psychologist; 4. psychology;
5. psychiatrist

Exercise N
Medical Terms Related to the Nervous System and Behavioral Health
1. cerebral; 2. neural; 3. psychogenic

Exercise O
Use Medical Terms in Clinical Statements
1. Depression; psychology; anxiety disorder; psychiatrist, psychologist
2. bipolar disorder; psychosis
3. Cephalgia; Migraine; Subarachnoid hemorrhage
4. electroencephalography; electroencephalograph; electroencephalogram; seizures; concussions; meningitis; encephalitis
5. stroke; aphasia; hemiplegia; cerebral; TIA
6. dementia; Alzheimer disease; Parkinson disease; hydrocephalus

Exercise P
Apply Medical Terms to A Case Study
Answers will vary and may include aphasia, dysphasia, hemiplegia, stroke, or cerebrovascular accident, along with their respective definitions.

Exercise Q
Use Medical Language in a Document
1. aphasia; 2. hemiplegia; 3. dementia;
4. dysphasia; 5. subarachnoid hemorrhage; 6. cerebrovascular accident (or stroke); 7. cerebral thrombosis;
8. cerebral angiography; 9. cerebral;
10. neurology; 11. neurologist;
12. transient ischemic attack;
13. dictionary/online exercise

Exercise R

Use Medical Language in Electronic Health Records on Evolve

Complete with online resources

Exercise S

Online Review of Lesson Content

Complete with online resources

Exercise T

Lesson Content Quiz

1. b; 2. c; 3. a; 4. b; 5. c; 6. b; 7. c;
8. b; 9. a; 10. c

LESSON 12

Exercise A

Build and Translate Terms Built from Word Parts

1. **Label:** Figure 12.2, (1) gland, aden/o;
(2) thymus gland, thym/o;
(3) thyroid gland, thyroid/o;
(4) adrenal gland, adrenal/o
2. **Match:** a. acr/o, extremities;
b. -ic, pertaining to; c. -itis, inflammation; d. -ectomy, excision;
e. -oma, tumor; f. -megaly, enlargement
3. **Build:** a. adrenal/itis;
b. adrenal/ectomy; c. aden/oma;
d. acr/o/megaly; e. adren/o/megaly
4. **Reading exercise**
5. **Label:** Figure 12.3, acr/o/megaly
6. **Translate:** a. thym/ic, pertaining to the thymus gland; b. thym/oma, tumor of the thymus gland;
c. thym/ectomy, excision of the thymus gland; d. thyroid/ectomy, excision of the thyroid gland;
e. thyroid/itis, inflammation of the thyroid gland
7. **Reading exercise**
8. **Match:** a. hyper-, above, excessive;
b. hypo-, below, deficient, under;
c. -emia, blood condition; d. -ism, state of; e. glyc/o, sugar
9. **Build:** a. hyper/thyroid/ism;
b. hypo/thyroid/ism
10. **Reading exercise**
11. **Translate:** gylc/emia, condition of sugar in the blood; b. hyper/glyc/emia, condition of excessive sugar in the blood; c. hypo/glyc/emia, condition of deficient sugar in the blood
12. **Reading exercise**

13. **Match:** a. poly-, many, much;
b. ur/o, urination, urine, urinary tract;
c. dips/o, thirst; d. -ia, diseased state, condition of
14. **Build:** a. poly/dips/ia;
b. poly/ur/ia
15. **Reading exercise**
16. **Match:** a. endo-, within; b. crin/o, to secrete; c. path/o, disease; d. -logist, one who studies and treats (specialist, physician), e. -logy, study of; f. -e, -y, no meaning
17. **Translate:** a. endo/crin/e, to secrete within; b. endo/crin/o/logy, study of the endocrine system;
c. endo/crin/o/logist, physician who studies and treats diseases of the endocrine system; d. endo/crin/o/path/y, (any) disease of the endocrine system
18. **Reading Exercise**
19. **Term Table: Review of Endocrine System Terms Built from Word Parts**

Exercise B

Pronounce and Spell Terms Built from Word Parts

1. Check responses with the Term Table in Exercise A, #19
2. Check answers with the online resources

Exercise C

Label

1. Graves disease
2. metabolic syndrome
3. goiter
4. Addison disease

Exercise D

Learn Medical Terms NOT Built from Word Parts

1. diabetes mellitus; fasting blood sugar; glycosylated hemoglobin; 2. goiter;
3. Graves disease; 4. Addison disease;
5. Fine needle aspiration; 6. Metabolic syndrome

Exercise E

Pronounce and Spell Terms NOT Built from Word Parts

1. Check responses with the Table for Terms NOT Built from Word Parts

2. Check answers with the online resources

Exercise F

Abbreviate Medical Terms

1. a. DM; b. T1DM; T2DM;
2. a. FBS; b. HbA1c; c. FNA

Exercise G

Signs and Symptoms

1. hyperglycemia; 2. hypoglycemia;
3. polydipsia; 4. polyuria;
5. adrenomegaly

Exercise H

Diseases and Disorders

1. endocrinopathy; 2. Addison disease;
3. adrenalitis; 4. Graves disease;
5. goiter; 6. hyperthyroidism;
7. hypothyroidism; 8. adenoma;
9. acromegaly; 10. thymoma;
11. thyroiditis; 12. diabetes mellitus;
13. metabolic syndrome

Exercise I

Diagnostic Tests

1. glycosylated hemoglobin;
2. fasting blood sugar; 3. fine needle aspiration

Exercise J

Surgical Procedures

1. adrenalectomy; 2. thymectomy;
3. thyroidectomy

Exercise K

Specialties and Professions

1. endocrinologist; 2. endocrinology

Exercise L

Medical Terms Related to the Endocrine System

1. endocrine; 2. glycemia; 3. thymic

Exercise M

Use Medical Terms in Clinical Statements

1. fine needle aspiration; endocrinologist;
2. FBS; HbA1c; 3. Polydipsia; polyuria;
4. hyperthyroidism; goiter; 5. Thymic;
6. adenoma; acromegaly; 7. adrenalitis; Addison disease

Exercise N

Apply Medical Terms to the Case Study

Answers will vary but may include polydipsia, polyuria, endocrinologist, fasting blood sugar, and their corresponding definitions

Exercise O

Use Medical Terms in a Document

1. 1. polyuria; 2. polydipsia; 3. Graves disease; 4. diabetes mellitus; 5. fasting blood sugar; 6. glycosylated hemoglobin; 7. hyperglycemia; 8. hypoglycemia; 9. endocrinology; 10. Answers will vary but may include nocturia, cyanosis, urinalysis; 11. Dictionary exercise.

Exercise P

Use Medical Language in Electronic Health Records Online

Complete with online resources

Exercise Q

Online Review of Lesson Content

Complete with online resources

Exercise R

Lesson Content Quiz

1. b; 2. a; 3. b; 4. c; 5. a; 6. b; 7. c; 8. a

Illustration Credits

Courtesy Rhoda Baer (Photographer). National Cancer Institute (NCI). **Unnumbered Fig. 1.6**

Courtesy Dr. Dale M. Levinsky. **Fig. 3.7**

Courtesy Nonin Medical Inc. Reprinted with permission of Nonin Medical Inc. **Fig. 4.5AB**

Adam, A et al: *Grainger and Allison's diagnostic radiology*, ed 5, Edinburgh, 2008, Churchill Livingstone. **Fig. 11.4**

Anderson KN: *Mosby's medical, nursing and allied health dictionary*, St Louis, 1998, Mosby. **Fig. 8.9**

Aspinall, RJ, Taylor-Robinson, SD: *Mosby's color atlas of gastroenterology and liver disease*, ed 1, St. Louis, 2002, Mosby. **Fig. 8.6**

Ballinger PW, Frank ED: *Merrill's atlas of radiographic positions and radiologic procedures,* ed 10, St Louis, 2003, Mosby/Elsevier. **Figs. 1.9B, 2.11, 5.4A, 5.13, 7.8, 7.10BC, 7.12A, 11.9, Unnumbered Fig. 10.11**

Barkauskas VH et al: *Health and physical assessment*, ed 3, St. Louis, 2002, Mosby. **Fig. 9.11**

Bontrager KL: *Textbook of radiographic positioning and related anatomy,* ed 5, St Louis, 2001, Mosby. **Figs. 2.5, 2.15, 8.17A**

Bontrager K, Lampignano J: *Textbook of radiographic positioning and related anatomy*, ed 6, St Louis, 2005, Mosby. **Figs. 5.5, 6.8, Unnumbered Fig. 10.7**

Bontrager KL, Lampignano J: *Textbook of radiographic positioning and related anatomy*, ed 7, St Louis, 2010, Mosby/Elsevier. **Figs. 2.2 and 2.17 (1.2, 5.6), 7.7**

Bontrager K, Lampignano J: *Textbook of radiographic positioning and related anatomy*, ed 8, St Louis, 2014, Mosby/Elsevier. **Fig. 8.14, Unnumbered Fig. 11.6**

Bork K, Brauninger W: *Skin diseases in clinical practice,* ed 2, Philadelphia, 1998, Saunders. **Fig. 7.22, Unnumbered Fig. 3.7**

Canale, ST, Beaty, JH: *Campbell's operative orthopaedics*, ed 11, Philadelphia, 2008, Mosby/Elsevier. **Fig. 10.17**

Cohen BA: *Pediatric dermatology*, ed 3, St. Louis, 2005, Mosby. **Figs. 3.8 (second from bottom, right) and 3.9A**

Damjanov I: *Pathology for the health professions*, ed 3, Philadelphia, 2006, Saunders/Elsevier. **Fig. 5.9**

Ball J et al: *Seidel's guide to physical examination,* ed 8, St. Louis, 2015, Mosby/Elsevier. **Fig. 12.3**

Dorland's illustrated medical dictionary, ed 32, Philadelphia, 2012, Saunders/Elsevier. **Fig. 11.5, Unnumbered Figs. 3.6, 3.8**

Eisenberg R, Johnson N: *Comprehensive radiographic pathology*, ed 5, St. Louis, 2012, Mosby/Elsevier. **Unnumbered Figs. 10.10, 11.13**

Ferri F: *Ferri's color atlas and text of clinical medicine*, ed 1, Philadelphia, 2009, Saunders/Elsevier. **Unnumbered Fig. 10.14**

Frank ED, Long B, Smith B: *Merrill's atlas of radiographic positions and radiologic procedures,* ed 11, St Louis, 2007, Mosby/Elsevier. **Figs. 10.14 and 10.16**

Frazier M: *Essentials of human disease and conditions,* ed 3, St. Louis, 2004, Mosby. **Fig. 3.3**

Goldman M, Weiss R: Sclerotherapy, ed 5, Philadelphia, 2011, Saunders/Elsevier. **Unnumbered Fig. 7.4**

Habif TP: *Clinical dermatology*, ed 4, St. Louis, Mosby/Elsevier. **Figs. 3.8 (top right) and 3.9B**

Haught JM, Patel S, and English JC: Xanthoderma: A clinical review, Journal of the American Academy of Dermatology; December 2007 57(6), Elsevier, 1051-1058. **Fig. 3.9C**

Ignatavicius D, Workman ML: *Medical-surgical nursing*, ed 6, Philadelphia, 2010, Saunders/Elsevier. **Fig. 7.12B, Unnumbered Fig. 11.9**

Jacob S: *Human anatomy*, ed 1, Edinburgh, 2007, Churchill Livingstone. **Fig. 10.6**

James S, Ashwill J: *Nursing care of children*, ed 3, Philadelphia, 2007, Saunders/Elsevier. **Unnumbered Fig. 5.4**

Jarvis C: *Physical examination and health assessment,* ed 5, Philadelphia, 2008, Saunders. **Figs. 9.6AB and 9.10**

Kamal A, Brockelhurst JC: *Color atlas of geriatric medicine*, ed 2, St. Louis, 1991, Mosby. **Figs. 3.8 (bottom right) and 3.10B**

Kowalczyk N: *Radiographic pathology for technologists*, ed 6, St. Louis, 2014, Mosby/Elsevier. **Fig. 8.11, 11.8, Unnumbered Fig. 8.5**

LaFleur Brooks M: *Exploring medical language,* ed 5, St Louis, 2002, Mosby. **Fig. 7.6**

LaFleur Brooks M: *Exploring medical language*, ed 9, St Louis, 2014, Mosby/Elsevier. **Figs. 5.16A, 8.12, 9.15, 12.5, and Unnumbered Figs. 1.5, 7.9, 8.2, 8.11, 9.2, 9.5, 10.5**

Lewis S et al: Medical-surgical nursing, ed 8, St. Louis, 2011, Mosby/Elsevier. **Fig. 3.8** (second from top, right)

Mace JD, Kowalczyk N: *Radiographic pathology for technologists*, ed 4, St Louis, 2004, Mosby/Elsevier. **Fig. 1.8**

Neville BW et al: *Oral and maxillofacial pathology*, ed 3, Philadelphia, 2009, Saunders/Elsevier. **Fig. 8.4**

Patton K, Thibodeau G: *Anthony's textbook of anatomy & physiology*, ed 19, St. Louis, 2010, Mosby/Elsevier. **Figs. 6.6, 10.21, Unnumbered Figs. 10.6, 10.12**

Paulino A: *PET-CT in radiotherapy treatment planning*, ed 1, Philadelphia, 2008, Saunders/Elsevier. **Fig. 4.14B, Unnumbered Fig. 4.2**

Perry PS, Potter PA, Elkin M: *Nursing interventions & clinical skills*, ed 4, St. Louis, 2008, Mosby/Elsevier. **Fig. 2.17 (3)**

Potter PA, Perry PS, Hall A: *Basic nursing,* ed 7, St. Louis, 2011, Mosby/Elsevier. **Fig. 4.2**

Potter PA, Perry PS: *Fundamentals of nursing: concepts, process, and practice,* ed 5, St Louis, 2001, Mosby. **Fig. 4.5C**

Regezi, JA et al: *Oral pathology,* ed 5, Philadelphia, 2008, Saunders/Elsevier. **Fig. 8.5**

Robertson B et al: *Polysomnography for the sleep technologist,* ed 1, St. Louis, 2014, Mosby/Elsevier. **Fig. 4.13B**

Ruppel GL: *Manual pulmonary function testing,* ed 7, St. Louis, 1998, Mosby. **Fig. 4.14A, Unnumbered Fig. 4.3**

Scheie HG, Albert DM: Textbook of ophthalmology, ed 9, Philadelphia, 1977, W. B. Saunders. **Fig. 9.7A**

Schwarzenberger K, Werchniak A, and Ko C: *General dermatology,* ed 1, Edinburgh, 2009, Saunders/Elsevier. **Fig. 3.14**

Seidel H et al: *Mosby's guide to physical examination,* ed 4, St Louis, 1999, Mosby. **Fig. 9.16**

Sorrentino S, Remmert L, and Gorek B: *Mosby's essentials for nursing assistants,* ed 4, St. Louis, 2010, Mosby/Elsevier. **Fig. 2.17 (4)**

Shiland B: *Mastering healthcare terminology,* ed 1, St Louis, 2003, Mosby. **Fig. 10.18**

Shiland B: *Mastering healthcare terminology,* ed 2, St. Louis, 2006, Mosby/Elsevier. **Figs. 3.5 (left), 11.11, Unnumbered Figs. 3.2, 3.3, 8.3**

Śliwa LS et al: A comparison of audiometric and objective methods in hearing screening of school children: A preliminary study, International Journal of Pediatric Otorhinolaryngology; April 2011 75(4), Elsevier, 483-488. **Fig. 9.13**

Stein HA, Skatt BJ, Stein RM: *The ophthalmic assistant: fundamentals and clinical practice,* ed 5, St Louis, 1998, Mosby. **Fig. 9.8**

St. John Sutton M, Wiegers S: *Echocardiography in heart failure,* ed 1, Philadelphia, 2012, Saunders. **Fig. 7.7**

Swartz M: *Textbook of physical diagnosis,* ed 5, St Louis, 2006, Saunders/Elsevier. **Fig. 1.6, Unnumbered Fig. 12.4**

Thomsen TW et al: Laceration Repair: Simple Interrupted Sutures, Procedures Consult; May 2017, Elsevier. **Unnumbered Fig. 3.9**

Turgeon M: Immunology & serology in laboratory medicine, ed 5, St. Louis, 2014, Mosby/Elsevier. **Fig. 7.16**

Wein A et al: *Campbell-Walsh urology,* ed 10, 2012, Saunders/Elsevier. **Unnumbered Fig. 5.5, 5.6, 5.9**

Wilson S, Giddens J: *Health assessment for nursing practice,* ed 9, St. Louis, 2009, Mosby. **Unnumbered Figs. 1.4, 3.5**

Yousem D, Grossman R: *Neuroradiology: the requisites,* ed 2, Philadelphia, 2003, Mosby. **Fig. 10.13**

Zitelli BJ, Davis HW: *Atlas of pediatric physical diagnosis,* ed 3, St Louis, 1997, Mosby. **Fig. 9.7B**

Zitelli BJ, Davis HW: *Atlas of pediatric physical diagnosis,* ed 4, St Louis, 2002, Mosby. **Figs. 3.8 (center right), 3.10A, 9.6C, Unnumbered Fig. 3.4**

THINKSTOCK:

AlexRaths (504033911). **Unnumbered Figs. 3.1, 3.10, Fig. 9.4**

BakiBG (482457871). **Unnumbered Fig. 4.9**

BakiBG (477510971). **Fig. 10.1**

Belchonock (480990487). **Unnumbered Fig. 5.3**

Ca-ssis (507513366). **Unnumbered Fig. 4.7**

Christopher Robbins (sb10063626cl-001). **Unnumbered Figs. 8.1 and 8.10**

Creatas (76753512). **Unnumbered Figs. 10.1 and 10.13**

Devilkae (818231774). **Fig. 4.13A**

Darrin Klimek (72991405). **Unnumbered Fig. 7.8**

diego_cervo (178131972). **Unnumbered Figs. 9.1 and 9.9.**

g-stockstudio (627673672). **Unnumbered Fig. 11.10**

John Foxx (71085840). **Fig. 6.1**

Eans (491917595). **Unnumbered Fig. 7.11**

Eraxion (116975927). **Unnumbered Fig. 1.2**

EyeMark (185509324). **Unnumbered Fig. 2.3**

Hemera Technologies (87527136). **Unnumbered Figs. 3.1 and 3.10**

Huntstock (144110254). **Unnumbered Fig. 9.10**

IHUAN (506133839). **Unnumbered Fig. 9.7**

JCPJR (670505394). **Unnumbered Fig. 1.7**

Jupiterimages (86516515). **Fig. 5.2**

KatarzynaBialasiewicz (478746499). **Unnumbered Figs. 7.1 and 7.10**

Keith Brofsky (MD000744). **Fig. 7.4**

Keith Brofsky (MD001576). **Fig. 11.2**

kolinko_tanya (186938642). **Unnumbered Figs. 4.1 and 4.8**

ktsimage (610234084). **Unnumbered Fig. 1.3**

LightFieldStudios (690043948). **Fig. 1.3**

Medioimages/Photodisc (56372462). **Unnumbered Fig. 3.11**

MEHMET CAN (489124493). **Unnumbered Fig. 12.7**

Mike Watson Images (77739125). **Unnumbered Figs. 6.1 and 6.9, Fig. 8.2**

Monkeybusinessimages (459128571). **Unnumbered Fig. 6.10**

natalie_board (613660104). **Unnumbered Figs. 1.1 and 1.9**

Norman Pogson (96769173). **Unnumbered Figs. 12.1 and 12.6**

pablohart (92282427). **Unnumbered Fig. 2.4**

Pixel_away (614979428). **Unnumbered Fig. 7.7**

Rakkogumi (109841260). **Unnumbered Figs. 11.1 and 11.12**

Siri Stafford (200488093-001). **Unnumbered Figs. 2.1 and 2.3**

StockPhotosArt (186908603). **Fig. 10.9**

Sukanya082 (512571793). **Unnumbered Fig. 7.5**

Tetsu/amanaimagesRF (102758125). **Unnumbered Fig. 9.8**

UberImages (518285048). **Fig. 9.3, Unnumbered Fig. 9.6**

Viafilms (138069439). **Unnumbered Figs. 5.1 and 5.8**

Wavebreakmedia (653910152). **Fig. 12.1**

Wavebreakmedia (599980560). **Unnumbered Fig. 11.5, 11.11**

XiXinXing (4746049570) **Unnumbered Fig. 1.10**

Zilli (168762373). **Unnumbered Fig. 7.2**

Index

A

-a, 53t–54t, 70t, 186t, 290t
A-, 83t, 87b, 120t, 151t–152t, 186t, 222t, 290t, 332t
AAAs. See Abdominal aortic aneurysms (AAAs).
Abbreviations
   for abdominopelvic quadrants, 42–43, 42f, 43t
   body structure-related, 8t–9t
   for cardiovascular terms, 207–208, 207t, 217t
   for digestive terms, 246–247, 246t, 256t
   for directional terms, 43, 43t
   for endocrine terms, 375, 375t, 383t
   for eye- and ear-related terms, 277–278, 277t
   for integumentary terms, 69–70, 69t, 79t
   for lymphatic terms, 207–208, 207t, 217t
   for musculoskeletal terms, 317t, 318, 328t
   for neurological terms, 352–353, 352t
   oncology-related, 8t–9t, 21t
   for reproductive terms, 171t, 172
   for respiratory terms, 103–107, 104b, 106t, 116t
   for urinary terms, 138t, 139
   for word parts, 3t, 8t–9t
Abdomen, 218–219
Abdominal aortic aneurysms (AAAs), 205, 205f
Abdominal cavity, 7t
Abdominal paracentesis. See Abdominocentesis.
Abdominal ultrasonography, 235f
Abdomin/o, 221t–222t
Abdominocentesis, 231, 231t
Abdominopelvic cavity, 7b, 13, 13f, 31
Abdominopelvic quadrants
   abbreviations related to, 42–43, 42f, 43t
   divisions of, 42, 42b, 42f
Abdominopelvic regions, 39–41, 39f–40f, 41b, 44, 50t
   pronunciation and spelling of, 39t, 42
Abscesses, 65t–66t
Absorption, 219
-ac, 186t, 290t
Achilles tendon, 310b
Acr/o, 53t–54t, 365t
Acrocyanosis, 63, 64t
Acromegaly, 367, 370t
Acronyms, 1, 2f, 3
Activities of daily living (ADLs), 352t
AD. See Alzheimer disease (AD).
-ad, 30t
Addison disease, 371t
Aden/o, 186t, 198b, 365t, 366–367
Adenomas, 367, 370t
ADLs. See Activities of daily living (ADLs).
Adrenal gland, 363–364, 366f
Adrenalectomy, 367, 370t
Adrenalitis, 367, 370t
Adrenal/o, 365t, 366–367
Adrenomegaly, 367, 370t
AGBs. See Arterial blood gases (AGBs).
Age-related macular degeneration (ARMD), 273t–274t, 277t
-al, 8t–9t, 13, 30t, 35–36, 54t, 56–57, 83t, 87b, 120t, 151t–152t, 186t, 222t, 261t, 266, 290t, 332t
-algia, 221t–222t, 290t, 332t
Alimentary canal. See Gastrointestinal (GI) tract.
Alveoli, 80–82, 81f, 103f
Alzheimer disease (AD), 2b, 3, 345t–346t, 352t
Amenorrhea, 159, 160t–161t
An-, 83t, 87b, 120t, 186t, 222t, 290t

Anal, 240t
Anal fissures, 239
Anatomic planes, 38, 38f, 40–41, 40f, 44
   definition of, 38, 38t
   pronunciation and spelling of, 38t, 42
Anatomic position, 29, 29f, 38
Anatomic structures
   of cardiovascular system, 7t, 182–183, 183f, 187–192, 187f, 194, 194f
   of digestive system, 7t, 218–219, 223, 223f, 232, 232f
   of ears, 258–259, 268–272, 268f
   of endocrine system, 7t, 363–364, 366, 366f, 372f
   of eyes, 257–258, 262, 262f
   of female reproductive system, 7t, 148–149, 152, 152f
   of integumentary system, 7t, 51–52
   of lymphatic system, 7t, 183
   of male reproductive system, 7t, 149, 162–165, 162f
   of musculoskeletal system, 7t, 287–288, 291, 291f, 302, 302f, 305, 305f
   of nervous system, 7t, 329–331, 330f, 331b, 333, 333f, 339, 339f
   of respiratory system, 7t, 80–82, 84f, 91–99, 91f
   of urinary system, 117–118, 121f, 125, 125f, 128f
Anemia, 201t–202t
Aneurysm, 201t–202t, 350f
Angi/o, 186t, 191, 194b, 242b, 332t
Angiography, 191, 192t–193t
Angioplasty, 191, 192t–193t
An/o, 221t–222t
Anterior, 31, 34b, 36, 43t
Anter/o, 30t
Anterolateral, 36
Anteromedial, 36
Anteroposterior (AP), 32, 36, 43t
Anterosuperior, 33, 37
Anuria, 124b, 126t–127t
Anus, 218–219, 220f
Anxiety disorder, 345t–346t
A1c. See Glycated hemoglobin (A1c).
AP. See Anteroposterior (AP).
Aphagia, 226, 231t
Aphasia, 342, 344t
Apnea, 88, 90t
Appendages of the skin, 51–52
Appendectomy, 236, 240t
Appendicitis, 236, 240t
Appendic/o, 221t–222t, 236
Appendix, 218–219, 236f
Append/o, 221t–222t, 236
Arachnoid, 331b
ARMD. See Age-related macular degeneration (ARMD).
Arterial, 190, 192t–193t
Arterial blood gases (AGBs), 106t
Arterial pulse palpation, 45–47, 45f
Arteries, 182–183, 190
Arteri/o, 186t, 190
Arteriogram, 190, 192t–193t
Arteriosclerosis, 190, 192t–193t
Arthr, 4t
Arthralgia, 308, 310t–311t
Arthritis
   definition of, 310t–311t
   types of, 308, 337
Arthr/o, 289t, 308–309, 332t
Arthrocentesis, 310t–311t
Arthrodesis, 308, 310t–311t
Arthrogram, 310t–311t
Arthroplasty, 308, 310t–311t

Arthroscopic, 310t–311t
Arthroscopy, 310t–311t
-ary, 83t, 87b
AST. See Astigmatism (AST).
-asthenia, 289t
Asthma, 101t
Astigmatism (AST), 266b, 273t–274t, 274f, 277t
Atherogenic, 213
Atrophy, 296, 300t–301t
Audi/o, 261t, 271
Audiologists, 271, 272t
Audiology, 271, 272t
Audiology technicians, 260b, 260f
Audiometers, 271, 272t
Audiometry, 271, 272t
Auricles, 258–260
Axial plane, 38f, 38t

B

Bacterium, 19f
Balloon angioplasty. See Percutaneous transluminal coronary angioplasty (PTCA).
Bar, 241b
Bariatric, 241b
Bariatric surgery, 241t–242t
Barium enema (BE), 241t–242t, 246t
Basal cell carcinoma (BCC), 65t–66t, 66f, 69t
BE. See Barium enema (BE).
Bedsores, 65t–66t, 67f
Behavioral health. See also Nervous system.
   aspects of, 331
   medical terms related to, 344t–346t, 347–349, 362t
      in case study, 357
      by clinical category, 353–356
      in clinical statements, 356–357
      quiz on, 361
   professionals who work with, 331b, 331f
   pronunciation and spelling of terms related to, 344–345, 351–352
   word parts for, 332t, 343, 362t
Benign, 12, 15, 18t
Benign prostatic hyperplasia (BPH), 167t, 171t
Benign tumors, 63
Bilateral, 158b
Bile ducts, 235
Billroth, Christian Albert Theodor, 87b
Biopsy (Bx), 18t, 21t
Bipolar disorder, 345t–346t
Birthmarks, 65t–66t
Bladder, 122b. See also Urinary bladder.
Bladder stones. See Cystolithiasis.
Blepharitis, 264, 266t–267t
Blephar/o, 261t
Blepharoplasty, 265, 266t–267t
Blepharoptosis, 265, 266t–267t
Blood, composition of, 182–184, 183f
Blood cells, 63, 64f
Blood pressure (BP), 201t–202t, 207t
Blood vessels
   anatomic structure of, 182–183, 187f, 194f
   ruptured, in stroke, 350f
BM. See Bowel movement (BM).
Body cavities, 7, 7t, 13, 13f
Body organs. See Organs, body.
Body structure
   abbreviations related to, 8t–9t
   categories of, 6, 6t, 10f
   medical language of, 16, 22
   professionals who work with terms related to, 8b
Body systems. See Systems, body.

Page numbers followed by "f" indicate figures, "t" indicate tables, and "b" indicate boxes.

Body tissues. *See* Tissues, body.
Bone marrow, 287–288
Bones, 287–288
Bowel movement (BM), 246*t*
BP. *See* Blood pressure (BP).
BPH. *See* Benign prostatic hyperplasia (BPH).
Brady-, 186*t*, 290*t*
Bradycardia, 189, 192*t*–193*t*
Bradykinesia, 300, 300*t*–301*t*
Brain
　anatomic structure of, 329–330, 330*f*, 333*f*, 339, 339*f*
　functions of, 331
Brainstem, 329–330
Breasts, 148–149
Bronchi (*s.* bronchus), 80–82, 81*f*, 91*f*, 93*b*
Bronchial tree, 80–81
Bronchitis, 99*t*–101*t*
Bronch/o, 83*t*, 94
Bronchopneumonia, 95, 99*t*–100*t*
Bronchoscope, 94, 94*f*, 99*t*–100*t*
Bronchoscopy, 94, 99*t*–100*t*
Bursae, 287–288
Bursectomy, 297, 300*t*–301*t*
Bursitis, 297, 300*t*–301*t*
Burs/o, 289*t*, 297
Bursotomy, 297, 300*t*–301*t*
Bx. *See* Biopsy (Bx).

C
CA, 21*t*. *See also* Cancer (CA); Carcinoma (CA).
CABG. *See* Coronary artery bypass graft (CABG).
CAD. *See* Coronary artery disease (CAD).
Cancer (CA)
　cervical, 170*b*
　colon, 237
　laryngeal, 93
　lymphatic, 198
　prostate, 163
　radiation therapy for, 18*t*
　of reproductive systems, 166*b*
　terms related to, 15
C&S. *See* Culture and sensitivity (C&S).
Capillaries
　anatomic structure of, 182–183
　function of, 82
Capn/o, 83*t*
Capnometer, 89, 90*t*
Carbon dioxide (CO_2), 106*t*
Carcin/o, 8*t*–9*t*
Carcinogenic, 15–16
Carcinoma (CA), 15–16, 65*t*–66*t*, 66*f*
Cardiac, 188, 192*t*–193*t*
Cardiac catheterization, 201*t*–202*t*, 205*f*
Cardi/o, 186*t*, 187, 189
Cardiologists, 188, 192*t*–193*t*
Cardiology, 188, 192*t*–193*t*
Cardiomegaly, 188, 192*t*–193*t*
Cardiomyopathy, 189, 192*t*–193*t*
Cardiopulmonary resuscitation (CPR), 201*t*–202*t*, 207*t*
Cardiovascular Perfusionists, 185*b*
Cardiovascular system. *See also* Lymphatic system.
　abbreviations related to, 207–208, 207*t*, 217*t*
　anatomic structures of, 7*t*, 182–183, 183*f*, 187–192, 187*f*, 194, 194*f*
　functions of, 7*t*, 183–184, 183*f*–184*f*
　medical terms related to, 192*t*–193*t*, 200*t*–202*t*, 202–206, 217*t*
　　in case study, 212
　　by clinical category, 208–211
　　in clinical statements, 211–212
　　in electronic health records, 214
　　in medical document, 212–214, 212*f*–214*f*
　　quiz on, 216
　professionals who work with, 185*b*, 185*f*
　pronunciation and spelling of terms related to, 193, 200–201, 206–207
　word parts for, 186*t*, 187–192, 188*b*, 194–200, 217*t*
Cardiovascular technicians and technologists, 185*b*
Carotid arteries, 45, 45*f*
Carpal, 295, 295*f*, 300*t*–301*t*, 324
Carpal tunnel syndrome (CTS), 312*t*, 317*t*
Carpectomy, 295, 300*t*–301*t*

Carp/o, 289*t*, 295
Cartilage, 287–288, 305*b*
　damage to, 305
Cataracts, 273*t*–274*t*, 276*b*
Catheterization, 138*t*
　cardiac, 201*t*–202*t*, 205*f*
　urinary, 135*t*
Catheters, intravenous, 195
Cauda equina, 333*b*
Caudad, 34, 37
Caudal, 34, 34*b*, 37
Caud/o, 30*t*, 33*b*
CBC. *See* Complete blood count (CBC).
CCPs. *See* Certified clinical perfusionists (CCPs).
CDEs. *See* Certified diabetes educators (CDEs).
Cecum, 236
-cele, 151*t*, 222*t*, 332*t*
Celiac disease, 241*t*–242*t*
Cells
　blood cells, 63, 64*f*
　definition of, 6*t*
Cellulitis, 65*t*–66*t*
-centesis, 83*t*, 96, 222*t*, 290*t*
Central nervous system (CNS)
　anatomic structure of, 329–330, 330*f*, 352*t*
　functions of, 331
Cephalad, 34, 37
Cephalalgia, 341, 344*t*
Cephalic, 34, 34*b*, 37
Cephal/o, 30*t*, 33*b*, 332*t*, 341
Cerebellum, 329–330
Cerebral, 338*t*
Cerebral angiography, 334, 338*t*
Cerebral embolus, 350*f*
Cerebral thrombosis, 334, 338*t*, 350*f*
Cerebr/o, 332*t*, 334
Cerebrospinal fluid (CSF), 329–330, 352*t*
Cerebrovascular accident (CVA), 345*t*–346*t*, 352*t*
Cerebrum
　anatomic structure of, 329–330
　functions of, 331
Certified clinical perfusionists (CCPs), 185*b*
Certified diabetes educators (CDEs), 364*b*–365*b*
Certified nurse midwives (CNMs), 150*b*
Certified nursing assistants, 53*b*
Certified polysomnographic technicians (CPSGTs), 82*b*
Cervical, 160*t*–161*t*
Cervical cancer, 170*b*
Cervical infections, 153
Cervical vertebrae (C1-C7), 317*t*
Cervicectomy, 157, 160*t*–161*t*
Cervicitis, 153, 160*t*–161*t*
Cervic/o, 151*t*, 153*b*
Cervix, 148–149, 171*t*
Chemotherapy (chemo), 18*t*, 21*t*
Chest cavity, 82, 91*f*, 96*f*
Chest computed tomography (CT), 101*t*, 102*f*
Chest radiograph (CXR), 32, 36*f*, 102*f*, 106*t*
Chiropractic, 312*t*
Chlor/o, 64*b*
Cholangiopancreatography, 242*b*
Chol/e, 235, 235*b*
Cholecystectomy, 235, 235*b*, 240*t*
Cholecystitis, 235, 240*t*
Cholelithiasis, 235, 240*t*
Chol/o, 221*t*–222*t*
Chondrectomy, 305, 310*t*–311*t*
Chondritis, 305, 310*t*–311*t*
Chondr/o, 289*t*, 305
Chondromalacia, 305, 310*t*–311*t*
Choroid, 257–258
Chrom/o, 64*b*
Chronic kidney disease (CKD), 135*t*, 138*t*
Chronic obstructive pulmonary disease (COPD), 101*t*, 106*t*
Circumcision, 167*t*
Cirrhosis, 241*t*–242*t*
CKD. *See* Chronic kidney disease (CKD).
Clostridium difficile, 238
CMV retinitis. *See* Cytomegalovirus (CMV) retinitis.
CNMs. *See* Certified nurse midwives (CNMs).

CNS. *See* Central nervous system (CNS).
Cochlea, 258–259
Colectomy, 238, 240*t*
Colitis, 238, 240*t*
Col/o, 221*t*–222*t*, 237
Colon, anatomic structure of, 218–219
Colon cancer, 237
Colon/o, 221*t*–222*t*, 237
Colonography, CT, 237, 240*t*
Colonoscopy, 237, 240*t*
Colors, 52, 53*t*–54*t*, 61, 64*b*, 79*t*
Colostomy, 238, 240*t*
Colp/o, 151*t*, 155
Colposcope, 155, 160*t*–161*t*
Colposcopy, 155, 160*t*–161*t*
Combining forms, 4–5, 4*b*, 8*t*–9*t*, 11, 15
　in behavioral health terms, 332*t*
　in cardiovascular and lymphatic terms, 186*t*, 187, 187*f*, 194, 194*b*, 194*f*, 197*f*, 217*t*
　in digestive terms, 221*t*–222*t*, 223, 223*f*, 232, 232*f*, 256*t*
　in directional terms, 30*t*, 31, 31*f*, 33–34, 33*b*, 33*f*–34*f*
　in ear-related terms, 261*t*, 268–272, 268*f*, 286*t*
　in endocrine terms, 365*t*, 366, 366*f*, 383*t*
　in eye-related terms, 261*t*, 262, 262*f*, 286*t*
　in integumentary and color terms, 53*t*–54*t*, 62, 79*t*
　in musculoskeletal terms, 289*t*–290*t*, 291, 291*f*, 302, 302*f*, 305, 305*f*, 327*t*
　in neurological terms, 332*t*, 333, 333*f*, 339, 339*f*
　in reproductive terms
　　female, 151*t*–152*t*, 152, 152*f*, 159, 181*t*
　　male, 151*t*–152*t*, 162–165, 162*f*, 181*t*
　in respiratory terms, 83*t*, 84, 84*f*, 115*t*
　in urinary terms, 120*t*, 121, 121*f*, 125, 125*f*, 128, 128*f*, 147*t*
Combining vowels, 3*t*, 8*t*–9*t*, 10*b*
　abbreviation for, 3*t*
　dermat and, 56*b*
　thorac and, 95*b*
Complete blood count (CBC), 201*t*–202*t*, 207*t*
Computed tomography, 38*t*, 101*t*, 102*f*, 105*b*, 106*t*
　chest, 101*t*, 102*f*
Computed tomography (CT) technologists, 30, 30*f*
Concussion, 345*t*–346*t*
C1-C7, 317*t*
Congestive heart failure (CHF). *See* Heart failure (HF).
Connective tissue, 6*t*, 11*f*
Constipation, 241*t*–242*t*
Continuous positive airway pressure (CPAP), 106*t*
Convulsion. *See* Seizure.
COPD. *See* Chronic obstructive pulmonary disease (COPD).
Cornea, 257–258, 258*f*, 260
Coronal plane, 38*f*, 38*t*
Coronary, 214
Coronary artery bypass graft (CABG), 201*t*–202*t*, 207*t*
Coronary artery disease (CAD), 201*t*–202*t*, 207*t*
Coronary stent, 214*f*
Cost/o, 289*t*, 304
Costochondral, 310*t*–311*t*
Costochondral joints, 305
CPAP. *See* Continuous positive airway pressure (CPAP).
CPR. *See* Cardiopulmonary resuscitation (CPR).
CPSGTs. *See* Certified polysomnographic technicians (CPSGTs).
Cranial cavity, 7*t*, 13, 31
Crani/o, 289*t*, 303
Craniomalacia, 303, 310*t*–311*t*
Cranioschisis, 303, 310*t*–311*t*
Craniotomy, 303, 310*t*–311*t*
Crin/o, 365*t*, 369*b*
Crohn disease, 241*t*–242*t*
CSF. *See* Cerebrospinal fluid (CSF).
CT. *See* Computed tomography.
CT colonography, 237, 240*t*
CT technicians. *See* Computed tomography (CT) technologists.
CTS. *See* Carpal tunnel syndrome (CTS).
Culture and sensitivity (C&S), 101*t*, 106*t*
Cutane/o, 53*t*–54*t*, 55*b*, 58

Cutaneous, 58, 60*t*
Cutaneous membrane, 52, 55*f*
CVA. *See* Cerebrovascular accident (CVA).
CXR. *See* Chest radiograph (CXR).
Cyan/o, 53*t*–54*t*
Cyanosis, 63, 64*t*
Cystitis, 122, 126*t*–127*t*
Cyst/o, 120*t*, 121–122, 151*t*–152*t*, 222*t*, 235*b*
Cystocele, 155, 160*t*–161*t*
Cystogram, 122, 126*t*–127*t*
Cystography, 122, 126*t*–127*t*
Cystolithiasis, 122, 126*t*–127*t*
Cystolithotomy, 123, 126*t*–127*t*
Cystoscope, 123, 126*t*–127*t*
Cystoscopy, 123, 126*t*–127*t*
Cystostomy, 123, 126*t*–127*t*
Cystourethrography, 123, 126*t*–127*t*
Cyt/o, 8*t*–9*t*, 10, 54*t*, 186*t*
Cytoid, 12, 16
Cytology, 10, 10*b*, 16
Cytomegalovirus (CMV) retinitis, 264

D
D&C. *See* Dilation and curettage (D&C).
Deep vein thrombosis (DVT), 207*t*
Dementia, 345*t*–346*t*
Dental assistants, 220*b*–221*b*, 221*f*
Dental hygienists, 220*b*–221*b*
Depression, 345*t*–346*t*
Dermal, 57, 60*t*
Dermatitis, 56, 56*b*, 60*t*
Dermat/o, 53*t*–54*t*, 55*b*–56*b*
Dermatologists, 56, 60*t*
Dermatology, 56, 56*b*, 60*t*, 69*t*
Dermatopathologists, 56, 60*t*
Dermatopathy, 56, 56*b*, 60*t*
Dermis, 51–52, 55*f*, 57
Derm/o, 53*t*–54*t*, 55*b*, 56–57, 61
-desis, 289*t*
Detached retina, 273*t*–274*t*
Diabetes mellitus (DM), 368–369, 371*t*, 372*b*, 375*t*
Diagnosis (Dx), 18*t*, 21*t*
Diagnostic imaging, 38*t*, 102*b*, 102*f*
Dialysis, 135*t*, 138*b*
Dialysis patient care technicians (PCTs), 119*b*, 119*f*
Diarrhea, 241*t*–242*t*
Dietetic technicians, 220*b*–221*b*
Digestion, 219
Digestive system
   abbreviations related to, 246–247, 246*t*, 256*t*
   anatomic structures of, 7*t*, 218–219, 223, 223*f*, 232, 232*f*
   functions of, 7*t*, 219, 220*f*
   medical terms related to, 231*t*, 240*t*–242*t*, 241*b*, 244–245, 256*t*
      in case study, 252
      by clinical category, 247–250
      in clinical statements, 251
      in electronic health records, 254
      in medical document, 252–253, 252*f*–253*f*
      quiz on, 255
   professionals who work with, 220*b*–221*b*, 221*f*
   pronunciation and spelling of terms related to, 232, 240–241, 246
   word parts for, 221*t*–222*t*, 223–240, 242*b*, 256*t*
Digestive tract. *See* Gastrointestinal (GI) tract.
Digital rectal examination (DRE), 167*t*, 171*t*
Digital subtraction angiography (DSA), 207*t*
Dilatation, 166*t*
Dilation and curettage (D&C), 166*t*, 171*t*
Dips/o, 365*t*
Directional terms
   abbreviations related to, 43, 43*t*
   building and translation of, 31–36, 31*f*–36*f*
   definition of, 29
   list of, 36, 36*t*–37*t*, 50*t*
   professionals who use, 30*b*, 30*f*
   pronunciation and spelling of, 37
   quiz on, 49–50
   word parts for, 30*t*, 31–36
Disc, 292*b*
Distal, 35, 35*f*, 37

Dist/o, 30*t*
DM. *See* Diabetes mellitus (DM).
Dorsal, 31, 34*b*, 37, 46*b*
Dorsal cavity, 13, 31
Dorsalis pedis artery, 45–47, 45*f*
Dors/o, 30*t*
DRE, digital rectal examination (DRE)
DSA. *See* Digital subtraction angiography (DSA).
Duodenal, 240*t*
Duodenal ulcers, 233
Duoden/o, 221*t*–222*t*
Duodenum, 233*b*
Dura mater, 331*b*
DVT. *See* Deep vein thrombosis (DVT).
Dx. *See* Diagnosis (Dx).
Dys-, 83*t*, 120*t*, 151*t*–152*t*, 222*t*, 226, 290*t*, 332*t*
Dysentery, 226, 231*t*
Dyskinesia, 300, 300*t*–301*t*
Dysmenorrhea, 159, 160*t*–161*t*
Dyspepsia, 226, 231*t*
Dysphagia, 226, 231*t*
Dysphasia, 342, 344*t*
Dyspnea, 88, 90*t*
Dystrophy, 296, 300*t*–301*t*
Dysuria, 124, 126*t*–127*t*

E
-e, 53*t*–54*t*, 186*t*, 365*t*
-eal, 83*t*, 87*b*, 222*t*, 290*t*
Eardrum. *See* Tympanic membrane.
Ears
   abbreviations related to, 277–278, 277*t*
   anatomic structures of, 258–259, 268–272, 268*f*
   disorders of, 269, 273*t*–274*t*, 274–276
   functions of, 259–260, 259*f*
   medical terms related to, 272*t*–274*t*, 274–276, 286*t*
      in case study, 281
      by clinical category, 278–280
      in clinical statements, 280–281
      in medical document, 281–282, 281*f*–283*f*
      quiz on, 285
   professionals who work with, 260*b*, 260*f*
   pronunciation and spelling of terms related to, 273, 277
   word parts related to, 261*t*, 268–272, 286*t*
ECG/EKG. *See* Electrocardiogram (ECG/EKG).
ECHO. *See* Echocardiogram (ECHO).
Ech/o, 186*t*
Echocardiogram (ECHO), 189, 192*t*–193*t*, 207*t*
Echocardiography technicians, 185*b*
-ectomy, 83*t*, 120*t*, 151*t*–152*t*, 186*t*, 222*t*, 261*t*, 290*t*, 365*t*
ED. *See* Erectile dysfunction (ED).
Edema, 65*t*–66*t*
EEG. *See* Electroencephalogram (EEG).
EGD. *See* Esophagogastroduodenoscopy (EGD).
Electr/o, 186*t*, 188, 290*t*, 332*t*
Electrocardiogram (ECG/EKG), 188, 192*t*–193*t*, 207*t*, 335*b*
Electrocardiograph, 188, 192*t*–193*t*
Electrocardiography, 188, 192*t*–193*t*
Electroencephalogram (EEG), 335, 335*b*, 338*t*, 352*t*
Electroencephalograph, 335, 338*t*
Electroencephalography, 335, 338*t*
Electromyogram (EMG), 299, 300*t*–301*t*, 317*t*, 335*b*
Elimination, 219
Embolism, 206*b*
Embolus, 201*t*–202*t*, 206*b*
Emesis, 253*b*
-emesis, 252, 253*b*
EMG. *See* Electromyogram (EMG).
-emia, 120*t*, 365*t*
Emphysema, 101*t*
Encephalitis, 335, 338*t*
Encephal/o, 332*t*, 334–335
Encephalopathy, 335, 338*t*
Endarterectomy, 190, 192*t*–193*t*
Endo-, 83*t*, 97, 153*b*, 186*t*, 365*t*, 369*b*
Endocrine, 369, 370*t*

Endocrine system
   abbreviations related to, 375, 375*t*, 383*t*
   anatomic structures of, 7*t*, 363–364, 366, 366*f*, 372*f*
   disorders of, 367–368, 372*b*, 374
   functions of, 7*t*, 364, 366*f*
   medical terms related to, 370*t*–371*t*, 373–374, 383*t*
      in case study, 378
      by clinical category, 376–377
      in clinical statements, 378
      in electronic health records, 381
      in medical document, 379, 379*f*–380*f*
      quiz on, 382
   professionals who work with, 364*b*–365*b*, 364*f*
   pronunciation and spelling of terms related to, 370–371, 374–375
   word parts for, 365*t*, 366–370, 369*b*, 383*t*
Endocrinologists, 369, 370*t*
Endocrinology, 369, 370*t*
Endocrinopathy, 369, 370*t*
Endometrial, 154, 160*t*–161*t*
Endometri/o, 151*t*, 153*b*
Endometriosis, 154, 160*t*–161*t*
Endometritis, 153, 160*t*–161*t*
Endometrium, 148–149
Endoscope, 97, 97*b*, 99*t*–100*t*
Endoscopic, 97, 97*b*, 99*t*–100*t*
Endoscopic retrograde cholangiopancreatography (ERCP), 241*t*–242*t*, 246*t*
Endoscopy, 97–98, 97*b*, 99*t*–100*t*
Endoscopy report, 252–253, 252*f*–253*f*
Endotracheal (ET), 99*t*–100*t*, 106*t*
Endotracheal intubation, 92
Endotracheal tube, 92, 92*f*
Enter/o, 221*t*–222*t*
ENTs. *See* Otolaryngologists (ENTs).
Epi-, 53*t*–54*t*
Epidermal, 57, 57*b*, 60*t*
Epidermis, 51–52, 55*f*
Epididymis, 149–150
Epidural nerve block, 345*t*–346*t*
Epigastric region, 39*f*, 39*t*
Epilepsy, 346*b*
Epithelial, 17
Epithelial tissue, 6*t*, 11*f*
Epitheli/o, 8*t*–9*t*
Epithelioma, 12, 17
Epithelium, 6*t*, 11*f*
Eponyms, 1, 2*b*, 2*f*, 3
ERCP. *See* Endoscopic retrograde cholangiopancreatography (ERCP).
Erectile dysfunction (ED), 167*t*, 171*t*
Erythema, 65*t*–66*t*
Erythr/o, 53*t*–54*t*
Erythrocytes (RBCs), 63, 63*b*, 64*f*, 64*t*, 69*t*, 184
Erythroderma, 61, 64*t*
Esophageal, 226, 231*t*
Esophagitis, 226, 231*t*
Esophag/o, 221*t*–222*t*, 226
Esophagogastroduodenoscopy (EGD), 233, 240*t*, 246*t*
Esophagus
   anatomic structure of, 218–219
   function of, 219, 220*f*
Estheticians, medical, 53*b*
ESWL. *See* Extracorporeal shock wave lithotripsy (ESWL).
ET. *See* Endotracheal (ET).
Eustachian tube, 258–259
Exfoliative dermatitis, 61
Exhalation, 81*f*, 82
External auditory canal, 258–260, 259*f*
External ear, 258–260, 259*f*
Extracorporeal shock wave lithotripsy (ESWL), 135*t*, 138*b*
Eyes
   abbreviations related to, 277–278, 277*t*
   anatomic structures of, 257–258, 262, 262*f*
   disorders of, 264–265, 266*b*, 273*t*–274*t*, 274–276
   functions of, 258–260, 258*f*
   medical terms related to, 266*t*–267*t*, 273*t*–274*t*, 274–276, 286*t*
      in case study, 281
      by clinical category, 278–280

Eyes (*Continued*)
    in clinical statements, 280–281
    in electronic health records, 284
    in medical document, 281–282
    quiz on, 285
    pathway of light through, 258*f*
    professionals who work with, 260*b*, 260*f*
    pronunciation and spelling of terms related to, 267, 277
    word parts related to, 261*t*, 262–266, 263*b*, 286*t*

F
Fallopian tubes. *See* Uterine tubes.
Fallopius, Gabriele, 152*b*
Farsightedness. *See* Hyperopia.
Fasting blood sugar (FBS), 371*t*, 375*t*
FBS. *See* Fasting blood sugar (FBS).
Female reproductive system
    abbreviations related to, 171*t*, 172
    anatomic structures of, 148–149, 152, 152*f*
    disorders, 153–154, 154*f*, 159, 166*b*
    functions of, 149–150
    medical terms related to, 160*t*–161*t*, 166*b*, 166*t*, 169–171, 181*t*
        in case study, 176
        by clinical category, 172–175
        in clinical statements, 176
        in medical document, 177, 177*f*–178*f*
        quiz on, 180
    pronunciation and spelling of terms related to, 162, 171
    word parts for, 151*t*–152*t*, 152–160, 153*b*, 156*b*, 158*b*, 181*t*
Femoral, 300*t*–301*t*
Femoral artery, palpation of, 45, 45*f*
Femor/o, 289*t*
Fine needle aspiration (FNA), 371*t*, 375*t*
Fissures, anal, 239
Flu. *See* Influenza (flu).
Fluoroscopy, 157*b*
FNA. *See* Fine needle aspiration (FNA).
Fowler position, 39*b*, 39*t*
Fractures (Fx), 312*t*, 317*t*, 325
Frontal plane, 38*f*, 38*t*
Fungal infections, 59, 59*f*
Fx. *See* Fractures (Fx).

G
Gallbladder, 235, 235*b*
    anatomic structure of, 218–219
Gallstones, 235
Garcia, Manuel, 87*b*
Gastrectomy, 228, 231*t*
Gastric, 228, 231*t*
Gastric ulcers, 228*f*, 241*t*–242*t*
Gastritis, 228, 231*t*
Gastr/o, 221*t*–222*t*, 227–228
Gastroenteritis, 228, 231*t*
Gastroenterologists, 228, 231*t*
Gastroenterology, 231*t*
Gastroesophageal, 228, 231*t*
Gastroesophageal reflux disease (GERD), 241*t*–242*t*, 246*t*
Gastrointestinal, 246*t*
Gastrointestinal (GI) tract, 219, 220*f*
Gastroscopes, 229, 231*t*
Gastroscopy, 229, 231*t*
Gastrostomy, 229, 231*t*, 233
-genic, 8*t*–9*t*, 14, 332*t*
GERD. *See* Gastroesophageal reflux disease (GERD).
GI tract. *See* Gastrointestinal (GI) tract.
Gingivalgia, 224, 231*t*
Gingivitis, 224, 231*t*
Gingiv/o, 221*t*–222*t*, 224
Glauc/o, 64*b*
Glaucoma, 273*t*–274*t*
Glossitis, 225, 231*t*
Gloss/o, 221*t*–222*t*, 225
Gluten enteropathy. *See* Celiac disease.
Glycated hemoglobin (A1c), 371*t*, 375*t*
Glycemia, 368, 370*t*
Glyc/o, 365*t*

Goiters, 371*t*
Gout, 312*t*
-gram, 83*t*, 120*t*, 151*t*–152*t*, 186*t*, 188*b*, 290*t*, 332*t*
-graph, 186*t*, 188*b*, 332*t*
-graphy, 83*t*, 120*t*, 151*t*–152*t*, 186*t*, 188*b*, 222*t*, 332*t*
Graves disease, 371*t*
Greek and Latin word parts, terms built from, 1, 2*f*, 3
Guillain-Barré syndrome, 337
Gums, 218–219
Gynec/o, 151*t*
Gynecologists, 150, 155, 160*t*–161*t*
Gynecology, 160*t*–161*t*

H
Hair, 51–52, 55*f*
Hair follicles, 55*f*
Hard of hearing (HOH), 277*t*
HbA1c. *See* Glycated hemoglobin (A1c).
HD. *See* Hemodialysis (HD).
Headache. *See* Cephalalgia.
Hearing, 259*f*, 260
Heart
    anatomic structure of, 182–183, 187*f*, 194*f*
    functions of, 184
Heart attack. *See* Myocardial infarction (MI).
Heart failure (HF), 4, 201*t*–202*t*, 207*t*
Hematemesis, 252
Hemat/o, 120*t*, 186*t*, 199
Hematologists, 199, 200*t*
Hematology, 199, 200*t*
Hematoma, 199, 200*t*
Hematuria, 124, 125*b*, 126*t*–127*t*
Hemi, 332*t*
Hemiplegia, 342, 344*t*
Hem/o, 120*t*, 186*t*, 199
Hemodialysis (HD), 138*b*, 138*t*
Hemoglobin A1c. *See* Glycated hemoglobin (A1c).
Hemolysis, 199, 200*t*
Hemorrhage, 201*t*–202*t*, 204*b*
    intracranial, 303
Hemorrhagic stroke, 350*f*
Hemorrhoids, 241*t*–242*t*
Hemostasis, 199, 200*t*
Hepatitis, 234, 240*t*
Hepat/o, 221*t*–222*t*, 234
Hepatomas, 234, 240*t*
Hepatomegaly, 234, 240*t*
Hernia, 312*t*
Herniated disc, 312*t*
Herpes, 65*t*–66*t*
HF. *See* Heart failure (HF).
HHD. *See* Hypertensive heart disease (HHD).
High Fowler position, 39*b*
Hist/o, 8*t*–9*t*, 10
Histology, 10, 10*b*, 17
History and physical form, 379*f*–380*f*
Hodgkin lymphoma, 198
HOH. *See* Hard of hearing (HOH).
Horizontal plane, 38*t*
Hormones, 363–364
Horny tissue, 55*f*
HPV. *See* Human papillomavirus (HPV).
HSG. *See* Hysterosalpingogram (HSG).
HTN. *See* Hypertension (HTN).
Human papillomavirus (HPV), 171*t*
    vaccine for, 170*b*
Hydr/o, 120*t*, 332*t*
Hydrocephalus, 341, 344*t*
Hydronephrosis, 129, 133*t*–134*t*
Hyper-, 83*t*, 87*b*, 290*t*, 365*t*
Hypercapnia, 89, 90*t*
Hyperglycemia, 368–369, 370*t*
Hyperopia, 265, 266*b*, 273*t*–274*t*, 274*f*
Hyperoxia, 89, 90*t*
Hyperpnea, 88, 90*t*
Hypertension (HTN), 201*t*–202*t*, 207*t*
Hypertensive heart disease (HHD), 207*t*
Hyperthyroidism, 368, 370*t*
Hypertrophic, 296, 300*t*–301*t*
Hypertrophy, 296, 300*t*–301*t*
Hypo-, 53*t*–54*t*, 83*t*, 87*b*, 365*t*
Hypocapnia, 89, 90*t*

Hypochondriac regions, 39*f*, 39*t*
Hypodermic, 57, 58*b*, 60*t*, 69*t*
Hypogastric region, 39*f*, 39*t*
Hypoglycemia, 368, 370*t*
Hypopnea, 88, 90*t*
Hypotension, 201*t*–202*t*
Hypothyroidism, 368, 370*t*
Hypoxia, 88*b*, 89, 90*t*
Hysterectomy, 157, 160*t*–161*t*
Hyster/o, 151*t*
Hysteropexy, 155, 157, 160*t*–161*t*
Hysterorrhaphy, 157, 160*t*–161*t*
Hysterorrhexis, 157, 160*t*–161*t*
Hysterosalpingogram (HSG), 157, 157*b*, 160*t*–161*t*, 171*t*
Hysterosalpingo-oophorectomy, 157, 160*t*–161*t*

I
-ia, 83*t*, 120*t*, 186*t*, 222*t*, 290*t*, 332*t*, 365*t*
-iasis, 120*t*, 222*t*, 290*t*
Iatr, 241*b*
IBS. *See* Irritable bowel syndrome (IBS).
-ic, 4, 30*t*, 54*t*, 87*b*, 151*t*–152*t*, 222*t*, 261*t*, 290*t*, 332*t*, 365*t*
Ile/o, 221*t*–222*t*, 298*b*
Ileostomy, 233, 240*t*
Ileum, 233*b*
Iliac, 300*t*–301*t*, 324
Iliac regions, 39*f*, 39*t*
Ili/o, 289*t*, 298*b*
Iliofemoral, 298, 300*t*–301*t*
Impetigo, 65*t*–66*t*
Incidentaloma, 12*b*
Incontinence, 135*t*
Infections, 18*t*
    bladder, 124
    cervical, 153
    kidney, 129
    respiratory, 101*t*, 104*f*
    urinary tract, 135*t*, 138*t*
Inferior, 33, 34*b*, 37, 43*t*
Infer/o, 30*t*
Inferolateral, 37
Inflammation, 18*b*, 18*t*
Influenza (flu), 101*t*, 106*t*
Ingestion, 219
Inguinal regions, 39*t*
Inhalation, 81*f*, 82
Inner ear, 258–260, 259*f*
Insulin resistance syndrome. *See* Metabolic syndrome.
Integumentary, 52
Integumentary system, 52
    abbreviations related to, 69–70, 69*t*, 79*t*
    anatomic structures of, 7*t*, 51–52
    functions of, 7*t*, 52
    medical terms related to, 60*t*, 64*t*–66*t*, 68, 79*t*
        in case study, 75
        by clinical category, 72–73
        in clinical statements, 74–75
        in medical document, 75–77, 75*f*–76*f*
        quiz on, 78
    professionals who work with, 53*b*, 53*f*
    pronunciation and spelling of terms related to, 60, 65, 69
    word parts for, 53*t*–54*t*, 55–64
Inter-, 289*t*
Intercostal, 304, 310*t*–311*t*
Intervertebral, 292–293, 300*t*–301*t*
Intervertebral disks, 292–293
Intra-, 4*t*, 53*t*–54*t*, 290*t*
Intracranial, 303, 310*t*–311*t*
Intradermal, 57, 60*t*, 69*t*
Intraocular pressure (IOP), 277*t*
Intravenous (IV), 4*t*, 195, 200*t*, 207*t*
IOP. *See* Intraocular pressure (IOP).
-ior, 30*t*
Iridectomy, 265, 266*t*–267*t*
Irid/o, 261*t*
Iridoplegia, 265, 266*t*–267*t*
Iris (in Greek mythology), 261*b*
Iris, anatomic structure of, 257–258, 260
Iritis, 264, 266*t*–267*t*

Ir/o, 261*t*
Irritable bowel syndrome (IBS), 241*t*–242*t*, 246*t*
Ischemic stroke, 350*f*
Ischial, 298, 300*t*–301*t*
Ischi/o, 289*t*
Ischiopubic, 298, 300*t*–301*t*
Islets of Langerhans, 363–364, 372*f*
-ism, 365*t*
-itis, 4*t*, 53*t*–54*t*, 56*b*, 83*t*, 120*t*, 151*t*–152*t*, 153, 186*t*,
    222*t*, 261*t*, 290*t*, 332*t*, 365*t*
IV. *See* Intravenous (IV).

J
Jaundice, 61, 65*t*–66*t*
Jejun/o, 221*t*–222*t*
Jejunostomy, 233, 240*t*
Jejunum, 233*b*
Joints, 287–288
    knee, 305*f*

K
Kerat/o, 261*t*
Keratometers, 263, 266*t*–267*t*
Keratoplasty, 265, 266*t*–267*t*
Kidney stones. *See* Nephrolithiasis.
Kidneys
    anatomic structure of, 117–118, 125, 125*f*, 128*f*
    disorders of, 129, 129*f*, 135*t*, 139*b*
    functions of, 118, 118*f*
    procedures related to, 130, 130*f*, 135*t*, 137*f*
Kinesi/o, 289*t*, 300
Knee joints, 305*f*
Kyph/o, 289*t*
Kyphosis, 300*t*–301*t*

L
Laboratory (lab), 21*t*
Laboratory technicians and technologists, 8, 8*f*
Labyrinth. *See* Inner ear.
Laceration, 65*t*–66*t*, 69*t*
Lapar/o, 221*t*–222*t*, 230
Laparoscopes, 230, 230*f*, 231*t*
Laparoscopic, 230, 231*t*
Laparoscopic surgery, 230, 230*f*
Laparoscopy, 230, 231*t*
Laparotomy, 231, 231*t*
Large intestine, anatomic structure of, 218–219, 220*f*
Laryngeal, 90*t*, 93
Laryngeal cancer, 93
Laryngectomy, 87*b*, 90*t*, 93
Laryngitis, 87, 90*t*
Laryng/o, 83*t*, 87, 261*t*, 271*b*
Laryngoscope, 87*b*, 90*t*, 92, 92*f*
Laryngoscopy, 90*t*
Larynx, 80–82, 81*f*, 84*f*, 87
Laser, 2*f*
Laser-assisted in situ keratomileusis (LASIK),
    273*t*–274*t*
LASIK, 273*t*–274*t*
Lateral, 35, 35*f*, 37, 43*t*
Later/o, 30*t*
Latin and Greek word parts, terms built from, 1, 2*f*, 3
Left lower quadrant (LLQ), 42, 42*f*, 43*t*
Left upper quadrant (LUQ), 42, 42*f*, 43*t*
Lens (eye), 257–258, 258*f*, 260
Lesions, 65*t*–66*t*
Leukemia, 201*t*–202*t*
Leuk/o, 53*t*–54*t*
Leukocytes (WBCs), 63, 63*b*, 64*f*, 64*t*, 69*t*, 184
Leukocytopenia, 197, 200*t*, 307*b*
Leukoderma, 61, 64*t*
Ligaments, 287–288
Lingu/o, 221*t*–222*t*, 225
Lip/o, 8*t*–9*t*
Lipoid, 12, 17
Lipoma, 12, 17
Lith/o, 120*t*, 125, 151*t*–152*t*, 222*t*
Lithotripsy, 126, 126*t*–127*t*
Liver, 218–219, 235
LLQ. *See* Left lower quadrant (LLQ).
-logist, 8*t*–9*t*, 13*b*, 54*t*, 83*t*, 120*t*, 151*t*–152*t*, 186*t*, 222*t*,
    261*t*, 332*t*, 365*t*

-logy, 8*t*–9*t*, 10, 54*t*, 56*b*, 83*t*, 120*t*, 151*t*–152*t*, 186*t*,
    222*t*, 261*t*, 290*t*, 332*t*, 365*t*
L1-L5. *See* Lumbar vertebrae (L1-L5).
Lord/o, 289*t*
Lordosis, 300*t*–301*t*
Low Fowler position, 39*b*
Lower GI series. *See* Barium enema (BE).
Lower respiratory tract, 82
    infections, 104*f*
LP. *See* Lumbar puncture (LP).
Lumbar puncture (LP), 345*t*–346*t*, 352*t*
Lumbar regions, 39*f*, 39*t*
Lumbar vertebrae (L1-L5), 317*t*
Lung ventilation/perfusion scan (V/Q scan), 106*t*
Lungs, 80–82, 81*f*, 91*f*
LUQ. *See* Left upper quadrant (LUQ).
Lyme disease, 312*t*
Lymph, 183, 186*t*
    function of, 185
Lymph nodes
    anatomic structure of, 183
    combining forms for, 197*f*
    function of, 198
Lymph vessels, 183
Lymphadenitis, 198, 200*t*
Lymphadenopathy, 198, 200*t*
Lymphatic system. *See also* Cardiovascular system.
    abbreviations related to, 207–208, 207*t*, 217*t*
    anatomic structures of, 7*t*, 183
    functions of, 7*t*, 183–185, 184*f*
    medical terms related to, 192*t*–193*t*, 200*t*, 204–206,
        217*t*
        in case study, 212
        by clinical category, 208–211
        in clinical statements, 211–212
        quiz on, 216
    professionals who work with, 185*b*, 185*f*
    pronunciation and spelling of terms related to, 193,
        200–201, 206–207
    word parts for, 186*t*, 194–200, 194*b*, 217*t*
Lymphatic vessels, 185, 194*b*
Lymph/o, 186*t*, 194*b*, 198*b*
Lymphoma, 198, 200*t*
-lysis, 53*t*–54*t*, 186*t*

M
Macular degeneration, 273*t*–274*t*
Magnetic resonance imaging (MRI), 38*t*, 102*b*, 312*t*,
    317*b*, 317*t*
Magnetic resonance (MR) technologists, 30
-malacia, 289*t*
Male reproductive system
    abbreviations related to, 171*t*, 172
    anatomic structures of, 149, 162–165, 162*f*
    disorders, 163–164, 166*b*
    functions of, 149–150
    medical terms related to, 165*t*, 167*t*, 169–171, 181*t*
        in case study, 176
        by clinical category, 172–175
        in clinical statements, 176
        in electronic health records, 179
        in medical document, 177, 177*f*–178*f*
        quiz on, 180
    pronunciation and spelling of terms related to,
        165–166, 171
    word parts for, 151*t*–152*t*, 162–165, 181*t*
Malignant, 12, 15, 18*t*
Malignant tumors, 63, 66*f*
Mamm, 159*b*
Mammary glands. *See* Breasts.
Mamm/o, 151*t*, 159
Mammogram, 15*f*, 159–160, 160*f*, 160*t*–161*t*
Mammographers, 150*b*, 150*f*
Mammography, 159–160, 160*f*, 160*t*–161*t*
Mammography technologists. *See* Mammographers.
Mammoplasty, 159–160, 160*t*–161*t*
Mastectomy, 159–160, 160*t*–161*t*
Mastitis, 160*t*–161*t*
Mast/o, 151*t*, 159
Mastopexy, 159–160, 160*t*–161*t*
MD. *See* Muscular dystrophy (MD).
Meatal, 133*t*–134*t*

Meat/o, 120*t*, 132
Meatoscopy, 132, 133*t*–134*t*
Meatotomy, 132, 133*t*–134*t*
Meatus, 132*b*
Medial, 35, 35*f*, 37, 43*t*
Medical assistants, 364*b*–365*b*, 364*f*
Medical documents
    cardiology, 212–214, 212*f*–214*f*
    emergency department record, 47, 48*f*
    for endocrine system, 379, 379*f*–380*f*, 381
    endoscopy report, 252–253, 252*f*–253*f*
    ENT clinic visit, 281–282, 281*f*–283*f*
    history and physical form, 379*f*–380*f*
    for integumentary system, 75–77, 75*f*–76*f*
    medical language in, 25–26, 47, 48*f*
    for musculoskeletal system, 324–325, 324*f*–325*f*
    neurology report, 358, 358*f*–359*f*, 360
    ophthalmology clinic visit, 281–282, 284
    for reproductive systems, 177, 177*f*–178*f*, 179
    for respiratory system, 112–113, 112*f*–113*f*
    for urinary system, 143–145, 143*f*–144*f*
Medical estheticians, 53*b*
Medical language
    of body structure, 16, 22
    in medical documents, 25–26, 47
    of oncology, 16, 23–24
    origins of, 1–2, 2*f*
Medical terms
    built from word parts, 3–5, 3*t*–4*t*, 9–17, 16*t*–17*t*
    not built from word parts, 3–4, 18*t*, 19*f*–20*f*, 20–21
Medical/surgical nurses, 119*b*
Medi/o, 30*t*
Mediolateral, 37
Megaly, 222*t*, 365*t*
-megaly, 186*t*
Melanin, 55*f*
Melan/o, 53*t*–54*t*
Melanoderma, 61, 64*t*
Melanoma, 63, 64*t*
Meninges, 329–331, 331*b*, 339
Mening/o, 332*t*, 339
Meningiomas, 340, 344*t*
Meningitis, 340, 344*t*
Mening/o, 332*t*, 339
Meningocele, 340, 344*t*
Meningomyelitis, 340, 344*t*
Men/o, 151*t*, 158, 158*b*
Menorrhagia, 159, 160*t*–161*t*
Menorrhea, 159, 160*t*–161*t*
Mental health. *See* Behavioral health.
Meta-, 8*t*–9*t*, 295
Metabolic syndrome, 371*t*
Metabolism, 363–364
Metacarpals, 295, 295*f*
Metastasis (mets), 15, 16*f*, 17, 21*t*
-meter, 83*t*, 89, 261*t*
Methicillin-resistant *Staphylococcus aureus* (MRSA), 3,
    65*t*–66*t*, 69*t*
Metr, 153*b*
-metry, 261*t*
Mets. *See* Metastasis (mets).
MI. *See* Myocardial infarction (MI).
Micro-, 332*t*
Microcephalus, 341, 344*t*
Microcephaly. *See* Microcephalus.
Middle ear, 258–260, 259*f*
Midline, 34*b*, 34*f*–35*f*
Midsagittal plane, 38*f*
Midwives, 150*b*
Migraine, 345*t*–346*t*
Modern language, 1, 2*f*, 3
Moles, 65*t*–66*t*
Mouth, 218–219, 220*f*
MR (magnetic resonance) technologists, 30
MRI. *See* Magnetic resonance imaging (MRI).
MRSA (methicillin-resistant *Staphylococcus aureus*).
    See Methicillin-resistant *Staphylococcus aureus*
    (MRSA).
MS. *See* Multiple sclerosis (MS).
Muc/o, 83*t*
Mucous, 86, 86*b*, 90*t*
Mucus, 86*b*

Multiple sclerosis (MS), 345t–346t, 352t, 360
Muscle tissue, 6t, 11f
Muscles, anatomic structure of, 287–288
Muscular dystrophy (MD), 296, 312t, 317t
Musculoskeletal system
　abbreviations related to, 317t, 318, 328t
　anatomic structures of, 7t, 287–288, 291, 291f, 302, 302f, 305, 305f
　disorders of, 294, 294f, 296–297, 299–300, 300t–301t, 305–308, 315–316
　functions of, 7t, 288
　medical terms related to, 300t–301t, 310t–312t, 315–316, 328t
　　in case study, 323
　　by clinical category, 318–322
　　in clinical statements, 322–323
　　in electronic health records, 325
　　in medical document, 324, 324f–325f
　　quiz on, 326–327
　professionals who work with, 288b–289b, 288f
　pronunciation and spelling of terms related to, 301, 311, 317
　word parts for, 289t–290t, 291–300, 298b, 302–310, 307b, 327t
Myalgia, 299, 300t–301t
Myasthenia, 299, 300t–301t
Myc/o, 53t–54t
Myel/o, 332t, 340–341
Myelogram, 341, 344t
Myelography, 341, 344t
My/o, 8t–9t, 186t, 290t, 299, 332t
Myocardial, 190, 192t–193t
Myocardial infarction (MI), 201t–202t, 207t
Myoma, 12, 17
Myopia, 265, 266b, 273t–274t, 274f
Myringitis, 269, 272t
Myring/o, 261t, 270
Myringoplasty, 270, 272t
Myringotomy, 270, 272t

N
Nails, 51t–52t, 52, 59, 59f
　definition of, 51–52
　disorders of, 59, 59f
Nasal, 90t
Nasal cavity, 86
Nas/o, 83t, 86
Nasopharyngitis, 90t
Nearsightedness. See Myopia.
Necr/o, 289t
Necrosis, 310t–311t
Neo-, 8t–9t
Neoplasms, 15, 17, 20
Nephrectomy, 130, 133t–134t
Nephritis, 129, 133t–134t
Nephr/o, 120t, 128, 130
Nephrolithiasis, 126, 126t–127t, 135t, 136f
Nephrologists, 133, 133t–134t
Nephrology, 133, 133t–134t
Nephrology nurses, 119b
Nephrostomy, 130, 133t–134t
Nephrotomy, 130, 133t–134t
Nerve endings, 51–52
Nerve tissue, 6t, 11f
Nerves, 329–331, 330f
Nervous system
　abbreviations related to, 352–353, 352t
　anatomic structures of, 7t, 329–331, 330f, 331b, 333, 333f, 339, 339f
　disorders, 334–337, 340, 342, 349–351
　endocrine system and regulation of, 364
　functions of, 7t, 330–331, 330f
　medical terms related to, 333b, 338t, 344t–346t, 346b, 349–351, 362t
　　in case study, 357
　　by clinical category, 353–356
　　in clinical statements, 356–357
　　in electronic health records, 360
　　in medical document, 358, 358f–359f
　　quiz on, 361
　professionals who work with, 331b, 331f

Nervous system (Continued)
　pronunciation and spelling of terms related to, 338, 344–345, 351–352
　word parts for, 332t, 333–344, 362t
Neural, 336, 338t
Neuralgia, 336, 338t
Neur/o, 8t–9t, 332t, 336–337
Neurodiagnostic technicians, 331b, 331f
Neurologists, 337, 338t
Neurology, 337, 338t
Neuroma, 11–12, 17
Neuropathy, 337, 338t
Nevus, 65t–66t
NM. See Nuclear medicine (NM).
Noct/i, 120t
Nocturia, 125, 126t–127t
Non-possessive form of eponyms, 2b
Nose, 80–82, 81f, 84f, 85
Nuclear medicine (NM), 38t, 102b, 312t, 317t
Nursing assistants, 53t, 53f

O
OA. See Osteoarthritis (OA).
OAB. See Overactive bladder (OAB).
OB/GYN techs. See Obstetric technicians (OB/GYN techs).
Obstetric technicians (OB/GYN techs), 150b
Obstetricians, 150
Obstetrics, 166t
Obstructive sleep apnea (OSA), 101t, 106t
Occupational therapy (OT), 317t
Occupational therapy assistants (OTAs), 288b–289b
Ocular, 282
-oid, 8t–9t
Olig/o, 120t
Oliguria, 125, 126t–127t
OM. See Otitis media (OM).
-oma, 8t–9t, 11, 54t, 186t, 222t, 290t, 332t, 365t
Onc/o, 8t–9t
Oncologists, 13b, 16–17
Oncology
　abbreviations related to, 8t–9t, 21t
　definition of, 6, 16–17
　medical language of, 16, 23–24
　professionals who work with terms related to, 8b
Onych/o, 53t–54t, 59
Onycholysis, 59, 60t
Onychomycosis, 59, 60t
Onychosis, 59, 60t
Oophorectomy, 157, 158b, 160t–161t
Oophoritis, 153, 160t–161t
Oophor/o, 151t
Oophoropexy, 157, 160t–161t
Operating room technicians. See Surgical technologists.
Ophth. See Ophthalmology (ophth).
Ophthalmic, 266, 266t–267t
Ophthalmic medical technicians, 260b
Ophthalm/o, 261t, 263, 263b
Ophthalmologists, 263, 266t–267t
Ophthalmology (ophth), 263, 266t–267t, 277t
Ophthalmometers. See Keratometers.
Ophthalmoscopes, 263, 266t–267t
Optic, 266, 266t–267t
Optic nerve, 257–258, 258f, 260
Opticians, 260b, 260f
Opt/o, 261t
Optometrists, 273t–274t
Optometry, 266, 266t–267t
Oral, 225, 231t
Oral cavity. See Mouth.
Orchiectomy, 164, 165t
Orchi/o, 151t, 164
Orchiopexy, 164, 165t
Orchitis, 164, 165t
Organs, body, 7t
　body cavities and, 7, 7t, 13f
　definition of, 6t
Or/o, 221t–222t, 225
Orth, 4
Ortho. See Orthopedics (ortho).
Orth/o, 39b

Orthopedics (ortho), 4, 312t, 317t
Orthopedists, 312t
Orthopnea, 39b
Orthopnea position, 39b, 39t
OSA. See Obstructive sleep apnea (OSA).
-osis, 53t–54t, 120t, 151t–152t, 186t, 222t, 290t, 332t
Ossicles, 258–260, 259f
Oste, 4t
Oste/o, 289t, 306–307
Osteoarthritis (OA), 4t, 308, 310t–311t, 317t
Osteochondritis, 306, 310t–311t
Osteomalacia, 307, 310t–311t
Osteonecrosis, 306, 310t–311t
Osteopathy, 307b, 310t–311t
Osteopenia, 310t–311t
Osteoporosis, 312t
Osteosarcoma, 308, 310t–311t
OT. See Occupational therapy (OT).
OTAs. See Occupational therapy assistants (OTAs).
Otitis, 269, 272t
Otitis media (OM), 273t–274t, 277t
Ot/o, 261t, 268, 271, 271b
Otolaryngologists (ENTs), 86, 271, 271b, 272t, 277t
Otolaryngology, 271, 271b, 272t
Otoplasty, 269, 272t
Otorhinolaryngologists, 271b
Otorhinolaryngology, 271b
Otorrhea, 269, 272t
Otoscopes, 269, 272t
-ous, 4t, 53t–54t, 83t, 87b, 186t
Ovaries, 148–150, 156, 158f
Overactive bladder (OAB), 138t
Ovum (pl. ova), 148–150
Ox/i, 83t
Oximeter, 89, 90t
Oxygen (O$_2$), 106t

P
PA. See Posteroanterior (PA).
PAD. See Peripheral artery disease (PAD).
Pallor, 65t–66t
Palpation of arterial pulses, 45–47, 45f
Pancreas
　anatomic structure of, 218–219, 363–364, 366f, 372f
　functions of, 236
　with islets of Langerhans, 372f
　word roots for, 236b
Pancreatic, 236, 240t
Pancreatitis, 236, 240t
Pancreat/o, 221t–222t, 236
Pap test, 166b, 166t
Papanicolaou, George N., 166b
Paralysis, 342t
Paralysis agitans. See Parkinson disease (PD).
Paranasal sinuses. See Sinuses.
Paraplegia, 342b, 345t–346t
Parenteral, 241t–242t
Parkinson, James, 346b
Parkinson disease (PD), 300, 345t–346t, 346b, 352t
PATH. See Pathology (PATH).
Path/o, 8t–9t, 54t, 186t, 290t, 332t, 365t
Pathogenic, 14, 17
Pathologists, 14, 17
Pathology (PATH), 14, 17, 21t
Patient care technicians (PCTs), 119b, 119f, 138t
Patient positions. See Positions, patient.
PCTs. See Patient care technicians (PCTs).
PD. See Parkinson disease (PD).
Ped, 4
PEG. See Percutaneous endoscopic gastrostomy (PEG).
Pelvic cavity, organs of, 7t
Pelvic inflammatory disease (PID), 154f, 166t, 171t
Pelvis, 298, 298f
-penia, 186t, 290t, 307b
Penis, 149–150
Peps/o, 221t–222t
Peptic ulcers, 233, 241t–242t
Per-, 53t–54t
Percutaneous, 58, 58b, 60t
Percutaneous endoscopic gastrostomy (PEG), 229, 246t

Percutaneous transluminal coronary angioplasty (PTCA), 191b, 192f, 207t
Peripheral artery disease (PAD), 207t
Peripheral nervous system (PNS), 329–331, 330f, 352t
Peritoneal dialysis, 138b
"Pertaining to", 4t, 87b
-pexy, 151t
PFTs. See Pulmonary function tests (PFTs).
Phag/o, 221t–222t
Phalangeal, 295, 295f, 300t–301t
Phalangectomy, 295, 300t–301t
Phalang/o, 289t, 295
Pharmacy technicians, 8
Pharyngeal, 90t
Pharyngitis, 87, 90t
Pharyng/o, 83t
Pharynx, 81f, 82
    anatomic structure of, 80–81, 84f, 218–219
    function of, 219, 220f
Phas/o, 332t, 342
Phlebitis, 196, 200t
Phleb/o, 186t, 196
Phlebotomists, 185b, 185f
Phlebotomy, 196, 200t
Physical therapist assistants (PTAs), 288b–289b, 288f
Physical therapy (PT), 317t
Pia mater, 331b
PID. See Pelvic inflammatory disease (PID).
Pituitary gland, 363–364
PKD. See Polycystic kidney disease (PKD).
Plantar fasciitis, 312t
-plasm, 8t–9t, 14b
Plasma, 182–184
-plasty, 120t, 151t–152t, 186t, 222t, 261t, 290t
Platelets. See Thrombocytes.
-plegia, 261t
Pleg/o, 332t, 342
Plural word endings, 70–71, 70t, 79t, 93b
Pne, 87b
-pnea, 39b, 83t, 87b, 88, 186t
Pneum/o, 83t, 95b
Pneumonectomy, 95, 99t–100t
Pneumonia, 95, 99t–100t
Pneumon/o, 95, 95b
Pneumothorax, 96, 99t–100t
PNS. See Peripheral nervous system (PNS).
Poli/o, 64b, 332t
Poliomyelitis, 340, 344t
Poly-, 83t, 332t, 337, 365t
Polyarthritis, 337, 338t
Polycystic kidney disease (PKD), 138t, 139b
Polydipsia, 369, 370t
Polymyalgia, 337, 338t
Polyneuritis, 337, 338t
Polyp, 241t–242t
Polysomnogram, 99t–100t
Polysomnography (PSG), 99t–100t, 106t
Polyuria, 369, 370t
Positions, patient, 39–41, 39b, 41f, 45, 50t
    MRI of, 40f
    pronunciation and spelling of, 39t, 42
    quiz on, 49–50
Possessive use of eponyms, 2b
Posterior, 31, 34b, 37, 43t
Posterior prolapse, 239
Posterior tibial artery, palpation of, 45, 45f
Poster/o, 30t
Posteroanterior (PA), 32, 37, 43t
Posterolateral, 37
Prefixes
    abbreviation for, 3t
    in behavioral health terms, 332t
    building with, 3, 3t–4t, 8t–9t
    in cardiovascular and lymphatic terms, 186t, 217t
    definition of, 3t, 8t–9t
    in digestive terms, 222t
    in endocrine terms, 365t
    in integumentary terms, 53t–54t, 79t
    in musculoskeletal terms, 289t–290t
    in neurological terms, 332t

Prefixes (Continued)
    in reproductive terms, 151t–152t
    in respiratory terms, 83t, 92, 115t
    in urinary system, 120t
Presbycusis, 273t–274t
Presbyopia, 266b, 273t–274t
Pressure injury/ulcer, 65t–66t, 67f
Primary adrenal insufficiency. See Addison disease.
Proct/o, 221t–222t
Proctoscopes, 238, 240t
Proctoscopy, 238, 240t
Prognosis (Px), 18t, 21t
Prolapses
    posterior, 239
    uterovaginal, 166t
Prone position, 39t
Pronunciation and spelling
    of abdominopelvic regions, 39t, 42
    of anatomic planes, 38t, 42
    of behavioral health terms, 344–345, 351–352
    of cardiovascular terms, 193, 200–201, 206–207
    of digestive terms, 232, 240–241, 246
    of directional terms, 37
    of ear-related terms, 273, 277
    of endocrine terms, 370–371, 374–375
    of eye-related terms, 267, 277
    of integumentary terms, 60, 65, 69
    of lymphatic terms, 193, 200–201, 206–207
    of musculoskeletal terms, 301, 311, 317
    of neurological terms, 338, 344–345, 351–352
    of patient positions, 39t, 42
    of reproductive terms, 162, 165–166, 171
    of respiratory terms, 91, 100, 105
    of terms built from word parts, 9t, 17
    of terms not built from word parts, 18t, 21
    of urinary terms, 127, 134, 138
Prostate cancer, 163
Prostate gland, 149–150
Prostatectomy, 163, 165t
Prostate-specific antigen (PSA) assay, 167t, 171t
Prostatic, 163, 165t
Prostatitis, 163, 165t
Prostat/o, 151t, 163
Prostatocystitis, 163, 165t
Prostatoliths, 163, 165t
Proximal, 35, 35f, 37
Proxim/o, 30t
PSA assay. See Prostate-specific antigen (PSA) assay.
PSG. See Polysomnography (PSG).
Psychiatric aides, 331b
Psychiatrists, 345t–346t
Psych/o, 332t, 343
Psychogenic, 343, 344t
Psychologists, 13b, 343, 344t
Psychology, 343, 344t
Psychopathy, 343, 344t
Psychosis, 343, 344t
PT. See Physical therapy (PT).
PTAs. See Physical therapist assistants (PTAs).
PTCA. See Percutaneous transluminal coronary angioplasty (PTCA).
Ptosis. See Blepharoptosis.
-ptosis, 261t
Puberty, 149–150
Pub/o, 289t
Pulmonary, 95, 99t–100t
Pulmonary function tests (PFTs), 106t
Pulmon/o, 83t, 94
Pulmonologists, 95, 98b, 99t–100t
Pulmonology, 95, 99t–100t
Pulse (P), 201t–202t, 207t
Pulse oximeter, 89
Pupils, 257–258, 258f, 260
Px. See Prognosis (Px).
Pyel/o, 120t
Pyelolithotomy, 126, 126t–127t
Pyelonephritis, 129, 133t–134t
Pyelos, 125b
Py/o, 120t
Pyuria, 124, 126t–127t

Q
Quadr/i, 332t
Quadriplegia, 342, 344t

R
RA. See Rheumatoid arthritis (RA).
Rachi/o, 289t, 293
Rachiotomy, 294, 300t–301t
Rachischisis, 294, 300t–301t
Radial artery, palpation of, 45, 45f
Radiation oncology. See Radiation therapy (XRT).
Radiation therapists, 30
Radiation therapy (XRT), 18t, 21t
Radical prostatectomy, 171t
Radi/o, 8t–9t
Radiograph, 32, 32f, 38t, 101t, 102b, 102f
Radiographers, 30
Radiologic technologists (RTs), 30
Radiologists, 14, 17
Radiology, 14, 17
Radiotherapy. See Radiation therapy (XRT).
Range of motion (ROM), 317t
RBCs. See Erythrocytes (RBCs).
RDs. See Registered dietitians (RDs).
Rectal, 239, 240t
Rect/o, 221t–222t, 239
Rectocele, 239, 240t
Rectum, 218–219
Red blood cells. See Erythrocytes (RBCs).
Refraction, 266b
Refraction errors, 266b, 274f
Registered dietitians (RDs), 220b–221b
Registered polysomnographic technologists (RPSGTs), 82b
Remission, 18t
Renal, 133t–134t
Renal calculi, 135t
Renal failure, 135t, 139b
Renal pelvis, 117–118, 118f, 125b, 125f
Renal transplant, 135t
Ren/o, 120t, 128
Reproductive systems
    abbreviations related to, 171t, 172
    components and functions of, 7t, 149–150
    female. See Female reproductive system.
    male. See Male reproductive system.
    professionals who work with, 150b, 150f
Respiratory system
    abbreviations related to, 103–107, 104b, 106t, 116t
    anatomic structures of, 7t, 80–82, 84f, 91–99, 91f
    functions of, 7t, 81–82, 81f
    medical terms related to, 90t, 93b, 99t–101t, 103–105, 116t
        in case study, 111
        by clinical category, 107–110
        in clinical statements, 110–111
        in electronic health records, 113
        in medical document, 112, 112f–113f
        quiz on, 114–115
    professionals who work with, 82b, 82f
    pronunciation and spelling of terms related to, 91, 100, 105
    word parts for, 83t, 84–99, 85b–88b, 95b, 97b
Respiratory therapists (RTs), 82b, 82f, 106t
Respiratory therapy technicians, 82b
Retina
    anatomic structure of, 257–258, 258f, 260
    detached, 273t–274t
Retinal, 266, 266t–267t
Retinitis, 264, 266t–267t
Retin/o, 261t
Rheumatoid arthritis (RA), 312t, 317t
Rhinitis, 85, 90t
Rhin/o, 85, 271b
Rhinorrhagia, 85, 90t
Rhinorrhea, 85, 90t
Right lower quadrant (RLQ), 42, 42f, 43t
Right upper quadrant (RUQ), 42, 42f, 43t
RLQ. See Right lower quadrant (RLQ).
ROM. See Range of motion (ROM).
RPSGTs. See Registered polysomnographic technologists (RPSGTs).

-rrhagia, 83t, 85b, 151t–152t, 156b, 204b
-rrhaphy, 151t, 156b
-rrhea, 83t, 85b, 151t–152t, 156b, 158
-rrhexis, 151t, 156b
RTs. See Radiologic technologists (RTs); Respiratory therapists (RTs).
RUQ. See Right upper quadrant (RUQ).

S
Sagittal plane, 38t
SAH. See Subarachnoid hemorrhage (SAH).
Salpingitis, 153, 160t–161t
Salping/o, 151t
Salpingo-oophoritis, 157b
Sarc/o, 8t–9t, 290t
Sarcoma, 12, 17
SCC. See Squamous cell carcinoma (SCC).
-schisis, 289t
Sciatica, 345t–346t
Sclera, anatomic structure of, 257–258, 258f, 260
Scleral, 266, 266t–267t
Scleritis, 264, 266t–267t
Scler/o, 261t
-sclerosis, 186t
Scoli/o, 289t
Scoliosis, 300t–301t
Scop, 97b
-scope, 83t, 97b, 151t–152t, 222t, 261t
-scopic, 83t, 97b, 120t, 222t, 290t
-scopy, 83t, 97b, 120t, 151t–152t, 222t, 290t
Scrotal, 164, 165t
Scrot/o, 151t, 164
Scrotoplasty, 164, 165t
Scrotum, 149, 164
Scrub techs. See Surgical technologists.
Sebaceous glands, 51–52, 55f
Seizure, 345t–346t
Semen, 149–150
Semen analysis, 167t
Semi-Fowler position, 39b
Seminal vesicles, 149–150
Sexually transmitted diseases (STDs), 167b, 167t, 171t
Sexually transmitted infections (STIs), 167b, 167t, 171t
Shaking palsy. See Parkinson disease (PD).
Shortness of breath (SOB), 104b, 106t
Sigmoid colon, 218–219
Sigmoid/o, 221t–222t
Sigmoidoscopy, 238, 240t
Sims position, 39t
Singular word endings, 70–71, 70t, 79t, 93b
Sinuses, 80–81, 84f, 86f
Sinusitis, 90t
Sinus/o, 83t
Sinusotomy, 86, 90t
Skeletal system. See Musculoskeletal system.
Skin, 51–52, 55f, 58f
    color, 61f
    disorders of, 61, 62f, 63, 65t–66t, 66f–67f
Sleep technicians, 82b
Sleep technologists, 82b
Small intestine, 218–219, 220f
SOB. See Shortness of breath (SOB).
Somn/o, 83t
Son/o, 151t
Sonographers, 30, 150b
Sonography. See Ultrasonography (US).
Sound, perception of, 259f, 260
Speech-language pathology aides, 331b
Spelling. See Pronunciation and spelling.
Sperm, 149–150
Sperm count/test. See Semen analysis.
Sphygmomanometers, 201t–202t
Spina bifida, 340
Spinal cavity, 7t, 31
Spinal cord
    anatomic structure of, 329–330, 330f, 333f, 339, 339f
    functions of, 331
    injuries, 342
Spinal stenosis, 312t
Spinal tap. See Lumbar puncture (LP).
Spir/o, 83t
Spirometer, 89, 90t

Spirometry, 82f
Spleen
    anatomic structure of, 183
    combining forms for, 197f
    function of, 185, 198
Splenectomy, 198, 200t
Splen/o, 186t, 198
Splenomegaly, 198, 200t
Spondylarthritis, 294, 300t–301t
Spondyl/o, 289t, 294
Sputum, 101t
Sputum culture and sensitivity (C&S), 101t
Squamous cell carcinoma (SCC), 65t–66t, 66f, 69t
Staphylococcus (staph), 18t, 21t
-stasis, 8t–9t, 14b, 186t
STDs. See Sexually transmitted diseases (STDs).
Sternal, 304, 310t–311t
Stern/o, 289t
Sternocostal, 304, 310t–311t
Sternum, 31, 304, 304f
Stethoscopes, 201t–202t
STIs. See Sexually transmitted infections (STIs).
Stoma, 241t–242t
Stomach, anatomic structure of, 218–219, 220f
-stomy, 83t, 120t, 222t
Streptococcus (strep), 18t, 21t
Stroke, 345t–346t, 350f
Sub-, 53t–54t, 222t, 290t
Subarachnoid hemorrhage (SAH), 345t–346t, 350f, 352t
Subcostal, 304, 310t–311t
Subcutaneous, 58, 58b, 60t, 69t
Sublingual, 225, 231t
Sudoriferous glands, 55f
Suffixes
    abbreviations for, 3t, 14b
    in behavioral health terms, 332t
    building with, 3, 3t–4t, 8t–9t, 9, 13
    in cardiovascular and lymphatic terms, 186t, 188b, 217t
    definition of, 3t, 8t–9t
    in digestive terms, 221t–222t
    in directional terms, 30t, 31, 35–36, 50t
    in ear-related terms, 261t
    in endocrine terms, 365t
    in eye-related terms, 261t
    in integumentary terms, 53t–54t, 79t
    in musculoskeletal terms, 289t–290t, 327t
    in neurological terms, 332t
    in reproductive terms
        female, 151t–152t, 153, 155–156, 156b, 159
        male, 151t–152t, 163–164
    in respiratory terms, 83t, 86, 92, 94–95, 115t
    in urinary terms, 120t, 130, 132, 147t
Superior, 33, 34b, 37, 43t
Super/o, 30t
Superolateral, 37
Supine position, 39t
Surgical nurses, 119b
Surgical technologists, 288b–289b
Sweat glands, 51–52
Syncope, 345t–346t
Syndrome X. See Metabolic syndrome.
Systems, body
    components and functions of, 7, 7t
    definition of, 6t

T
Tachy-, 186t
Tachycardia, 190, 192t–193t
Tachypnea, 190, 192t–193t
TAH/BSO. See Total abdominal hysterectomy/bilateral salpingo-oophorectomy (TAH/BSO).
TB. See Tuberculosis (TB).
Temporal artery, 45, 45f
Tendinitis, 310, 310t–311t
Tendin/o, 289t, 310
Tendons, 287–288, 310
Ten/o, 289t, 310
Tenodesis, 310, 310t–311t
Tenoplasty, 310, 310t–311t
Testes/testicles, 149, 164

THA. See Total hip arthroplasty (THA).
Thoracentesis, 95b, 96, 99t–100t
Thoracic, 99t–100t
Thoracic cavity, 13, 31, 80–82
    organs of, 7t
Thoracic surgeon, 98, 98b
Thoracic vertebrae (T1-T12), 317t
Thorac/o, 83t, 95, 95b, 97
Thoracoscope, 98, 99t–100t
Thoracoscopic, 98, 99t–100t
Thoracoscopic surgery, 98
Thoracoscopy, 98, 99t–100t
Thoracotomy, 96, 99t–100t
Thorax, 80–81
-thorax, 83t, 95
Throat. See Pharynx.
Thromb/o, 186t, 332t
Thrombocytes, 184, 197, 200t
Thrombocytopenia, 197, 200t
Thrombophlebitis, 196, 200t
Thrombosis, 196, 200t
Thrombus, 206b
Thymectomy, 368, 370t
Thymic, 368, 370t
Thym/o, 365t
Thymomas, 368, 370t, 381
Thymus
    anatomic structure of, 183, 363–364
    functions of, 185
Thyroid gland, anatomic structure of, 363–364
Thyroidectomy, 368, 370t
Thyroiditis, 368, 370t
Thyroid/o, 365t, 368
TIA. See Transient ischemic attack (TIA).
Tinnitus, 273t–274t
Tissues, body
    categories of, 6, 6t, 11, 11f
    definition of, 6t
TKA. See Total knee arthroplasty (TKA).
-tomy, 83t, 120t, 151t–152t, 186t, 222t, 261t, 290t
T1-T12. See Thoracic vertebrae (T1-T12).
Tongue, 218–219
Total abdominal hysterectomy/bilateral salpingo-oophorectomy (TAH/BSO), 171t
Total hip arthroplasty (THA), 317t
Total knee arthroplasty (TKA), 317t
Total parenteral nutrition (TPN), 246t
TPN. See Total parenteral nutrition (TPN).
Trachea, 80–82, 81f, 91f
Trache/o, 83t, 92
Tracheostomy, 93, 93b, 93f, 99t–100t
Tracheotomy, 93, 93b, 99t–100t
Trans-, 53t–54t
Transdermal, 57, 57b–58b, 60t, 69t
Transient ischemic attack (TIA), 345t–346t, 352t
Transrectal ultrasound (TRUS), 171t
Transurethral resection of the prostate gland (TURP), 167t, 171t
Transverse plane, 38t
Trendelenburg position, 39t
-tripsy, 120t
Troph/o, 289t, 296
True skin. See Dermis.
TRUS. See Transrectal ultrasound (TRUS).
Tuberculosis (TB), 101t, 106t
Tumors, types of, 11–12, 15
TURP. See Transurethral resection of the prostate gland (TURP).
Tympanic, 270, 272t
Tympanic membrane, 258–260, 259f
Tympan/o, 261t, 270
Tympanoplasty, 270, 272t

U
UA. See Urinalysis (UA).
UC, se ulcerative colitis (UC)
UGI series. See Upper GI (UGI) series.
Ulcerative colitis (UC), 241t–242t, 246t
Ulcers
    gastric, 228f, 233, 241t–242t
    pressure, 65t–66t, 67f

Ultrasonography (US), 38t, 102b, 159–160, 160t–161t
    abdominal, 235f
Ultrasound technicians. *See* Sonographers.
Umbilical region, 39f, 39t
Upper GI (UGI) series, 241t–242t, 246t
Upper respiratory infections (URIs), 101t, 104f, 106t
Upper respiratory tract, 82
Uremia, 125, 125b, 126t–127t
Ureter, 118, 118f, 131
Ureterectomy, 131, 133t–134t
Ureter/o, 120t, 131
Ureterolithiasis, 131, 133t–134t
Ureterolithotomy, 131, 133t–134t
Ureteroplasty, 131, 133t–134t
Ureteropyelonephritis, 131, 133t–134t
Ureters, 117–118, 118f, 128f
    procedures related to, 131
Urethra, 122f–123f, 150
    anatomic structure of, 117–118, 121, 121f, 128f
    function of, 118, 118f
    male, 149
Urethr/o, 120t, 123
Urethrocystitis, 123, 126t–127t
Urethroplasty, 123, 126t–127t
Urethroscope, 123, 126t–127t
Urinalysis (UA), 135t, 138t
Urinary bladder, 122f–123f
    anatomic structure of, 117–118, 121, 121f
    function of, 118, 118f
    infections, 124
Urinary catheterization, 135t
Urinary meatus, 117–118, 118f, 128f, 132
Urinary system
    abbreviations related to, 138t, 139
    anatomic structures of, 7t, 117–118, 121f, 125, 125f,
        128f
    functions of, 7t, 118, 118f
    medical terms related to, 124b–125b, 126t–127t,
        133t–135t, 137–138, 139b, 147t
        in case study, 143
        by clinical category, 139–142
        in clinical statements, 142
        in electronic health records, 145
        in medical document, 143–144, 143f–144f
        quiz on, 146
    professionals who work with, 119b, 119f
    pronunciation and spelling of terms related to, 127,
        134, 138
    word parts for, 120t, 121–126, 128–133, 147t
Urinary tract, 117–118
Urinary tract infections (UTIs), 135t, 138t
Urine, 117–118, 118f, 124

URIs. *See* Upper respiratory infections (URIs).
Ur/o, 120t, 124, 132, 365t
Urogram, 132, 133t–134t
Urologists, 132, 133t–134t
Urology, 132, 133t–134t
Urology technicians, 119b
Urostomy, 132, 133t–134t
US. *See* Ultrasonography (US).
-us, 332t
Uterine fibroids, 166t
Uterine tubes, 148–150, 152b, 156, 158f
Uterovaginal prolapse, 166t
Uterus, 148–150, 156, 158f
UTIs. *See* Urinary tract infections (UTIs).

V
VA. *See* Visual acuity (VA).
Vaccine
    for human papillomavirus (HPV), 170b
    for polio, 340
Vagina, 148–150
Vaginal, 160t–161t
Vaginal sprays, 153
Vaginitis, 153, 160t–161t
Vagin/o, 151t
Varicose veins, 201t–202t
Vas deferens, 149–150, 164
Vasectomy, 164, 165t
Vas/o, 151t
Vasovasostomy, 164, 165t
VCUG. *See* Voiding cystourethrogram (VCUG).
Veins, anatomic structure of, 182–183
Venipuncture, 185b, 185f, 196, 200t
Ven/o, 4t, 186t, 194
Venogram, 195, 200t
Ventral, 31, 34b, 37
Ventral cavity, 13, 31
Ventricles, 329–330
Ventr/o, 30t
Vertebrae, 292–293, 293f
Vertebral, 292–293, 300t–301t
Vertebral column, 292–293, 294f, 340
Vertebrectomy, 292–293, 300t–301t
Vertebr/o, 289t, 292
Vertebroplasty, 292–293, 300t–301t
Virtual colonoscopy, 237
Visceral, 17
Viscer/o, 8t–9t
Vision, 258, 258f
Visual acuity (VA), 277t
Vital signs (VS), 207t
Voice box. *See* Larynx.

Void, 135t
Voiding cystourethrogram (VCUG), 138t
V/Q scan. *See* Lung ventilation/perfusion scan (V/Q
    scan).

W
WBCs. *See* Leukocytes (WBCs).
West Nile virus, 2f
White blood cells. *See* Leukocytes (WBCs).
Windpipe. *See* Trachea.
Word parts
    abbreviations for, 3t
    for behavioral health, 332t, 343, 362t
    for cardiovascular system, 186t, 187–192, 188b,
        194–200, 217t
    for digestive system, 221t–222t, 223–240, 242b,
        256t
    for directional terms, 30t, 31–36
    for ear-related terms, 261t, 268–272, 286t
    for endocrine system, 365t, 366–370, 369b, 383t
    for eye-related terms, 261t, 262–266, 263b, 286t
    for integumentary system, 53t–54t, 55–64
    list of, 8t–9t
    for lymphatic system, 186t, 194–200, 217t
    medical terms built from, 3–5, 3t–4t, 9–17, 16t–17t
    for musculoskeletal system, 289t–290t, 291–300,
        298b, 302–310, 307b, 327t
    for nervous system, 332t, 333–344, 362t
    for reproductive systems
        female, 151t–152t, 152–160, 153b, 156b, 158b,
            181t
        male, 151t–152t, 162–165, 181t
    for respiratory system, 83t, 84–99, 85b–88b, 95b,
        97b
    for urinary system, 120t, 121–126, 128–133,
        147t
Word roots
    abbreviation for, 3t
    building from, 3, 3t–4t, 4b, 8t–9t, 10
    definition of, 8t–9t
Wrong-side errors, preventing, 41b

X
Xanth/o, 53t–54t
Xanthoderma, 61, 64t
Xanthoma, 63, 64t
Xanthosis, 63, 64t
X-ray. *See* Radiograph.
XRT. *See* Radiation therapy (XRT).

Y
-y, 53t–54t, 186t, 222t, 290t, 332t, 365t

COMMON TERMINOLOGY

Acronym: A term formed from the first letter of several words that can be spoken as a whole word; usually contains a vowel.

<u>EXAMPLE</u>: MRSA (methicillin-resistant *Staphylococcus aureus*)

Build: Constructing a medical term from its definition using Greek and Latin word parts as a learning exercise.

<u>EXAMPLE</u>: the term meaning "inflammation of the kidney" may be constructed from nephr/o (kidney) and -itis (inflammation) to arrive at the term nephritis.

Combining form: Combination of a word root and a combining vowel.

<u>EXAMPLE</u>: therm/o. Often referred to as a word part.

Combining vowel: Usually an **o**. Used between word parts to ease pronunciation.

<u>EXAMPLE</u>: therm/o/meter

Eponym: Medical term named for a person or a place.

<u>EXAMPLE</u>: Parkinson disease

Etymology: Origin and development of a word.

<u>EXAMPLE</u>: Cadaver, denoting a corpse or dead body, is derived from the Latin word *cadere*, which means to fall. The term literally means fallen and originally described those who fell dead in battle.

Implied meaning: Requires a more precise definition than literal translation.

<u>EXAMPLE</u>: an/emia. The literal translation is without blood; the implied meaning is a condition characterized by the deficiency of red blood cells and hemoglobin.

Literal translation: Translation of the word parts that make up a medical term to arrive at its meaning.

<u>EXAMPLE</u>: therm/o means heat, -meter means instrument used to measure; therefore, thermometer means instrument used to measure heat. In some medical terms literal translation does not define the current use of the term.

<u>EXAMPLE</u>: The literal translation of meta/stasis is beyond control; the implied or current definition is transfer of disease from one organ to another.

Medical language or medical terminology: A professional language made up of medical terms used mostly by those engaged directly or indirectly in the art of healing.

Medical term: Word(s) used to describe anatomic structures, medical diagnoses, diagnostic procedures, surgical procedures, and signs and symptoms of illness and disease. Medical terms originate from Greek and Latin word parts, such as gastr/itis; eponyms such as Alzheimer disease; acronyms such as MRSA; and modern language, such as bone marrow transplant.

Medical term building or word building: Using Greek and Latin word parts and a set of rules to combine them into meaningful medical terms.

Prefix: Attached at the beginning of a word root to modify its meaning.

<u>EXAMPLE</u>: re/play

Suffix: Attached at the end of a word root to modify its meaning.

<u>EXAMPLE</u>: play/er

Translate: Using the meaning of the word parts that comprise the medical term to arrive at its meaning.

<u>EXAMPLE</u>: nephr/o means kidney, -itis means inflammation, nephritis means inflammation of the kidney.

Word part: Consists of Greek and Latin prefixes, suffixes, word roots, and combining vowels.

Word root: Core of the word giving the medical term its primary meaning.

COMMON PLURAL ENDINGS FOR MEDICAL TERMS

In the English language plurals are often formed by simply adding *s* or *es* to the word. Forming plurals in the language of medicine is not so simple. Use the table below to learn the standard plural formation of medical terms.

SINGULAR ENDING	PLURAL ENDING	EXAMPLE SINGULAR	PLURAL
-a	-ae	vertebra	vertebrae
-ax	-aces	thorax	thoraces
-ex	-ices	cortex	cortices
-is	-es	pubis	pubes
-ix	-ices	cervix	cervices
-ma	-mata	sarcoma	sarcomata
-nx	-nges	pharynx	pharynges
-on	-a	ganglion	ganglia
-sis	-ses	diagnosis	diagnoses
-um	-a	ovum	ova
-us	-i	bronchus	bronchi